The Crime of Poison in the Middle Ages

The Crime of Poison in the Middle Ages

FRANCK COLLARD

Translated by Deborah Nelson-Campbell

PRAEGER

Westport, Connecticut
London

Library of Congress Cataloging-in-Publication Data

Collard, Franck.
[Crime de poison au Moyen Âge. English]
The crime of poison in the Middle Ages / Franck Collard ; translated by Deborah Nelson-Campbell.
p. ; cm.
Includes bibliographical references and index.
ISBN 978–0–313–34699–6 (alk. paper)
1. Poisoning—History—To 1500. I. Title.
[DNLM: 1. Poisoning—history. 2. Crime—history. 3. Crime—psychology. 4. History, Medieval. QV 11.1 c697c 2008a]
HV6552.C6513 2008
364.152'30940902—dc22 2008022062

British Library Cataloguing in Publication Data is available.

Library of Congress Catalog Card Number: 2008022062
ISBN: 978–0–313–34699–6

English edition first published in 2008

Original French edition, *Le crime de poison au Moyen Âge,* by Franck Collard first published in 2005. © Presses Universitaires de France, 2005.

Praeger Publishers, 88 Post Road West, Westport, CT 06881
An imprint of Greenwood Publishing Group, Inc.
www.praeger.com

Printed in the United States of America

The paper used in this book complies with the Permanent Paper Standard issued by the National Information Standards Organization (Z39.48–1984).

10 9 8 7 6 5 4 3 2 1

Contents

Preface ix
Acknowledgments xi
Introduction xiii

1 An Elusive Crime? 1
The Crime as Event: The Emergence of the Crime in Narrative 1
Narrations of Poisonings by the Chroniclers 2
Criminal Poisoning in Literary Fiction 6
Stories about Poisoning: Are They a Model for Behavior or Simply for Moral Instruction? 9
The Crime and Its Description: Its Existence in the Judicial Code 11
The Crime of Poisoning in Its Prescriptive Sources 11
The Relative Lack of Interest in Poisoning in Judicial Writings 16
The Lack of Clarity in Judicial Documents 17
The Difficulty in Quantifying Cases of Poisoning 20
The Challenge of Measuring the Frequency of the Crime 20
Evaluations and Indications of the Frequency of the Crime 21

2 A Unique Weapon 39
The Poison "Market" 39
Areas of Production and Distribution Points 39
Producer and Provider: Separate Worlds? 43
Products That Were Used and the Instructions 46

Simple Poisons 46
Compound Poisons 48
Consistency, Media, and Methods of Administering Poison 50
The Effects and the Marks 54
The Effects 55
The Marks 57
Confusing Symptoms 59
An Invincible Weapon? How to Prevent and to Recover from Poisoning 61
Prevention 61
Remedies 67

3 The Sociology of Poisoning 87
Profiles of the Victims of Poisoning 87
Gender and Age 88
From the Emperor to the Beggar, from the Pope to the Vicar 90
The Faces of the Poisoners 94
A Shared Crime 94
A Favorite Activity of Clerks? 96
An Affair of Women? 97
A Crime of the Other 101
The Crime of Poisoning in the World of Relationships 106
Murder within the Family 106
The Involvement of Servants in the Crime of Poisoning 110
Poison in Relationships Based on Power 112

4 *Horrendum scelus*. An Abominable Crime 127
A Crime Described in Superlatives 127
A *terribilis casus* between the Extreme and the Unspeakable 128
The Worst Kind of Treason 130
The Reasons for an Abomination: How to Kill 132
An Insidious and Secret Crime 132
Premeditated Homicide 134
Poisoning and Villainous Associations 137
Poisoning and Criminal Practices 139
The Reasons for the Abomination: Objectives and Effects of Poisoning 142
The Destruction of Basic Social Units 142
The Corrosion of the Political Body 144
The Poisoning of Christianity 151

5 Pursuit and Punishment 171
Theoretical Bases and Effective Practice 171
Permanence of Principles and the Extension of the Field of Repression 172

Which Courts? Which Procedures? 173
An Outburst of Repression? 179
The Poisoner on Trial 180
The Origins and Beginning of Prosecutions 181
Ways to Search for the Truth 183
"*Ferme prove e certa verità.*" The Consistency of Proof 189
Sentences and Sanctions 195
When Doubt or Mercy Benefits the Defendant 195
Providential, Symbolic, or Informal Punishments 198
Sentences and Punishments within the Judicial System 200

6 Beyond Crime: Issues and Uses of Poison 221
Poisonous Aggression, Heroism, and Sainthood 221
Poisoned Beverages and Certificates of Sainthood 222
Heroic Poison? 224
The Accusation of Poisoning, Regulation, and Catharsis 226
A Political Regulator 227
The Accusation of Poisoning and Social Regulation 234
Poison, Propaganda, and Identity 238
The Use of Poison: A Theme of Propaganda 238
The Crystallization of an Identity Crisis 248

Conclusion 265
Glossary 273
Major Sources 277
Selected Bibliography 283
Index of Major Historical Figures 289

Preface

This work is the revised, amended, and substantially abbreviated result of research that started a long time ago and was presented in January 2003 as an unpublished dissertation in order that I might be authorized to supervise research at the University of Paris I-Panthéon-Sorbonne. Support for two years from the CNRS contributed greatly to its completion. The project was inspired by the research of Bernard Guinée, who noticed the importance of the accusation of poisoning in the posthumous proceedings investigating the death of the Duc Louis d'Orléans, who was murdered on November 23, 1407. Claude Gauvard was instrumental in the final stages of the project not only by providing intellectual and moral support but, in addition, by generously agreeing to publish it in the collection she edits. Naturally, the author wishes to express his profound gratitude to her. And since medieval poisons have kept this historian away from his family for long periods, he wishes to dedicate this book *pueris matrique eorum*.

Acknowledgments

This project has been a fascinating challenge that led me into a medieval world that I had never experienced: the culture of ambition, greed, and jealousy that motivated men and women to take the lives of individuals who trusted them. I did not make this journey entirely alone but was helped along by friends and colleagues who were able to contribute from their areas of expertise. First of all, I with to thank Elodie Bouvet, who prepared preliminary translations for the Foreword, the Introduction, and Chapters II and V. Maher Awad, Lecturer in Arabic at Rice University, clarified some Arabic expressions that mystified me. Hilary Mackie, Associate Professor of Classical Studies at Rice University, translated several passages from Latin. My colleague, Madeleine Alcover, Professor Emerita of French Studies at Rice University, consulted with me on some of the particularly mysterious French expressions. Katherine Drew, Autrey Professor Emerita of History at Rice University, helped with information about Frankish law and legal language. I wish to thank in particular Janet Vrancken, a dear friend of many years, who possesses a broad knowledge of history and literature and who generously consented to proof the entire text.

I feel very fortunate to belong to a community of scholars who are so generous with their time and knowledge. Of course, any errors that remain are entirely my responsibility.

Introduction

It is with a completely distorted sense of the Middle Ages that our contemporaries consider cruelty and bloody violence as typical of the period, but associate poisoning with times thought to be more refined if not less brutal,[1] such as the eras of the Caesars or the Renaissance. One of the persons who is responsible for this false conception is the Italian historian Guichardin, who claimed that poisonings were well known in his country in the sixteenth century but virtually unknown in the lands beyond the Alps.[2] However, well-informed medievalists have described the Anglo-Norman twelfth century and the Iberian fourteenth century as being the "centuries of poison."[3] As early as the middle of the nineteenth century, J. Michelet was convinced of the importance of accusations of poisoning in major trials of the 1300s.[4] In truth, in the field of criminality, as in many others, the medieval era is in no way a break between Nero and the Borgias.

In comparison with other periods and/or to other areas that have been more closely examined, the historiography of the crime of poisoning in the occidental Middle Ages is very sketchy. When historical documents have deigned to consider it, they have been content to refer to enigmatic deaths or have tried to explain these deaths with the science of their time. At the beginning of the twentieth century, Dr. Brachet and Dr. Cabanès placed the mysterious deaths of the past under the blunt light of legal medicine. Their retro-diagnostics without appeal were a literal operation of the detoxification of history: among the twelve medieval sovereigns whose deaths Cabanès analyzed, he found none who could have been poisoned.[5] As far as Brachet is concerned, he came to the conclusion that all possible poisonings belonged to myth: such suppositions are simply "the pathology of history professors."[6] Positivist rigor considered the only events worthy of being examined to be those that had actually occurred. This approach was also limited to establishing the "truth" of the events not without denouncing the terrible judicial mistakes committed by the king's judge or the church's inquisitor. After being closely examined through such a lens, the matter of the crime of poisoning did not deserve a historical analysis.

However, historical criminal poisoning inspired the publication of a voluminous book in 1920: *Die Gifte in der Weltgeschichte* by L. Lewin. Lewin had come to the topic by means of chemistry, an extremely important science at that time in Germany. The author certainly does not escape from the positivism of his time or from the mind-set of his discipline, even though he does not systematically cast doubt on the cases he treats.[7] Nevertheless, most of the time, he limits himself to the establishment of the likelihood and also the material conditions surrounding the possible realization of the crime. His greatest merit is the gathering of numerous "facts of poison" coming from the wide perusal of mostly German chronicles, which he sometimes quotes word for word. The medieval period occupies an important place in this colossal collection. In addition, L. Thorndike's voluminous synthesis of the history of science must not be forgotten since, even if it does not approach poison solely from a scientific point of view, it provides numerous references and analyses from fundamental sources.[8]

The most recent historiography has contributed little to the topic. The general history of poison includes the medieval era in vast studies that are rarely the work of professional historians. In a pleasant and light review of celebrated poisoners, R. Villeneuve grants the medieval epoch only about twenty very descriptive pages that link, with little explanation, poisons to alchemy.[9] Faithful to Guichardin's conceptions, Jean de Maleyssie looks at the Middle Ages as a dark time of a "poisons' fair," where everything can be found.[10] Limiting his research to the domain of political murder, G. Minois begins his study of the knife and poison [two different ways of killing] in the year 1400, without raising the question of any alternative methods available to criminals. The surge of interest in historical demography and in the history of mores and private life, as well as the amazingly rapid development of the history of medieval criminality, have not included until now a specific and thorough examination of the crime of poisoning. The same observation can be made concerning the prolific historiography of witchcraft. R. W. Ireland is the only scholar who has sketched out his very suggestive ideas in a short article.[11] On the other hand, the topic of poison has inspired both ethnologists and anthropologists.[12] The facts that have been gathered concerning the making of poisons, their uses, or the social characteristics of those who mastered the skill, as well as the conspicuous position of an imaginary of poison, offer great interest to the historian, provided that medieval society is not likened to primitive societies. Poison has recently given rise to an "occidental" anthropological inquiry in a quest for current perceptions of poison in literature (including medieval), in lexicology and in psychoanalysis.[13] If this perspective tends naturally to diminish in importance the historicity of the subject (to the benefit of the kind of collective psychology dear to G. Bachelard), the work of C. Boujot is no less suggestive about the rapport between the body and poison or about the social imaginary of poison.

The lack of a rich bibliography is balanced by an abundance of documents. Narrative sources and sources from judiciary practice form two dissymmetrical poles of documentation: the first covers the entire medieval period and the second is limited to the late medieval centuries. Only sources from occidental historiography have been taken into account in this study (including works written from overseas in the tradition of Roman Christianity) since my purpose is to examine the perception of the crime of poisoning in the West in medieval times. To accomplish this goal, it was necessary to take into account Byzantine and Islamic documents in order to more accurately portray in contrast the "culture" of murder by poisoning in the Occident. It was also necessary to include some ancient texts since the Scriptures as well as Roman historians provide narrative outlines that are constantly used in the Middle Ages. (The prose of Thomas Basin can be understood only in the light of that of Suetonius.) The sources of judicial practice emanating from diverse medieval jurisdictions, mainly French, constitute the second source of data. This latter source is just as inexhaustible as the previous one but more difficult to exploit, even if excellent editions of documents and trials along with analytical inventories are sometimes available.

These two important sets of sources supply more than three hundred and forty cases and do not exhaust the documentation that is likely to shed light on the topic. The normative sources inherited by or created during the Middle Ages offer a set of fundamental indications on the status of the crime of poisoning. Judicial commentaries as well as procedural tracts also conceal important facts. As far as the scientific and medical literature is concerned, treatises on poison written or translated in the Occident, the general medical surveys, or the more specialized treatises on epidemics, surgery, or pharmacology, include material on deliberate poisonings and permit a grasp of poison as a material substance, as well as representations of poisonings linked to the Creation. Linked to theology, this last aspect makes the consultation of works on "natural philosophy" equally useful. There exists an imaginary of poison that the documents describing the "states of the world" and the functioning of the Terrestrial City do not ignore. In the primary sense of the term, the imaginary originates with the observation of images. Despite the interest of such diverse and numerous texts, this study has deliberately neglected to take systematically into account artistic representations of a crime that is more difficult to picture than aggression with a sharp weapon. The imaginary of the words of literary fiction has been privileged. It was necessary to select from a wealth of material and to choose one path among many possibilities.

The study of the crime of poisoning in the medieval Occident is inevitably grounded on a limited number of documents and therefore the subject needs to be carefully defined. The geography that has to be taken into consideration is unified by the culture and civilization of a world very different from Byzantine and, especially, Muslim centers. During the last medieval centuries, from Palermo to London and from Lisbon to Berlin, the same products and the same treatises circulated, and the same values and the same beliefs prevailed. Despite the similarities, there existed important differences in judicial traditions and in the medical cultures between the lands near the Mediterranean, which were better provided with toxic material and theoretical knowledge than were northern zones such as England, which was protected from dangerous contact with the Muslims. The chronological definition of the subject is more arbitrary. The decision to begin with modern times, about 500, is justified by judicial and political transformations then taking place, despite the desire of those in power to prolong the Roman Empire. The *terminus ad quem* is less obvious since in the time of Pierre de l'Estoile and Ambrose Paré, the matters of poison were hardly different from what they were one or two centuries earlier.[14] And, as far as France is concerned, this state of affairs remained valid until the time of Louis XIV, perhaps even beyond, since the conditions surrounding poison in the Middle Ages can be stretched until the 1830s, when it became possible to detect traces of arsenic scientifically.[15] The main reason for selecting the arbitrary date of 1500 is that one must end research at some point. Others will be able to continue it.

This book deals with criminal actions that involve poison and in no way does it concern poison as such. Strictly toxicological subjects are addressed only when they shed light on the crime. That said, it can be assumed that the intention of this project is not to establish a list of known criminal poisonings. It has been a long time since historical research consisted only in establishing events that really occurred. Even if it is not useless to know that an individual died of poisoning, what is important is an examination of the ways that the alleged crime was perceived in contemporary minds. Such a study must avoid a purely psychological approach based on the premise of some kind of "consistent context associated with poison," which merges the author of the poisoned letter sent to Alexander VI with the senders of the letters containing anthrax to members of the American Senate, or with the distributor of poisoned meat, or the merchants who sold the allegedly toxic pepper in 1245, or the serial fourteenth-century poisoner named Alice Kyteler[16] and the "good lady from Loudun." The examination of the crime of poisoning in medieval society is not confined to demonstrating the timeless darkness of the human soul. The matter can be treated only in relation to the values and descriptions from a time that is profoundly different from ours. It has to be dealt with in connection with important issues that were brought up by specialists in the history of criminality who are mindful of the very definition of the crime as well as of its extent and its sociology (imaginary or real), and also of its judicial and juridical dimensions that are closely linked to the political and ideological aspects.

The general structure of the project has to be narrowed down to the particular perspective of murder by poisoning. This criminal act goes beyond the ordinary paths of medieval criminality and, as such, it clashes completely with the values of Western medieval civilization. This crime avoids the use of violence, but it implies some kind of preparation, in a society in which spontaneous violence or homicide was often the result of an impulse. It was committed without a drawn weapon or bloodshed in a world in which wounds, swords, knives, and clubs represented aggression and in which the flow of blood determined the gravity of the crime.[17] It was often perpetrated treacherously during a meal, that is to say, often in a universe that was united by the companionship of a meal and the sociability of drinking.[18] It was an insidious and abstract homicide that was quite different from the physical fights led by loyal opponents driven by the ethics of "killing well." Such fights almost always ended in violent death that deprived the victim of the possibility of confessing and therefore condemned him to the terrible *mors repentina*.

Such accounts lead us to think that poisoning had taken an odd turn in the medieval West if not in fact, at least in the discourse. A British historian amusingly wrote that in Chaucer's time, poisoning someone took on a completely different dimension from stealthily pouring some powder into a glass of champagne, as is the case in detective novels.[19] Let us check that opinion by setting out on a quest for that "other dimension."

NOTES

1. "When the dagger shines less and the blood scarcely flows, it is then that the method was poison" (*Quand le poignard brille moins, que le sang coule plus rarement, c'est alors que la mode est au poison*) (Ch. Leleux, *Les poisons à travers les âges*, Foreword). Please refer to the bibliography for works and authors mentioned without a precise reference.

2. Guichardin, *Storia d'Italia*, I, 13, ed. S. Seidel Menchi, Turin, 3 vol., 1971, t. 1, p. 92.

3. J. C. Russell, Allegations of Poisoning in the Norman World; for the fourteenth century, opinion of Catalan Miret y Sans, cited by M. McVaugh, p. 158.

4. J. Michelet, *Histoire de France*, V, 5, t. 5 of the *Œuvres complètes*, Paris, 1975, p. 135.

5. A. Cabanès, *Les morts mystérieuses de l'histoire*, Paris, 1901.

6. A. Brachet, *Pathologie mentale des rois de France, Louis XI et ses ascendants, une vie humaine étudiée à travers six siècles d'hérédité (852–1463)*, Paris, 1903.

7. L. Lewin, *Die Gifte in der Weltgeschichte*. The author criticizes, for example, the rejection of the principle of the hypothesis concerning the poisoning of John Lackland (*Jean sans Terre*) such as he found it in the writings of Petit-Dutaillis (p. 479).

8. L. Thorndike, *An History of Magic and Experimental Science*, in particular t. 3, pp. 525–545: chap. XXXI on the treatises on poison of the fourteenth century, and t. 4, p. 180 and sq.

9. R. Villeneuve, *Poisons et empoisonneurs célèbres*, pp. 44–67.

10. J. de Maleyssie, *Histoire du poison*, chap. 7, entitled appropriately considering the organization of its content. One reads consistently that "the art of poison (...) was revealed to the French during the wars in Italy" (p. 260).

11. R. W. Ireland, Medicine, Necromancy and the Law: Aspects of Medieval Poisoning.

12. M. Mauss, *Sociologie et anthropologie*, Paris, PUF, 1950, 1re partie: "Esquisse d'une théorie générale de la magie"; E. E. Evans-Pritchard, *Sorcellerie, oracle et magie chez les Azandé*, Paris, PUF, tr. into French, 1972, pp. 307–404; A. Retel-Laurentin, *Sorcellerie et ordalies: l'épreuve du poison en Afrique noire*, Paris, Anthropos, 1974.

13. C. Boujot, *Le venin...*

14. G. Vigarello, *Le sain et le malsain*, Paris, Le Seuil, 1993, pp. 78–79, asserts incorrectly that a more "rational" approach toward poisons characterized the end of the sixteenth century.

15. J. de Maleyssie, *Histoire du poison*, chap. 9.

16. *Contemporary narrative*, p. 2 and sq.

17. J-M.Carbasse, *Introduction historique au droit pénal*, p. 279; C. Gauvard, "*De grace especial...*," p. 791, cites an ordinance of 1381 in which the *magna effusio sanguinis* holds an important place among the reasons for automatic intervention by judges.

18. Gauvard C., Cuisine et paix aux xive–xve siècles, *Sociabilité et conduites alimentaires, 3e colloque sur la sociabilité*, Rouen, 1990, ed. M. Aurell, O. Dumoulin et F. Thélamon, Rouen, 1993, III, 2.

19. R. W. Ireland, Chaucer's toxicology, p. 81.

1

An Elusive Crime?

The historic visibility of a phenomenon such as a crime is entirely dependent on the perceptions of the contemporary writers and thinkers upon whom we depend for information. Criminal poisoning, however, risks being doubly concealed from us. Its very nature makes it inherently secret and inaccessible to the authorities of the time, and consequently, to the historian. Unseen and not apprehended, the poisoner has no historic existence. In addition, poisoning constitutes a form of homicide whose recognition and conceptual identity were far from obvious during the medieval period. For us to succeed in understanding this crime and in measuring its frequency (if not actual, at least alleged), it is necessary to see first how the people of the Occidental Middle Ages understood poisoning as a fact and also as a judicial concept.

THE CRIME AS EVENT: THE EMERGENCE OF THE CRIME IN NARRATIVE

Criminal poisoning is considered today a noteworthy manner of dying or killing, a concrete fact. Was this the case in the medieval West? Was it important to an ordinary narrator to specify that a person had been poisoned when simply mentioning his demise would ordinarily suffice? We will examine, in succession, historical and literary sources as well as moral tales.

Narrations of Poisonings by the Chroniclers

One of the most important responsibilities of the medieval chroniclers was to record the deaths of the powerful. The authors were expected to mention the *manner of death*, as pointed out by the translator of Guillaume de Tyr.[1] They did not all approach this duty in the same way. In the index of Volume VII of the *Anthology of the Historians of the Gauls and of France* (*Recueil des historiens des Gaules et de la France*), the heading "Death of Charles the Bald" (*le Chauve*) refers to twenty-three passages from contemporary or posterior works.[2] Out of the twelve that give the cause of the death, ten attribute it to poison. But eleven of the texts limit themselves to recording the passing away of the emperor, without considering it necessary to describe the circumstances. Wasn't the crime of poisoning worthy of mention?

Indifference must be distinguished from censorship. The first requires a certain lack of understanding of the remarkable nature of the crime of poisoning and even a lack of interest in the causes of recorded deaths, the causes being secondary to the spiritual dimension of death, which remains more important in the clerical historiography of the early periods. In contrast, censorship reflects such a strong apprehension that it silences writers, either because the crime appears so shameful that it must not be part of the recorded account, or because the author has such a high opinion of his work that he wishes to dispense with gossip or suppositions.

Unlike his model Suetonius, Eginhard doesn't breath a word of any story of poison in the *Vita Karoli*. While possibly the result of a lack of information, this silence is more likely related to the high opinion the author had of his work. Suger's account, three centuries later, can certainly be explained by this reason. Concerning the toxic intrigues of Bertrade de Montfort against her stepson, related in detail by Orderic Vital, the Abbot of Saint-Denis is silent, as if he wanted to avoid tarnishing his *Vita Ludovici* with information worthy only of vague allusion.[3]

There is strong reason to believe that among the chroniclers of the fourteenth and fifteenth centuries, who were quick to exalt the chivalric life, the complete absence of any mention of criminal poisoning corresponds to a conception of history that was dedicated to the glorification of feats of arms. There is no place for poison. In his *Chronicle of the Good Duke Louis de Bourbon* (*Chronique du bon duc Louis de Bourbon*), Cabaret d'Orville mentions twice that the King of Castile Pierre le Cruel "caused the death" of his wife Blanche (Louis' sister) without ever explaining how.[4] Poison exists outside the historical field of vision of the herald Berry as well as of Olivier de la Marche.[5] Poison has also been banned for the most part from pontifical historiography: neither the *Liber pontificalis*, nor the *Martiniane*, nor Platina, in the fifteenth century spends much time on stories that contradict the glorious reputation of the head of the Christian church.[6] The discretion of the Roman diarist Burchard, who was quite capable of distinguishing among the ways that individuals met death,[7] is all the more remarkable since he wrote at the time of Alexander VI Borgia.

The negligence that results from a lack of perception is not easy to prove or to link to the problem of *toxicatio*. The fact that Flodoard in his *Annales* omits the cause of the death of the Archbishop of Reims Séulfe is linked to the inherent brevity of the history genre, also perhaps to political reasons. The proof is that he indicates clearly in his more complete *History of the Church of Reims* (*Histoire de l'Eglise de Reims*) that the prelate died from poison administered by Herbert de Vermandois.[8] In certain monastic chronicles, the mention of deaths appears to take on an importance removed from all details about their circumstances. Raoul Glaber mentions no poisonings; for him these are simply anecdotes from the terrestrial world without interest compared to the significance of the last moments.[9] In a later work such as the *Chronique de Bury Saint-Edmond*, which covers the thirteenth century, the characters die often but never from poison, even when other sources say that the pontiffs were poisoned.[10] Guillaume de Puylaurens reports a number of deaths, sometimes described as sudden; he relates the obscure circumstances surrounding the death of Louis VIII, but the possibility of poison seems to remain outside his field of vision.[11]

In any case, in a great majority of cases, the authors are quite aware of a death worthy to be remembered, such as death in combat, or of a crime that needs to be recognized. It is certainly probable that progress in medical knowledge inspired questions on the causes of death or illness, resulting in criminal hypotheses,[12] while before this time the mere observation of death or illness sufficed. In his long chronicle written in the thirteenth century, Rodrigo Jimenez de Rada is very careful to distinguish la *mors propria*, or natural death, from other types of death.[13] Froissart states precisely that he knows nothing about the cause of the death of Barnabo Visconti as if, in his time, this sort of ignorance had become the exception and needed to be pointed out.[14] But historians of previous eras also wondered why people died. And this preoccupation permitted the emergence of death by poisoning as a fact to be noted. Grégoire de Tours does not hesitate to give the reason for the deaths of several bishops.[15] Orderic Vital points out poisonings each time that such an occasion presents itself. In reality, for a number of chroniclers, the crime of poisoning constituted an obviously memorable event, reported in a multitude of ways.

Cornelius Zantfliet of Liège relates the criminal poisoning of Jean de Bavière, a former Bishop of Liège (1425), as a blunt fact. At just about the same time, the author of the *Annales de Brabant*, Edmond de Dynter, inserts into his account of the same event a formula that is quite common: *ut dicitur*, "as they say."[16] While other criminal acts are usually related more directly, narrators often distance themselves from poisoning in diverse ways. This phenomenon is not at all systematic or specific to one era. In a majority of cases, the information is given directly. "This king Louis reigned only one year and was poisoned" (*Cils roys Loeys ne regna que I an et fu empoisonné*), one reads for example in *The History and Chronicles of Flanders* (*L'Istore et croniques de Flandres*), concerning the successor of Philippe le Bel.[17] Of eight references taken from the works of Grégoire de Tours, four are direct statements. The relationship is twelve out of seventeen in the chronicle of Orderic Vital. Nicole Gilles presents directly eight out of eleven cases of poisoning, a proportion similar to that of Philippe de Vigneulles (sixteen out of twenty). However, while he often narrates facts by citing the opinions of his contemporaries, the Religieux de Saint-Denis does not hesitate to state directly a third of the crimes of poisoning he mentions, as in the case of the Duchesse de Bar.[18] Jacques du Clercq writes unequivocally that Agnès Sorel "died by poison" (*mourut par poison*): it is the identity of the murderer that is not made clear, not the crime itself.[19]

In about 30 percent of the cases taken from this type of source, the reference to a poisoning is expressed indirectly. Authors report less the act than the discourse or the rumors that it caused, the *fama de veneno*.[20] It would be tempting to attribute this approach to the later medieval centuries, considered as the time of the formation of a public opinion that produced a discourse about people's deaths.[21] But this later period does not monopolize the references of authors to rumors. Two of the four instances taken from Grégoire de Tours are presented in that way.[22] In the twelfth century, William of Malmesbury relates the disappearance of Richard III of Normandie based on *opinio incerta*, which had arisen on the subject.[23] In the thirteenth century, the *Chronica majora* of Matthieu Paris introduced fourteen out of twenty-one references to poisoning with the words *ut dicitur* (they say). The same narrative technique predominates in the work of the Religieux de Saint-Denis: even the references to the supposed poisoning of the Cardinal de Laon or that of Jean de Touraine.[24] The turn of phrase *non sine suspicione veneni* (not without suspicion of poison) is another way, a little less obvious, to point out a crime with the aid of discourse. The chroniclers in the vulgar language sprinkle their references to poisoning with similar formulas. Froissart normally uses this type of language: Jehan Lyon of Ghent was poisoned as "some say and maintain; It was true according to rumors that the King of Navarre from the time that he was in Normandy and that the King of France was Duc de Normandie, that he wanted to have him poisoned" (*aulcuns veulent dire et maintenir; Vérité fut, selon la fame qui couroit, que le roi de Navarre du temps qu'il se tenoit en Normandie et que le roi de France étoit duc de Normandie, il le voult faire empoisonner*).[25] Chastellain's account of the death of the wife of Philippe le Bon was based on "rumors" heard in the streets of Ghent.[26]

The crime of poisoning is thus feared as discourse as much as it is as an act and this reality became more pronounced at the end of the Middle

Ages, when rumors proliferated. The language emphasizes the doubts, even the incredulity—normally selective—of the authors about what they report as the fruit of the imagination of the common people or of the fantasy of jongleurs.[27]

Even though the crime of poisoning created the fear revealed in these accounts, it was an event that demanded a discourse, even if only because of a desire for an explanation. The vocabulary selected for these accounts privileges certain terms and neglects others. In the works of Latin authors, the words *veneficium* and *veneficus*, plentiful in classical historiography,[28] do not appear as often as one might expect because of their magical connotation. In the *Vulgate* from which the chroniclers borrowed, the *venefici* are indeed Pharaoh's magicians[29] and the *veneficia* of Queen Jezebel are enchantments.[30] This term with the double meaning pointed out by Giovanni Balbi's *Catholicon* (about 1286)[31] is ambiguous. Adam Usk prefers the term *intoxicatio*, which is absent from classical Latin works.[32] The verbal constructions formed on a verb meaning "to give" or "to present" (*propinare*), "to infect" (*inficere*) or "to kill" (*extinguere* and *interficere, occidere, tollere, suffocare,* or *necare*) and the words *venenum, potio(nes), toxicum,* even *virus,* accompanied (especially before 1300) by an adjective indicating their effect or nature are used with abandon. Without fearing redundancy, the anonymous author of the Chronicle of Tours presents a good sampling of terms when he writes concerning Frederick II that he was *potione veneni noxia intoxicatus.*[33] In the vulgar language, the words meaning "to poison" are numerous: *enherber, toxioner, faire entosche,* and *empoisonner,* a verb of much more common use than *envenimer,* which Froissart prefers. Other common expressions with the same meaning are *donner poisons, faire mourir par poison, and occire par venin.* Finally, writers sometimes select images to express the same idea: *bailer la corme verte*[34] (to give the green fruit) or *faire manger quelque mauvais morceau* (to have someone eat a bad morsel).[35]

Although authors are sometimes content with a few words,[36] because of their distance from the event or because of the type of work they are writing, criminal poisoning, in many cases, provides material for rather long accounts. In the early Middle Ages, it is not rare for authors to devote several lines to the narration of a poisoning. Grégoire de Tours lingers over the death of the Bishop of Coutances.[37] Orderic Vital gives many details in his description of the poisonings committed among the nobility of Normandie and Sicily and at the court of Philippe I.[38] This tendency becomes more pronounced after 1200, to the point of leading authors to copious development of their stories. The distant poisoning of Thierry of Austrasie by Brunehaut occupies an entire chapter of the *Grandes chroniques de France.*[39] The death of Henri VII in 1313, the story of the lepers of 1321, the cases concerning the King of Navarre or the Comte de Foix (see Froissart's long account[40]) are told with a luxury of detail that often betrays a desire to show off. Chastellain devotes no less than eight chapters of his Book

VI to the Coustain affair.[41] Philippe de Vigneulles goes on at length in his account of an event that affects an entirely different milieu.[42]

To draw attention to the murder, the victim is described in detail: his age or his seniority in his position, his physical well-being, the context and the circumstances in which he received or was supposed to have received the fatal poison, his words and subsequent reactions to the criminal attempt, his suffering, the marks left by the substance on him, and, especially at the end of the period, the lavish care that he receives. The figure of the poisoner takes on importance only after the thirteenth century. Sometimes remaining anonymous or vague, sometimes more or less suggested,[43] the criminal himself is identified by his social condition, which is often linked to his murderous motivations. In the writings of Orderic Vital, there is not one poisoner without motivation. His fate as well as his criminal act is normally indicated. On the other hand, the substance used doesn't receive much attention. The principal information that is furnished concerns its consistency, not its exact nature, and only occasionally its properties. Finally, the crime of poisoning presents an opportunity to analyze rumors and their sources. At the beginning of the thirteenth century, William of Newburgh devotes a long critical passage to the *fama* (rumor)of the alleged poisoning of the Archbishop of York.[44] Chastellain comments with much disbelief on the charges made against the Sire de Robays implicated in the death of the Duchesse de Bourgogne in 1422.[45]

On the whole, the historiographic concept of *veneficium* does not seem to have changed much over the course of time. Historians at the end of the Middle Ages who tell about crimes based on sources from previous eras stay very close to their model; note the various accounts of the poisoning of Charles the Bald (*le Chauve*) from the one in the *Annales de Saint-Bertin* to that of Robert Gaguin. One slight difference is that the accused occupies center stage in the later versions while the victim receives the focus of the authors' attention in the earlier medieval centuries. This is probably the result of a developing social approach to the crime of poisoning. Another question that arises is whether the historical sources reserve a place for the appreciation of the *scelus venenacionis* as such, apart from consideration of the veracity of the cases. Ferretus Vincentinus delivers some moral and historical reflections on the subject after presenting the case of Benoît XI, but his digression is exceptional.[46]

Criminal Poisoning in Literary Fiction

The existence of Apuleius' *L'Ane d'or* proves that classical fiction did not ignore the theme of poisoning.[47] At the beginning of the seventeenth century, this theme occupied a solid place in the French novel. In order to appear more realistic, authors gave preference to plots based on poison instead of sorcery.[48] During the medieval centuries, such plots linked to the process of the "disenchantment of the world" evidently could not prevail. Whether the crime of poisoning constituted a major theme in medieval literature is an important question.

The Index of Narrative Motifs in French Arthurian Verse Romances (*L'Index des motifs narratifs dans les romans arthuriens français en vers*)[49] indicates that for the twelfth and thirteenth centuries the crime of poisoning is not an important theme. Out of the fifty-six works considered, poison appears in only seven, including three versions of the *Tristan*. It is important to note that the crime of poisoning appears less often than the antidotes destined to prevent the effects of poison smeared on weapons rather than poison slipped into a dish or a drink.[50] An attentive examination of the fifteen texts and excerpts of texts contained in the volume entitled *The Arthurian Legend* (*La légende arthurienne*) leaves a similar impression of scarcity even though this literature is rich in potions and magic beverages.[51] In any case, the adaptations in verse of sources from Greece or from Bretagne naturally reproduce stories about poison. *Le Roman d'Alexandre* echoes, in its last branch, the crime of poisoning that resulted in the death of the conqueror.[52] *Le Roman de Brut* by Wace, an adaptation of Geoffrey of Monmouth's *History of the Kings of Britain* (*Historia regum Britannie*), mentions diverse cases of poisoning.[53] The French sources are not outdone by the Merovingian or Carolingian cycles nor by the accounts of the crusades. In all, about fifteen literary works of this type present stories of murder by poison where the word *enherbement* and its derivatives play a role, sometimes exclusively (*Godefroid de Bouilon*).

These stories are rarely the center of the plot. In the opinion of C. Boujot, the successive attempts to poison the hero constitute the drama of the story of Tristan.[54] In fact, this scenario is rare. In Chrétien de Troyes' *Chevalier de la Charrette*, the secondary plot of evil doctors who intentionally poison Kei's wounds is not significant.[55] In the same way, the poisoning of Yder by Kei is a marginal test in his (Kei's) quest.[56] *Li Roman de Dolopathos*, in its rhymed version given to Louis VIII, describes a banquet where a poisoned trap is set. Although developed at length, the scene is not crucial in the plot of the novel, which is organized around the enmity, not involving poison, of a stepmother queen toward her stepson.[57] The poisoning of the hero of *Guillaume de Palerme* is only a detail at the beginning of the story.[58] The same observation can be made for *Florent et Octavien*, a fourteenth-century epic poem, or the *Chanson d'Hugues Capet*, composed at the same time.[59]

In some works of chivalric literature, however, poisoning serves as a pivotal point of the story or occupies an important place. *La mort le roi Artu* gives a fair amount of importance to the story of Queen Guinevere whose innocence must be proved for a murder by poison that she did not intend to commit.[60] A bit earlier, *Gaydon* opens with a long narration about the poisonous schemes of the hero's enemies.[61] A similar story begins *Parise la Duchesse*.[62] Close to *La mort le roi Artu*, these two works give a more significant place to the poisoning episode.[63] Adapted about 1320–1350 from an earlier work, *Godefroid de Bouillon* devotes long verses to the poisoning of the hero.[64] A contemporary work, *Ciperis de Vignevaux*, reports the misfortunes of Dagobert's son-in-law who has been made to believe that he killed the king's son at a banquet.[65]

Poisoning adds vital material to a story. The moment of the ingestion of poison and the suffering that it causes are stimulating to the drama. Poison is almost always a test that afflicts the hero either physically (Lucinien in the *Dolopathos*) or compromises his reputation and his honor, when he is wrongly accused as with Ciperis de Vignevaux, Gaydon, or even the son of Charles the Bald (*le Chauve*) (*Dieudonné de Hongrie*).[66] The theme of the woman falsely accused is one of the most frequent motifs of the invocation of poison in literary works, as Guinevere in *La mort le roi Artu* or *Parise la Duchesse* illustrates.[67] Does the crime itself, which creates this kind of plot, therefore inspire a certain kind of mindset? Toward the middle of the fourteenth century, the author of *Li bastard de Bouillon* does not really separate death by poisoning from other homicides: the bastard, to whom his half-brother Ourry reveals his intention of poisoning their father so that they can divide the kingdom, describes the crime as follows: "with a sword or a knife or poison" (*d'espée ou de coutel ou par enherbement*).[68] In literature, however, death by poison linked to treason is given status by default: it does not occur in combat, the normal site of a knight's death. That is the meaning of the epitaph of a knight of the Round Table: "Here lies Gaheriz the White of Karaheu, the brother of Mador de la Porte whose death by poisoning the queen caused" (*Icy gist Gaheriz le blans de Karaheu, li freres Mador de la Porte que la reine fist morir par venim*).[69]

Investigations into other literary genres give only meager results. Death by poisoning does not exist in the fabliaux[70] : evidently *toxicatio* is a subject that does not inspire laughter. But surely it can deliver a moral, for example, concerning the dangers of naïveté.[71] *Le Roman de Fauvel*, whose hero in the middle of a court populated by allegories of various vices, names them "Murder" or "Treason" but ignores "Poison," with the exception of the poison of slander, which is another problem entirely.[72] Short stories or other forms of brief fiction provide few examples.[73] Chaucer's *Canterbury Tales* are inspired by collections of *exempla*, which tell the story of companions who poison each other in order to run off with a treasure and the work invokes, among the misfortunes of great men, the fates of the various poisoned men.[74] In the fifteenth century, neither the French *Cent nouvelles nouvelles* nor German short stories contain any episodes based on poisoning.[75] Those same stories recounted in Italian, however, turn out to be a bit richer. Boccaccio tells the story of the Florentine Simona, a poor wool weaver who is accused of the death of her fiancé who, in reality, was the victim of poison from a toad that was spread on the sage with which the unfortunate man had rubbed his gums.[76] The structure of the story of the twenty-third day of *Il pecorone* is similar.[77] These stories emphasize less the crime itself than the accusation of the act. Poisoning is easily attributable to a vulnerable hero, who must then prove his innocence: a test of his reputation more than of his body. Poisoning is not unknown in the universe of literary fiction, but it holds only a secondary position, and its characteristics are not easily separated from other treacherous and disloyal acts.

Stories about Poisoning: Are They a Model for Behavior or Simply for Moral Instruction?

At the end of the thirteenth century, Jacques de Voragine collected in his *Légende dorée* hagiographic material accumulated since the beginnings of Christianity. In this work, there are several saints who were victims of criminal poisoning including Saint Benedict,[78] whom the *Vita Benedicti*, incorporated into the *Dialogues* of Grégoire le Grand, presented as a victim of toxic traps. Several examples from hagiographic literature focus on the intervention of a saint who rendered a poison ineffective: an episode having to do with Benoît de Nursie,[79] two stories from the *Vita* of the Bishop of Dol in the sixth century, Saint Samson,[80] and an account by Guibert de Nogent about Saint Marcel.[81] These examples demonstrate that poisoning is not rare in hagiographic literature, but in each case, the crime itself matters less than the symbolism of a type of murder committed by enemies of the Faith.

Miraculous literature established a clear distinction among the methods of killing. A passage from the *Miracles de Notre-Dame par personnages* presented in Paris during the fourteenth century contrasts bloodshed to the use of herbs and poisons.[82] However, the works of Pierre-André Sigal reveal no special interest in miraculous accounts of the curing of people suffering from criminal poisoning.[83] The origin of the suffering of those cured miraculously is less important than the effect of their prayers and also less important than the power of the saint's intercession. Compiled a short time after his martyrdom, the *Miracles de Thomas Becket* do not ignore the victims of poison.[84] But the motif is quite marginal (less than 0.5 percent of the miracles) and the method of murder has very little importance in contrast with the exaltation of the miracle-working power of the Archbishop of Canterbury. As for Saint Catherine of Fierbois, she cures only an accidental poisoning.[85] The only case to note among the 126 miracles of Our Lady of Rocamadour collected around the year 1172 concerns an alleged *venefica* saved from the flames by the Virgin. Once again, it must be pointed out that the exact meaning of the word that designates the person who was miraculously cured is so vague that the translator hesitates between "poisoned" and "enchanted."[86]

Neither do the *exempla* pay much attention to this crime, in contrast with others, such as evil spells.[87] The collections or the indices of narrative themes furnish at best[88] a few stories in which no appreciation is ever shown for what remains a simple element of the story. While the *Dialogus miraculorum* by Césaire de Heisterbach features the demise of numerous personages, the cause of their deaths does not interest him: the distinctions that he makes among the types of death are not founded on the reasons for death.[89] Out of slightly more that 500 short stories published in the old partial edition of the *Tractatus de diversis materiis praedicabilibus* by Etienne de Bourbon, only one features a female poisoner of her parents, whose salvation results from her contrite tears.[90] The preacher is totally indifferent to the way in which the unworthy girl killed her father and mother; he wishes to emphasize only the idea that all sins can be purified by tears. None of the 314 *exempla* in the collection of Jacques de Vitry features criminal poisoning. At best, it is a question of a more or less deliberate poisoning of the digestive system.[91] The *Scala Coeli* recounts the story of the Italian Bishop Sabin, who overcame the poison put into his cup by a rival, a plot probably taken from the *Dialogues* of Grégoire le Grand.[92] The collection *Ci nous dit* compiled about 1320 includes the story of four valets, also used by Chaucer.[93] The method of killing is not important; the point of the tale is to show the consequences of covetousness and greed. With 1,375 *exempla*, the *Speculum exemplorum* written and printed at the end of the Middle Ages in the Empire presents two stories about poison, one emphasizing envy, and the other the virtues of communion.[94] The crime in the story is only a pretext for inspiring the souls of the faithful and causing them to turn away from sin which, curiously, is never that of *gula* (gluttony).[95]

The origins of such discretion are partially rhetorical. It is indeed doubtful that an account of *poculum mortis*, one of the authors' favorite expressions, could have struck the imagination of the faithful as much as a crime soaked in blood. On this subject, a little story reported by Jean Gobi is significant. A bishop envied by an ambitious archdeacon succumbed to wounds caused by the fall of a stone, intentionally balanced over a door often used by the victim. The vision of the bloody head of the prelate reveals the crime to a clerk.[96] A less bloody death would not have readily revealed the deed. For the preachers, poison exists essentially as a symbol of sin or of heresy.[97] The *venenum invidiae*[98] is more decisive as an idea than as a concrete weapon. Seldom the subject of interpretative discussions, the *veneficium* is somewhat stripped of its criminal identity in order to draw attention to its spiritual meaning.

Thus, poisoning does occupy a place in narrative medieval sources. A particular criminal act, separated from common murders, is an event worthy of mention, even of a story. Even so, it does not seem to possess a very marked identity. Is this the consequence of a lack of conceptual visibility?

THE CRIME AND ITS DESCRIPTION: ITS EXISTENCE IN THE JUDICIAL CODE

If, in our day, the definition of poisoning can be the subject of intense debates concerning whether the contaminated blood or the infected meat was conveyed intentionally or accidentally, the accusation of poisoning enjoys a clear existence defined by the penal code.[99] In France, its legal existence goes back to the edict of July 1682, issued the day after the Poison Affair.[100] In the Empire, the process of a similar emergence began with the *Carolina* of 1532.[101] The previous year, Henry VIII of England had proclaimed a judicial statute on criminal poisoning, before the English monarchy got around to categorizing it as a felony.[102] This reversal illustrates the fact that before the modern era, *toxicatio* remained in a sort of formalized limbo. Let us examine this lack of a statute by looking for the reasons, the manifestations, and the consequences.

The Crime of Poisoning in Its Prescriptive Sources

Influenced by the coexistence of the tradition of law inherited from Rome and the laws that evolved over the course of centuries, the medieval era reconsidered, clarified, or forged specific judicial categories. In the seventh century, Isidore of Seville excluded *veneficium* from his list of crimes inscribed in law.[103] Does this fact indicate that the crime of poisoning as such did not exist in law?

The starting point for understanding how the Middle Ages perceived the crime of poisoning legally is an examination of the legacy from Roman law, which was at first diffuse and then clarified in the eleventh century. The codification begun by Theodosius then completed by Justinian divides crimes into large categories such as theft, rape, arson, adultery, or homicide. This codification does not ignore the crime of poisoning (*extinguere veneno*), but it is not given a separate category.[104] The references to it are dispersed in various parts of the code treating particular cases (murder of parents, polluting the water, causes of renouncement) or of procedure (appeals, torture, penalties).[105] The stipulations of the two imperial texts repeat a law promulgated during the time of Sulla (82–80 B.C.) the *Lex Cornelia de sicariis et veneficis* of which article 5 was devoted specifically to *venefici* (understood as users, preparers, and suppliers of toxic substances) and to the jurisdiction charged with prosecuting them.[106] Differentiated from *homicidium*, with a more restrained meaning, *veneficium* included, as well, the administration of dangerous substances diverted from their therapeutic purpose. But it was the object of only one article among others, not of a special law. In 385, the *Lex Cornelia* was provided with an addition integrated into the ninth book of the *Justinian Code* devoted to crimes and accusations.[107] If the *crimen veneficii* thus benefited from judicial recognition, as Quintilian states,[108] its attachment to homicide in general deprived it of independent status. In the Roman Empire, crimes were not classified according to the weapon used, but whether force was used in their accomplishment.[109] This approach attaches *veneficium* to another type of misdeed.

Two titles after the reference to the *Lex Cornelia* appears a decree of Antonin, which incorporates the crime of poisoning into the sphere of magic, astrology, and divination. It is under the title *De maleficis et mathematicis et ceteris similibus* that an adage on the seriousness of poisoning appears. Its placement marks the connection of this crime to legislation against evil spells.[110] Roman law gives *venefici* a mixed definition. The *Digeste* explains that one must understand by *venefici* "those who kill men using odious arts, whether by poisons or by magic invocations."[111] Thus, the poisoner leaves the orbit of hired assassins only to enter that of astrologers and witches. The syntax of the codes brings together the two categories, notably in the enumeration of criminals.[112] This tradition was to hinder the emergence of a special category for the crime of poison in the Medieval West.

In the Germanic codes pertaining to secular legislation, the judicial visibility of *veneficium* seems muddled. The legislative work of the barbarous monarchies does not ignore the crime of poisoning. The law of the Alamans then of the Bavarians devotes an article to the *potiones mortiferae*.[113] The edict of the Lombard Rothari includes four articles on the crime of poisoning.[114] Book VI of Visigoth law includes the case of *venefici* considered to be those who make poison. A law of King Chindasvind (642–653) condemns those who make an attempt against royal power with a sword or with a deadly potion.[115] Inspired by Roman law, the equivalence sword/poison establishes clearly a distinction between two methods of killing. From Rome also comes the association of the crime of poisoning and evil spells. Salic law perceives a close relationship between these two methods of murder.[116] The article entitled *De maleficio* of the law of those Franks who lived on the banks of the Rhine (*la loi ripuaire*) describes the individual who kills another man *per venenum seu per aliquod maleficium*.[117] From association, one sometimes passes to confusion. When, according to the *Theodosian Code*, the *Lex romana* of the Burgundians stipulates the diverse causes that can justify repudiation, it substitutes *veneficium* for *maleficium* in the text of reference, as if the accusations were interchangeable.[118] Likewise, at the time of the revision of the Salic text in the eighth century, the scribe wrote, instead of *maleficium facere* as in the Merovingian version, the formula *herbas dare*.[119] In the Carolingian era, the assimilation becomes more pronounced because of the influence of the Scriptures on the prescriptive mode. Citing the Epistle to the Galatians, which gives a meaning more magic than toxic to *veneficium*, the *Admonitio generalis* links the crime of poisoning with evil spells.[120]

The legislative texts of the following era do nothing to refine the perception of the two concepts. In the area of an initial resurgence of imperial law in Italy, the Sicilian legislation enacted by Frederick II in 1231 does not improve on its glorious model. Lost in the middle of articles devoted to various infractions, the few clauses (stemming essentially from the laws of King Roger) that concern *veneficium* and *venefici* involve the sale and possession of toxic substances as well as the suitable procedure of inquiry for the *scelus*.[121] The consultation of several statutes of peninsular towns produces nothing solid. For some hints of a separate understanding of *veneficium* in the sense of a crime of poisoning (statutes of Aosta, 1188–1253; of Forli, 1359–1373[122]), nothing is found in the statutes of Modena, Udine, Novara, Imola,or even of Faenza that presents a fine discussion of objects used to attack others.[123] The *Siete Partidas* of Alphonso X of Castile (1265) emphasizes especially the sale of toxins that threaten the public good.[124] And, in the Roman tradition, an act of the King of Aragon still includes in the fourteenth century, in the same disapproving clause, magic and poisoning[125] linked as equals in the legislation of the Holy Land.[126]

Away from the Mediterranean area, the judicial visibility of the crime of poisoning is neither worse nor better. The *veneficium* present in a law of the Anglo-Saxon King Edgar (about 970) is characterized as much more magic than toxic.[127] Anglo-Norman penal law assembled at the beginning of the twelfth century does contain an article entitled *De veneficio*, but the laws ascribed to Henry I merge it into the article *De homicidio vel aliis*.[128] The texts of the thirteenth century treat poisoning in a variety of ways. Bracton omits it in his list of crimes, but *Britton* devotes a few lines to it and *Fleta* presents some interesting procedural considerations.[129] During the Empire, the *Miroirs* of the Saxons and the Swabians clearly link *Vergiftung* to enchantments.[130] The *Weistümer* present nothing interesting even though these texts contain special cases of penal justice, and the statutes of the cities probably do not include very different elements.[131]

French royal legislation ignores poisoning as such. Limited to summary classifications, the decrees that enumerate unpardonable crimes, such as the one of 1357, do not mention it. An adaptation of civil law in vulgar language, the *Book of Justice and Pleas* (*Livre de jostice et de plet*)remains faithful, in the thirteenth century, to the conception of the *Digeste* in the article entitled *De homecides et envenimeors*.[132] Texts of common law give very little space to the crime of poisoning when they mention it at all. At the end of the fourteenth century, Jacques d'Ableiges does not mention poisoning in his enumeration of cases relevant to high justice while his *Grant coutumier de France* gives details on the range of penalties to apply according to the parameters of a murder. *The Comprehensive Rural Survey* (*Somme rurale*) of Jean Boutillier, which concerns the laws in Artois, Flanders, and Hainault, does not mention the crime of poisoning among the nineteen capital crimes listed.[133] There are exceptions, however, to this absence. The *Advice to a Friend* (*Conseil à un ami*), a manual of common law of the Vermandois region from the years 1253 to 1259, devotes a brief passage to "poisoners" (*envenimeurs*).[134] Somewhat later, the *Customs of the Beauvais region* (*Coutumes de Beauvaisis*) of Philippe de Beaumanoir also mentions the crime of poisoning, but, by chance, as if it scarcely deserved to be mentioned: "There are two more cases of crime: the first case is to poison another and the second case is to kill oneself, if one does it knowingly" (*Encore sont-il dui cas de crime: li premiers cas si est d'autrui empoisonner et li second cas si est d'estre homicides de lui-meisme, si comme de celui qui se tue a escient*).[135] *Toxicatio* is not the focus of the author's interest. The *Penalties of the Duchy of Orleans* (*Poines de la duchié d'Orliens*) attempts especially to clarify exactly what the *Lex Cornelia* means by "*dard*" (Latin for knife), "hired assassins" being more interesting than "*envenimeurs*," defined elsewhere as those "who kill men with poisons or enchantments" (*qui ocient homes par venins ou enchantemanz*).[136] In the first half of the fifteenth century, the *Coutumes d'Anjou et de Maine* considered briefly the poisoners of wells and fountains after treating individual poisoning in a paragraph entitled *Concerning Magic Spells and Soothsayers* (*De sortileges et devins*).[137] The confusion continues.

The tropism of the evil spell is even stronger in canon law and its related documents fed by the Scriptures, the laws of the Church Fathers, and by Roman law. In the Bible, poisoning is a rare crime and does not call for any special punishment. A clear distinction is made between homicide and *veneficium*, but it is because poisoning continues to connote enchantment, a link clearly expressed in the writings of Saint Augustine.[138]

The canons of the church councils make no attempt to distinguish a crime that blends into other categories. *Veneficium* is not mentioned in the Merovingian texts. Canon 23 of the Synod of Pavia (850) groups together witches and *venenariae*. A canon from the Council of Tribur (895)[139] follows the same format. When the large canonical collections were put together, poisoning was not recognized as a separate crime. At the beginning of the eleventh century, Burchard of Worms considered the *veneficium* of a spouse who murdered her husband, but it is difficult to discern the exact details of this crime.[140] Taking from imperial law the mixed definition of *veneficium*, the *Decree* (*Décret*) of Yves de Chartres distinguishes *venenarii* from *homicidae* (the poisoned from the murdered); he is quite capable of perceiving the difference in the methods necessary to carry out poisoning and evil spells.[141] But when he or his predecessors speak of *veneficium sine idololatria*, one must not think that they are referring to poisoning that does not involve magic: they are focusing only on superstitions that do not involve the invocation of pagan gods or the devil.[142] Although Gratian's Decree considers them separately, the criminal association of the *venefici* with enchanters remains the dominant conception,[143] and this conception continues in the *Summa theologiae* in the thirteenth century.[144]

Following the same logic, the synodical statutes of the last three medieval centuries tend to associate *sortilegia* and *veneficia*, when they separate them from the category of murder, which is far from always being the case. In the statutes of Guiard de Laon for the diocese of Cambrai, about 1240, *veneficus* is linked with the witch or the disciple of the Devil.[145] If the Cambraisian statutes of 1277 mention separately the *propinatio veneni* and those of Tournai (1300) list *homicida venenans*,[146] numerous texts of the fifteenth century return to a conception that connects or even confuses *veneficium* and *maleficium*.[147]

As articulators of standards linked to canon law and of the *capitalia crimina* to be punished, the penitentials [book or set of church rules concerning the Christian sacrament of penance] that became in the thirteenth century *sommes de confession*, proceed sometimes to a *distinctio homicidiorum*.[148] Poisoning, however, does not receive any particular attention from them. In the texts of the early Middle Ages, the "sin of poison" (*homicidium per poculum*) appears only furtively, as a simple variant of homicide, or in the unsurprising company of witches, enchanters, and other soothsayers.[149] The famous *Corrector* of Burchard of Worms is, at the same time, discreet and embarrassed about this material. If one refers to the editions, which are probably unreliable, one observes that going back to the same canon of the Fifth Council of Elvira (310) as did Reginon de Prüm, Burchard calls "*veneficium*" what his predecessor called "*maleficium*," as if the two terms were the same.[150] In the thirteenth century, Alain de Lille takes into account premeditated murder by poisoning particularly in the context of conjugal disagreements but, according to a long tradition, the crime confuses poisoning, as such, and the administration of potions to make people fall in or out of love, which is related more to an evil spell.[151] When they mention it, and that happens infrequently, the surveys of confessions of the last centuries of the Middle Ages always give poisoning a meaning more magic that toxic. In the table of contents of an edition of a treatise (1472) by Bartholomew of Pisa, *veneficium* is given this cross-reference that says it all: *inquire maleficium, item sortilegium*.[152]

A survey of the rulebooks in monasteries and convents does not reveal any specific reference to this crime, which was certainly far from being unknown to the cloistered life, as we will see later. Neither the Rule Book of Saint Augustine nor that of Saint Benedict nor other less well-known Rule Books includes any reference to the possible use of poison by a bad monk. The Rule of Saint Francis makes no reference to poisoning; neither do the early Dominican constitutions, which mention only in a very general way the case of brothers rising up against their superior. It is necessary to wait until the beginning of the sixteenth century to find a clear reference to poisoning in the Rule Books of the Dominicans.[153]

The Relative Lack of Interest in Poisoning in Judicial Writings

As a substance, poison was the focus, as we will see, of significant attention during the two last centuries of the Middle Ages; as a category of homicide, the crime of poisoning did not inspire any particular treatises, despite the flourishing and prolific judicial writings on other criminal matters, such as witchcraft or ideas such as *animus occidendi*.

Obsessed with the importance of civil law, medieval jurists were not interested in refining the Roman conception of poisoning, which was complex, diluted, and confused. About 1286, the *Tractatus de maleficiis* of Albertus Gandinus purely and simply ignores poisoning. In the fourteenth century, Jean Faber (or Faure) wrote a commentary on Book IX of the Code that totally neglects *veneficium*.[154] No one wondered about the somewhat problematic inclusion of poisoners in the title *De mathematicis*. Those who had a vague interest in the question of *venenatio* remained faithful to the *Lex Cornelia* and linked criminal poisoning to homicide without comment.[155] Rainierus Perusinus (thirteenth century) was content to place the *venefici* in the same category as murderers, killers of parents, the debauched, enemies of the public good and of the sovereign, thieves, enchanters, sellers of bad medicine, forgers, and other such criminals.[156] Accurse and Azon limit themselves to furnishing the strict etymological definition of the word *veneficus*[157]; Balde defines it broadly and cites, without commentary, the adage concerning the extreme seriousness of homicide by poisoning. He examines the *Lex Cornelia de sicaiis* at length, but ignores *venefici*, for it is homicide in general that interests him.[158] As part of his *Consilia*, he takes up certain characteristics that Roman law had labeled *veneficium*, but he does not have much to say on the subject.[159]

The crime of poisoning, however, is not totally ignored. In his commentary on the *Digeste*, Bartole lingers for some time on the subject of the production of poison in the *Lex Cornelia* in order to discuss the question of murderous intention and its relationship to the effective accomplishment of the crime that consists of "giving poison." He takes up attempted poisoning, one of the most important judicial dimensions of *veneficium*, as does Placentinus as early as the twelfth century, but the subject doesn't hold him long. The same situation arises with Angelus Gamblione who limits himself to *est casus singularis*.[160] Two other important aspects are emphasized by Italian jurists: the link between *veneficium* and treason (*proditio*), which Butrigario, Balde, Barbazza, and, at the beginning of the sixteenth century, Hippolite de Marsiliis emphasize, even explore, along with the long process of the distinction between murder and a simple homicide.[161] The qualification of poisoning as a secret and hidden crime (*crimen occultum*) is noted by the same Balde.[162] These two particular traits are not exclusive to poisoning since they are also characteristics of other forms of homicide.

Legal scholars who wrote commentaries on the *Decretum Gratiani* (décrétistes) and legal scholars who wrote commentaries on papal documents that offered legal advice to papal judges-delegate (décrétalistes) do not define the crime of poisoning with more clarity nor with more attention than the specialists in civil law. Bernard of Pavia ignores it despite his reference to the *Lex Cornelia* and his enumeration of various forms of crime.[163] Glossing the term *sicarii* that is present in Cornelian law, Hostiensis neglects the second term of this law as do his colleagues who treat civil law.[164] The *Summa decretorum* by Rufin neglects the crime of poisoning even though he comments on the passage from *Gratian's Decree* that mentions it.[165] The commentaries on the decrees of Pietro d'Ancharano (fourteenth century) are limited to reproducing an adage from the *Corpus juris civilis*.[166] The doctor *in utroque* Felino Sandeo, in a work dedicated to Innocent VIII, takes up without comment the relationship between treason and the crime of poisoning.[167] In summary, Felino Sandeo has the outlook of the jurists but not their power of reflection, which could have clarified his vague statute. And the proliferation of works devoted to witchcraft in the fourteenth and fifteenth centuries does not compensate for this deficit. The *veneficium* of witches, which is often concerned more with evil spells than with poisoning,[168] does not preoccupy the theoreticians except to the extent that they are related to the relationship of the guilty parties with the Devil. Powders and harmful salves attract more attention than the homicidal act itself and their diabolic source leads to linking poisoning with evil spells, conforming to the *Lex de mathematicis* that inspires the ***juge-mage*** Claude Tholosan of Briançon.[169] The situation is increasingly confusing.

The process of refining criminal casuistry, linked to the progress accomplished by the clerks in the exploration of consciences, has not benefited *veneficium* very much, because of the failure to clearly separate poisoning from evil spells. It is necessary to wait for Bodin for poisoning to be clarified, in the rank of crimes *exceptez* (separated) from witchcraft, assassination, and high treason.[170]

The Lack of Clarity in Judicial Documents

No one any longer sees medieval judicial practice as the mechanical application of prescriptive literature and judicial thinking. Acts of medieval justice seldom invoke the theoretical foundations on which they are supposed to be based.[171] Nevertheless, it is not unreasonable to wonder if the rather vague judicial anxiety associated with the crime of poisoning influenced the judges' ability to recognize and understand it.

Before claiming a lack of judicial concern with criminal poisoning, one must consider diverse factors unrelated to this crime. They have to do with the nature of the documents as well as the general anxiety associated with the documents linked to judicial cases. A demand for inquiry, a ***lettre***

de commission or brief verbal processes do not have to be as detailed as a sentence or a defense. The supplicant of a ***lettre de rémission*** will avoid using certain words. To speak about reconciliation powders or of drugs while carefully avoiding the term of poisoning reflects judicial strategy; it does not indicate in any way a misunderstanding of the crime.[172] Besides, the lack of precision in judicial documents is general. Behind generic words like "homicide" or "murder" are hidden crimes that it is not useful to qualify more precisely,[173] even though these terms have only a distant relationship with the facts.[174] About 1275, the criminal register of Saint-Maur mentions a man detained for the death of his spouse, without giving further details.[175] In Parlement, documents mention inquiries *pro suspicione mortis* or *homicidii* without further specifics.[176] It is likely that poison was not absent from the minds of the judges, but the author of the document did not feel the need to indicate it. The archives where explicit poisoning cases are described without any attempt to catalogue them or to characterize them similarly follow a general tendency that makes the narration of a crime more important than its conceptualization. The trial of Hugues Géraud, Bishop of Cahors, in the papal court (1317) avoids the word *veneficium* in favor of circumlocutions such as *propinatio veneni*.[177] ***Lettres de rémission*** that present the case of the poisoner who asks for mercy describe the crime more than they define it: that is why this type of document exists.

Nevertheless, the lack of judicial visibility of the crime of poisoning evidenced in the two incriminations seen above provokes questions. In Roman Antiquity, this visibility was strong enough for the rhetorical treatises to give defense models adapted to *veneficium*.[178] This is no longer the case in the Middle Ages. Guillaume de Drogheda presents formulas to be used in court by an accuser in cases of crimes: theft, abduction, fire, property damage, slander, violation of burial grounds. One would look in vain for the mention of the accusation of poisoning.[179] In collections of cases used to set precedents, poisoning is rarely encountered. The *Decisiones* of Gui Pape from the province of Dauphiné do not cite any cases of poison as examples, while many other types of crimes are treated.[180] The author of the criminal register of the Châtelet included the case of the well poisoners of 1390 only to furnish an example of the rigors of justice against crimes of high treason,not for the specific interest that the use of poison presents.

Judicial practice is, however, in a position to define the crime. At the time of the case of the parents of the late Guillaume de Flavy against his wife, the one who pled against the widow was satisfied with describing the poisoning attempt but knew very well how to invoke *crimen paricidii* in order to characterize the murder that was finally carried out with a knife.[181] Nowhere is it a question of *crimen veneficii*, as if this accusation lacked strength. Under the pen of the authors of the acts of justice, criminal poisoning appears characterized by the terms "murder" or "evil spell." In 1357, Etienne *de Vallibus* from Toulouse was accused of causing several deaths. After speaking about the use of poisonous potions, the clerk of Parlement no longer designates the crimes alleged against the accused with any word but "murders."[182] The nearness of the crime of poisoning to evil spells caused another kind of confusion. In 1319, the clerk of Parlement, Etienne de Giens notes at the beginning of a deposition of an accomplice of Guichard de Troyes: "confession of the old woman taken for the poisoning of the Queen Jehanne" (*confession de la vielle prinse pour l'empoisonnement de la reine Jehanne*). However, the confessions of the accused mention only witchcraft.[183] If a slip of the pen explains the label of infamy committed against the wife of Philippe le Bel, it is very revealing about the judicial inclination to blend two crimes that are poorly defined. The criminal register of the Châtelet leaves the same impression. In July 1390, Margot de la Barre was apprehended on "suspicion that she was participant and consenting party in sorcery or poisons made and given" (*souspeçon que elle ne soit faisante et consentante des ensorcelemens ou poisons faites et données*). But the continuation of the trial treats exclusively witchcraft.[184] Following the example of the legal writers,the judges connect quite easily *veneficium* and *maleficium*. Is it because of the lack of the ability or the will to distinguish between them?

In witchcraft trials, the link of the crime of poisoning to evil spells is less indicative of a consistency in the treatment of toxic homicide than of a very conscious judicial strategy on the identity of *veneficium*. The trial of a certain Périssone Gapit, from the diocese of Lausanne, presents the toxic schemes of the accused without ever explicitly accusing her of poisoning (1464).[185] Only the term "evil spell" is used to describe all the crimes of Pierre Menetrey, witch and poisoner, held by the inquisition in Lausanne in 1498.[186] The justice of the Inquisition focuses the accusation on witchcraft so as not to let the case out of its hands. It is not a question of legal myopia but, on the contrary, of a perfect perception of the jurisdictional stakes present in these affairs, as we will see later. Inversely, certain lay judges do succeed in disengaging the crime of poisoning from the realm of evil spirits, where the witchcraft trials put it. A case brought before the ***juge mage*** Claude Tholosan in 1443 qualifies the accused as *venefficus* using *venenis venefficis*.[187] Being associated with *homicida, mathematicus, negromanticus*, the word isolates a particular category of criminal, a poisoner operating with the aid of evil spells. The strange expression *venenum venefficum* is not linked to the natural redundancy of judicial language but to the desire to designate a particular category of poisons linked to evil spells and different from ordinary poisons. Tholosan isolates, therefore, a crime that could be called poisoning by witchcraft. As an indirect consequence, he separates "ordinary" poisoning from its association with evil spells without, however, this demarcation definitively defining poisoning without witchcraft.

The judges were perfectly capable of identifying poisoning as a precise accusation. The archdeacon of the church of York, Osbert, was indeed accused in court *super crimine veneficii* in 1154.[188] In 1321, Jacques Fournier interrogated a leper *super potionibus*.[189] In 1354, the trial that opposed Jean de Jaux, Prévôt de Compiègne, to Denis Chiertemps, Baillif of Senlis, resulted from a formal accusation of "poisoning" (*enherbement*).[190] In August 1408, a woman and a man appeared before Parlement under suspicion of *facto mortis et intoxicationis defuncti Olivertii de Bernezay*: the accusation was worded with the help of a term which, with the French "*empoisonnement*," gained the favor of the clerks of the royal court who avoided the word *veneficium*, which they found too Roman and too ambivalent.[191] In the documents of proceedings conducted in 1391 against the doctor of Amédée VII de Savoie, it was, on the other hand, a question of *veneficiis* committed by Jean de Grandville.[192] The crime was very clearly described with a Roman vocabulary that is found unsurprisingly in the brief that Alexander VI addressed to the Florentine authorities.[193]

In the judicial and juridical sources, the crime of poisoning was assuredly considered special in several ways, but it did not constitute a specific accusation. Its identity appears fleeting. Toward the end of the Middle Ages, it evolved from criminal poisoning as murder, of which it certainly was a form: it was a category on the way to being identified but still far from being clearly constituted in comparison with *homicidium* and *maleficium*.

THE DIFFICULTY IN QUANTIFYING CASES OF POISONING

The impression left by *toxicatio* on the medieval West is not just an affair of stories or of judicial texts. If the filter of the documents determines and deforms the perception of the crime of poisoning for the historian of today, it does not reduce his or her responsibility to ask about the frequency of this crime despite the enormous difficulty of the task. How precise an idea of the practice of the crime of poison can be acquired from the available evidence? Are statistics of medieval criminal poisoning attainable in any way?

The Challenge of Measuring the Frequency of the Crime

The instances of the crime of poison are harder to quantify than any other crime, especially in distant historical periods, during which neither statistics nor records were kept that would enable later historians to reconstruct the figures. Is it even possible to estimate statistics of medieval poisoning?

Contemporary criminologists have spoken of the hidden statistics (*chiffre noir*) of criminality that make this group of crimes difficult to evaluate because not being subject to repression, they often escaped recognition. These crimes were probably quite frequent in ancient societies where the pursuit of criminal acts was not systematic and where the settling of conflicts, including the most serious, did not necessarily occur by judicial action or even in written form.[194] As A. Soman writes, "From medieval times to the death of the Sun King, apparent criminality is only tangentially related to real criminality."[195] Archives reveal not crimes but criminal justice. Poisoning is even more complicated since different from murder, it hid from view both the act and the evidence while violent murder was usually made obvious by a wound or blood. In other respects, as shown above, poisoning could be ignored or silenced. It could also be alleged rightly or wrongly since the proof of its accomplishment was thin and muddled and since a *lapsus calami* was always possible.[196] Because of the distance in time and also because of the scarcity of medical evidence about those who were poisoned, it is impossible to be sure about what really happened. Therefore, the desire to count the authentic crimes, accomplished or only projected, quickly reaches an impasse. The only measurable reality is perceived reality, necessarily subjective, and the only reality that can be perceivable and of interest to the historian. Even effectively carried out, a crime known only to its perpetrator is of little interest. On the other hand, an alleged poisoning, even an imagined one, brought to the attention of a court of justice or the readers of a chronicle, enjoys a social existence that can contribute to calculations. It is necessary, however, to consult a wide database with full consciousness of its limitations.

The global measure of reported instances of poisoning is founded only in one uncertain collection. It has no pretension of being exhaustive, and this collection gives only a sample that further research could surely enrich. The total information on hand is not greatly useful. On the other hand, statistics by century or even by decade present more interest, for they permit the perception of the stages without losing sight of the unequal chronological distribution of the sources. A measure can also be made by types of documents, even of a particular document. The measure makes sense only in relation to other crimes and other historical periods. We must attempt to measure to what degree Occidental medieval society was affected by the crime of poisoning according to specific time periods.

Evaluations and Indications of the Frequency of the Crime

The narrative and judiciary documents that we have consulted indicate that the crime of poison mentioned in documents occurred 342 times between 500 and 1500, to which can be added seventy-eight instances known by the intermediary of contemporary historians. The result of chance research, this total of 420 cases obviously has no meaning. This is the aspect of this kind of crime and its chronological evolution that needs to be examined. Modern criminal statistics reveal that the proportion represented by poisoning among the homicides or attempted homicides brought to justice is limited in the eighteenth century and declining in the nineteenth century in France as elsewhere.[197] Even in our day there are few cases.[198] For the end of the medieval period, the impression is the same. In the fifteenth century, authors of narrative sources that give great importance to news items, pay little attention to poisonings. Le Bourgeois de Paris contributes only one interesting passage; Jean de Roye mentions four cases (except for interpolations) and Philippe de Vigneulles, in the contemporary part of his account, points out only three, of which only one occurs in Metz, the rest based on events described by other authors. His account of the period 1500–1525, so rich in murders and executions of all sorts, is totally lacking in crimes of poisoning. Among numerous accounts of deaths, the *Chronicon Angliae* (1328–1388) includes very few examples of *toxicatio*.

A study of the violence in Cistercian convents, founded on the study of the acts of the general chapters of the order, revealed only four cases of poisoning, whereas stabbings and beatings abound. Poison is a factor in only one case out of fifteen.[199] Similar documents for the order of Cluny researched in cycles of five years gave a similar result: only one case surfaced.[200] Therefore, it is understandable why the prescriptive texts of the Church normally ignored the problem. Secular judicial registers for the ecclesiastic domains of Paris and surrounding areas do not reveal that poisoning was widespread among the populace just as there are few murders recorded for this group. The criminal register for Saint-Martin-des-Champs (1332–1357) contains only one very vague accusation of the fabrication of poison.[201] None of the thirty homicides mentioned, assuredly with very few details, by the register of Saint-Maur seems to implicate any poisoners.

The impression is the same with urban law. The cases of poisoning treated by the judicial system in Rheims are limited; there seem to be almost none.[202] The justice system of Abbéville, whose register (1184–1516) is regrettably brief about the exact circumstances of the homicides it records, leaves the same impression.[203] A study of criminality with statistical pretensions in Nuremburg between 1285 and 1400 does not mention one crime of poisoning. However, the judicial records of the same town, which consistently designate homicide with the word *Tötung*, communicates a general understanding of the *modus operandi* of the criminals.[204] The criminal sentences of the podestat [first magistrate of the cities of the center and the north of Italy] of Milan punished a single female poisoner among a total of sixty-eight homicides reported in the registers covering the period 1385–1429.[205] In Ferrara, the register of executions records 185 executions for nonpolitical crimes between 1441 and 1500. In this total, only two poisoners are included, curiously executed the same year

1465.[206] Finally, in Freiburg, the criminal registers of the chancellery, called *Black Books* (*Livres noirs*, 1475–1505), which record sixty-three homicides (according to the French sources) mention only one poisoning.[207]

At a high level of jurisdiction, the harvest is not much more plentiful. In the case of France, an examination of the registers of Parlement from its formation to 1423 brought to light barely thirty cases (twenty-eight to be exact) extracted from thousands of pages. Of course, such a result is not the fruit of exhaustive research; analytical indices and inventories are not totally trustworthy. But a thorough examination of register X2a 10 confirmed the information furnished by the corresponding inventory. For the modern period, a study of the types of crimes involved in appeals to the Parlement of Paris between 1539 and 1542 gave the same kind of result: not more than two appellants out of 561 are presumed poisoners.[208] The presence of criminal poisoning in the ***lettres de rémission*** is very slight if compared with the innumerable cases of mortal blows. Although perfectly within their rights to request a pardon for such a crime in the fifteenth century, the requests are rare, probably, in the first place, because the crime is rare. Analytical inventories and publications covering the fourteenth and fifteenth centuries and an extensive part of the kingdom of France including territorial principalities contribute only about ten poisonings at most that were pardoned by the prince. The ***lettres de rémission*** submitted to Philippe le Bon include only one interesting case lost in the middle of a multitude of cases of brawls and mortal blows[209]; the 538 ***lettres de rémission*** in Poitou issued between 1483 and 1502 include only two cases; the 1,080 ***lettres de rémission*** from the middle Loire Valley between 1380 and 1450 include none.[210] In Lorraine, *toxicatio* appears in only two ducal letters.[211]

Some investigations undertaken in the English registers of the king's bench in the years 1327–1422 convey the same impression of few instances of the crime of poisoning, at least in its discovery and pursuit. For the first half of the fourteenth century, B. Hanawalt confirms that poisoning was extremely rare in the rural communities of the kingdom of England. Out of 10,555 cases brought before the courts of the counties of Norfolk, Yorkshire, and Northamptonshire from 1300 to 1400, she found only one accusation of poisoning and that one was unfounded.[212] Finally, the "pope's attorneys" do not seem to have often treated cases of poisonings but perhaps the sources hide them from the historian's view.[213]

In the jurisdiction of the Church, research comes up against the very nature of the transgressions pursued and punished by canonical penalties. However, one could expect that among the causes of judicial separation of spouses, poison would put in an appearance or that among clerks who commit murder, certain ones would be poisoners and brought before the bishop. But that is not the case. In the partial edition of the register of the principality of Cérisy (fourteenth to the beginning of the fifteenth century) there appear a few references of attacks committed by clerks with a sharp weapon, but there is no mention of poison.[214] The excellent editions of the registers of sentences from the principalities of Brussels and Cambrai[215] (fifteenth century) and Troyes[216] contain almost no cases of poison. In the registers of the Inquisition, poisoners appear only in so much as they belong to the categories of heretics and/or witches. Scarcely richer than the register of Bernard Gui (1308–1323), that of Jacques Fournier (1318–1325) reveals only three cases.[217] Among the male and female witches, the use of poisons concerns far from the majority of the defendants. Hansen's collection, with its 334 cases, does not contain more than about ten that also involve crimes of poisoning. The eight cases in Florence during the years 1375–1430 studied by G. A. Brucher contain none at all.[218] Out of nineteen trials of male and female witches from the banks of Lake Geneva between 1448 and 1498, only five connect the two crimes of poisoning and witchcraft.[219]

Sources from the last centuries of the Middle Ages demonstrate the relatively low numbers of crimes of poisoning brought to justice. Poisoning is a method of murder that is either so discrete that it leaves very little trace in documents or so scarce that it holds a much more limited place than the dagger or the club used in front of witnesses. Let us add that in contrast with ancient times, poisoning in the Middle Ages was an extremely rare means of suicide: out of 750 cases of suicide reported by A. Murray, only 4 were from poison.[220]

The historians who have plotted the trajectory of witchcraft trials begin their graph only with the appearance of judicial documents that attest the pursuits without necessarily initiating them. For the crime of poisoning one can go back further in time. If archives from ancient periods are missing or never existed, the practice of poisoning is well represented, as narrative sources attest. Sixty percent of the cases belong to the fourteenth and fifteenth centuries; nearly 75 percent to the last three centuries of the Middle Ages, whereas the remaining 25 percent belong to the preceding seven centuries. The turning point can be placed between 1240 and 1300: after this date no number by decade is ever less than the highest value attained between 500 and 1240, i.e. seven. After the decade 1240–1250, the elevated numbers that characterize the end of the Middle Ages continue to rise. Poisoning is a crime invoked and flushed out especially at the end of the Middle Ages, slightly more frequently in the fourteenth century. The increase in frequency in the thirteenth century results from the first cases of mass poisoning that occurred along with the first repeated allegations of poisoning. Earlier centuries have many fewer examples. The eighth century records none: consultation of the detailed indices from Volumes V to VII of the *Anthology of French Historians* (*Recueil des historiens de la France*) confirms this observation.[221] Criminal poisoning in the great Carolingian period seems to have been almost unknown, and it is necessary to wait for the decade 1051–1060 to see the maximum figure of the previous period surpassed—i.e. five. The eleventh and twelfth centuries present a few more examples but clearly fewer than the thirteenth. Certain periods have more cases because of the contributions of chroniclers and verbose historians like Grégoire de Tours (eight cases), Benno (seven cases), and Orderic Vital (seventeen cases), who are the source of the elevated numbers of some decades between 1000 and 1200.

The distribution of the cases is thus clear. But it is risky to consider the documentary transformations as more important than the evolution of perceived and denounced criminality. If one subtracts from the 342 cases the seventy-four that come uniquely from sources lacking possible equivalents in the centuries before 1200 (essentially legal texts), the last three medieval centuries do not contribute more than two-thirds of the cases instead of three-quarters, and the last two centuries 50 percent instead of 60 percent. In any case, this corrective measure does not suffice to counteract the predominance of the fourteenth and fifteenth centuries. The overrepresentation of narrative documents from the end of the Middle Ages introduces another bias that is more difficult to correct: for one Grégoire de Tours covering the Frankish sixth century, how many authors are there for the fourteenth and fifteenth centuries? In the chronicles from the beginning to the end of the fifteenth century, the cases are distributed conforming to the global scheme. One can certainly object that authors pay more attention to recent periods than to more distant ones, but that doesn't prevent that in the writings of Robert Gaguin, Nicole Gilles, Alain Bouchart, or Philippe de Vigneulles, there is a clear imbalance in favor of the late Middle Ages.[222]

During the thirteenth, fourteenth, and fifteenth centuries, the evolution by decades reveals a first phase of increase in the number of documents between 1240 and 1260, a more pronounced second phase from 1301 to 1330, then another from 1371 to 1410, before a last phase with numerous cases covering the second half of the fifteenth century. A period of a reduction in numbers, the years 1331–1370 include nevertheless a decade of increase whereas the decline is more marked between 1411 and 1450. Covering the phase of decline, the chronicle of Jean Chartier is clearly less rich, with only one case noted, than the chronicles of Froissart, Michel Pintoin, or Enguerrand de Monstrelet.

Beside these objective data, other indications point to an increase in the crime of poison, or at least an impression of an increase about 1300. In the middle of the sixteenth century, Jacques Grevin links the compiling of his treatise on toxicology to the fact that the "evil deeds" of men have increased.[223] At the end of the Middle Ages, the same reasoning seems to be followed. The Cardinal of Auch and the patriarch of Jerusalem, Philippe d'Alençon, orders a work from Franciscus of Siena because of his fear of being poisoned.[224] The "mental" presence of *toxicatio* is in evidence by the end of the thirteenth century by the multiplication of specialized treatises. From the 1280s, numerous works are translated or produced (a good thirty before 1500) for the princes of the Church or for secular princes, who were curious about poison and especially concerned about *prolongatio vitae*.[225] At the forefront of this aspiration—the exact opposite of *abbreviatio vitae* that poisoning causes—the popes seem fascinated by a knowledge of toxicology with both practical and intellectual motivations. The most significant author, Pietro d'Abano, writes his work for a pontiff, who has the bad luck to be John XXII (Jacques Duèze), who experienced an attempted poisoning in 1317. His editorial legacy is immense.[226] Armangaud Blaise translated Maimonides for Clement V as early as 1307 after this treatise had been translated into Latin for the first time by Jean de Capoue for Boniface VIII.[227] Arnaud de Villeneuve composed a *Tractatus de arte cognoscendi venena*. The *Sertum papale de venenis* by Guillaume de Marra was offered to Urban V when the plague, which was compared to poisoning, reinforced the interest of the elite population in the subject of poison.[228]

Princes also sought this kind of text, alone or included in broader works, such as the one that Guido da Vigevano composed for Philippe VI in 1335. At the beginning of the 1340s, Giacomo Albini di Moncalieri combined a toxicological development with a health regimen written for the count of Savoie.[229] In 1402, the translation into the vulgar language of the work of Pietro d'Abano was carried out at the request of Maréchal Boucicaut, governor of Genoa, by his Carmelite chaplain Philippe Ogier. A Latin copy of the work was made by Antoine Astesan for his master Charles d'Orléans, another for Charles VIII, so that he might thwart traps set by traitors.[230] After 1471, the doctor Baptista Massa da Argenta offered *De venenis* to Hercule d'Este, master of Ferrara.[231] The feeling of insecurity had become so strong that legends spread easily. A chronicler claimed that Boniface VIII was so worried about being poisoned that he fasted for three days, a scenario repeated in 1461 concerning Charles VII, who died, in fact, from an abscess in his mouth.[232]

The feverish accumulation of objects of detection and other amulets noted in various inventories from the end of the thirteenth century (see Chapter II) corresponds directly to this same feeling of the rapid development of criminality. From 1295 on, these detectors can be found among the popes' treasures, and, in the fourteenth and fifteenth centuries, in the inventories of princes, whose meals involved numerous precautions.

Assuredly, the number of poisonings among murders that came to the attention of judges or chroniclers is quite low. But the quantitative data is so sparse that it is better not to jump to conclusions. The scarcity of toxic criminality does not exclude a great disparity between the periods before and after 1240. Although still very marginal, the crime of poison became more important in people's minds, if not in fact.

To grasp and to measure are the most important tasks of the historian of criminality. On the subject of medieval poisoning, the work is difficult and the results are unsure. This *modus necandi* is not totally elusive because from the beginning to the end of the Middle Ages, poisoning was a category of homicide that was considered separately. Its description in the sources appears to be reliable. Nevertheless, the crime of poison has never enjoyed a totally distinct identity. Familiar to other cultures,[233] its vocabulary is unstable because of the semantic instability of *veneficium*. This fact has led to certain confusion. Even though worried minds considered poisoning to be rapidly increasing in frequency toward the end of the Middle Ages, *venenatio* did not play a major role in the records kept on murders. Nevertheless, poisoning did appear in chronicles and in courts of justice and preoccupied, even haunted, those in powerful positions. It is now time to explore its many dimensions.

NOTES

1. Guillaume de Tyr, XV, 17, p. 686.
2. *Recueil des historiens des Gaules et de la France*, t. 7, Paris, 1749.
3. Suger, *Histoire de Louis VI le Gros*, ed.-tr. H. Waquet, Paris, 1929, pp. 84–85. In the severe portrait that he gives of the stepmother of the successor to the throne (p. 123), he doesn't say a word about her attempts to poison him.
4. Jean Cabaret d'Orville, *Chronique du bon duc Louis de Bourbon*, ed. Chazaud, Paris, 1876, pp. 30, 110.
5. Gilles le Bouvier, *Chroniques du roi Charles VII*, ed. L. Célier, H. Courteault, and M.-H. Julien de Pommerol, Paris, 1979; Olivier de la Marche, *Mémoires*, ed. H. Beaune and J. d'Arbaumont, Paris, 4 vol., 1883–1888.
6. Platina, *De vitis pontificum*, ed. de Cologne, 1540, adds only Clement II to Victor III (pp. 143 and 155).
7. Burchard, *Diarium*, ed. L. Thuasne, Paris, 3 vol., 1883–1885, t. 2 p. 36. The ritual of giving condolences is adapted to each death according to its cause, *morte naturali* or *ex infortunio et sinistro eventu*.
8. Flodoard, *Historia ecclesie remensis*, ed. M. Stratmann, *MGH SS*, XXXVI, Hanovre, 1998, IV, 19, then 35, p. 411 et 429, and *Annales (919–966)*, ed. Bandeville, Reims, 1855, p. 32. See M. Sot, *Un historien et son Église*, Paris, Fayard, 1993, pp. 259–260.
9. Raoul Glaber, *Histoires*, ed.-tr. M. Arnoux, Turnhout, 1996; the Burgundian monk makes no mention of the stories about poison concerning Queen Emma, Lothaire's wife.
10. *The Chronicle of Bury St Edmund, 1212–1301*, ed. A. Gransden, Londres, 1964, see p. 62 concerning the deaths of three popes in 1276.
11. Guillaume de Puylaurens, *Chronique*, ed.-tr. J. Duvernoy, Paris, 1976, pp. 122–123 for Louis VIII.
12. Example: Matthieu, Paris, t. 4 p. 61: *utrum morbo eventuali vel spiritu tristiae, vel peste, vel potione lethifera ignoratur*.

13. Rodrigo Jimenez de Rada, *Historia de rebus hispanie sive historia gothica*, ed. J. Fernandez Valverde, Turnhout, 1987, II, 10, p. 57 or IV, 5, p. 122.

14. Froissart, ed. Buchon, t. 2, p. 311.

15. Grégoire de Tours, III, 17, t. 1, p. 162 et V, 36, t. 1, p. 300 of R. Latouche's translation.

16. Zantfliet, col. 417/Edmond de Dynter, t. 3, p. 441.

17. *Istore et croniques de Flandres*, ed. Kervyn de Lettenhove, Bruxelles, 2 vol., 1879–1880, t. 1, p. 324.

18. *Chronique du Religieux de Saint-Denis*, XXV, 19, t. 3, p. 210.

19. Du Clercq, III, 4 and 5, pp. 618–619, ed. Michaud and Poujoulat.

20. Gilles li Muisit, *Chronique et annales*, ed. H. Lemaître, Paris, 1906, p. 225 (*Chr.*) and p. 222 (*Ann.*).

21. See in the last place B. Guenée, *L'opinion publique à la fin du Moyen Âge d'après la "Chronique de Charles VI" du Religieux de Saint-Denis*, Paris, Perrin, 2002.

22. Example, Grégoire de Tours, IV, t. 1 p. 226 of Büchner's edition: poisoning, *ut aiunt*, of Gondebaud, son of Gontran, by Marcatrude.

23. Guillaume de Malmesbury, t. 1, p. 211.

24. *Chronique du Religieux de Saint-Denis*, IX, 12, t. 1, p. 563: *oppinantur nonnulli eum veneno dato interisse* et XXXVII, 11, t. 6, p. 60.

25. Froissart, t. 9, p. 190 from the SHF edition and t. 2, p. 110 of Buchon's edition.

26. Chastellain, t. 1, p. I, 111, 341.

27. Mathias von Neuenburg, *Cronica*, ed. A. Hofmeister, *MGH, ss rr g in us. sch.*, n. série (4), Berlin, 1924, p. 160: *hystriones*.

28. Tite-Live, *Histoire romaine*, ed. A. Baillet, Paris, Les Belles Lettres, 1971–1986, 8, 18 and 40, 37, 4; 40, 43, 2 et 40, 44, 6; Ammien Marcellin, *Histoires*, ed.-tr. G. Sabbah, J. Fontaine, and E. Galletier, Paris, 3 vol., 1968–1977, XIX, 12, 13 or XXVI, 3, 1–3 or also XXVIII, 1, *passim*.

29. *Ex.*, VII–11.

30. II *Rois*, 9, 22.

31. Giovanni Balbi, *Catholicon*, Lyon edition, 1503, *sv.* At the end of the item *venefico*, Balbi adds: *unde veneficium – cii, tale maleficium*; the proximity of the two words goes beyond simply formal analogy.

32. Adam Usk, *Chronique, 1377–1421*, ed.-tr. C. Given-Wilson, Oxford, 1997, p. 204.

33. *Chronicon turonense*, ed. *MGH SS*, XXVI, Hanovre, 1882, p. 470.

34. Jean de Roye, t. 2, 281 of Mandrot's edition. The "corme" is the fruit of the domestic service tree (mountain ash or juneberry).

35. Bouchart, IV, 234, t. 2, p. 379.

36. Bernard Itier, *Chronique*, ed.-tr. J.-L. Lemaitre, Paris, Les Belles Lettres, 1998, p. 37: *pocionatur*.

37. Grégoire de Tours, t. 2, p. 206 of Büchner's edition.

38. Orderic Vital, III, t. 2, p. 28 then 73, VII, t. 3, pp. 181–182 and t. 4, pp. 196–197.

39. *Grandes Chroniques de France*, t. 2, p. 78 of Viard's edition.

40. Froissart, t. 12, pp. 81–88 from the SHF edition.

41. Chastellain, VI, 76 to 83, t. 4, pp. 235–269.

42. Vigneulles, t. 3, pp. 301–302.

43. Example Gaguin, p. 262: poisoning of Charles de Guyenne *non inscio, ut creditum est, rege.*

44. Guillaume de Newburgh, *Historia rerum anglicarum*, ed. H. C. Hamilton, Londres, 1856, t. 1, p. 71 and sq.

45. Chastellain, I, 111, t. 1, p. 34.

46. Ferretus Vicentinus, *Historia*, ed. Muratori, *RIS*, IX, Milan, 1726, col. 1013.

47. Apulée, *L'âne d'or*, tr. P. Grimal, Paris, Gallimard, 1975, pp. 67 and 251.

48. E. Henein, "Les poisons dans le Roman (1607–1628)," *Marseille*, 95 (Oct.–Dec. 1973), pp. 151–158. We owe this reference to Ph. Hamon whom we thank.

49. A. Guerreau-Jalabert, *Index des motifs narratifs dans les romans arthuriens français en vers (xii*[e]*-xiii*[e] *siècle)*, Genève, 1992.

50. As seen in *Les fragments du Roman de Tristan, poème du xii*[e] *siècle*, ed. B. H. Wind, Genève, 1960, v. 1046 et sq., pp. 127–128: Tristan poisoned by the sword of Morholt et v. 2250 and sq.: Tristan touched by the poisoned weapon of Estout l'Orgueilleux. See C. Cahné, *Le philtre et le venin dans* Tristan et Iseut, Paris, 1975.

51. *La légende arthurienne. Le Graal et la Table Ronde*, ed. D. Régnier-Bohler, Paris, 1989.

52. *Roman d'Alexandre*, pp. 735–840.

53. Wace, *Roman de Brut*, ed. I. Arnold, Paris, 1938–1940, v. 8957 and sq.

54. C. Boujot, p. 70.

55. Chrétien de Troyes, *Le chevalier de la charrette (Lancelot)*, ed.-tr. C. Mela, Paris, 1992, v. 4029 and sq.

56. *Yder (Der altfranzösische Yderroman)*, ed. H. Gelzer, Dresde, 1913, v. 5705–6016 then 6210 and sq.

57. Jean de Haute-Seille, *Li romans de Dolopathos*, ed. A. de Montaiglon, Paris, 1856, pp. 54–64, v. 1527–1801.

58. *Guillaume de Palerne*, ed. H. Michelant, Paris, 1876, p. 2, v. 53 and sq.

59. *Florent et Octavien, chanson de geste du xiv*[e] *siècle*, ed. N. Laborderie, 2 vol., Paris, Champion, 1991, laisse 226, v. 8865–8866 et 8875–8881, t. 1 p. 286; *Hugues Capet, chanson de geste du xiv*[e] *siècle*, ed. N. Laborderie, Paris, 1997, v. 509 and sq., p. 94.

60. *La mort le roi Artu*, § 62 à 84, p. 75 and sq.

61. *Gaydon*, v. 1–1892, pp. 1–58.

62. *Parise la Duchesse*, pp. 1–21.

63. Y. de Pontfarcy, Sources et structure de l'épisode de l'empoisonnement dans *La mort Artu*, *Romania*, 99 (1978), pp. 246–255, believes that the episode, which represents only 23 out of 204 lines, is minor.

64. *Le Chevalier au Cygne et Godefroid de Bouillon*, t. 3, p. 290 and sq.

65. *Ciperis de Vignevaux*, pp. 80–117.

66. *Roman de Charles le Chauve*, ou *Dieudonné de Hongrie*, BNF, ms fr. 24372.

67. J. Frappier first thought he saw a relationship between the two texts but later was no longer sure: *Étude sur la mort le roi Artu*, Paris, 1936, pp. 196–198. See also the ed. Plouzeau of *Parise la duchesse*, p. 126, on the theme of the unjust accusation of poisoning in literature of this genre.

68. *Li bastard de Bouillon*, v. 4369.

69. *La mort le roi Artu*, p. 78.

70. Research based on the *Nouveau recueil complet des fabliaux*, ed. W. Noomen and N. van den Boogaard, 10 vol., Assen, 1983–1998. For France, see M.-Th. Lorcin,

Façons de sentir et de penser: les fabliaux français, Paris, 1979: his catalogue of the principal themes and motifs omits poison. Nothing could be found in an examination of Branches II–VI and X–XI of the *Roman de Renart*.

71. *Renart le Contrefait*, ed. G. Raynaud and H. Lemaître, Paris, 2 vol., 1914, t. 1, p. 309: Érius embarks in the company of a certain Malpansant who flatters him; but when they are far from Érius's country, "Maupansant prepares the poison / That he always had ready beside him / One evening he put it in his meat / So that he killed him" (*Maupansant la poison apreste / Qu'il avoit tourjours lez li preste; / An sa viande un soir l'an mist/Tant que de mort morir le fist*).

72. Gervais du Bus, *Le roman de Fauvel*, ed. A. Langfors, Paris, 1914–1919, v. 1661 and 1507–1530.

73. For Italy, the research was based on D. P. Rotunda, *Motif-index of the Italian Novella in Prose*, Bloomington, IN, 1952.

74. Chaucer, *Pardoner's Tale, Canterbury Tales*, pp. 558–565; *Monke's Tale*, pp. 531–542.

75. For Germanic literature, J. Fuhrmann, *La représentation de la femme dans la nouvelle allemande du Moyen Âge Tardif: description de quelques schémas normatifs de l'imaginaire masculin et patriarcal*, Berne-Berlin-Florence, 2 vol., 1996, gives summaries of 126 stories, none of which make any reference to poison.

76. Boccace, *Decameron*, tr.-ed. C. Beck, IV, 3 and 7, pp. 363 and 386.

77. Ser Giovanni Fiorentino, *Il pecorone*, pp. 212–218: a stepmother wishing to kill her stepson, who had rejected her advances, is punished for her plan by the accidental death of her own son who by mistake drank the poisoned beverage destined for the victim whom she then accused of the crime.

78. Jacques de Voragine, *Legenda aurea*, chap. 9, 45, 49 and 58, pp. 85, 219, 237 and sq., 299 from the translation of the stories concerning Saints Benedict, John, George et Mathias.

79. Grégoire le Grand, *Dialogues, Vita Benedicti*, 27, 3.

80. *La vie ancienne de saint Samson de Dol*, I, 16 à 19 and I, 55.

81. Guibert de Nogent, *De vita sua*, ed.-tr. E. R. Labande, Paris, 1981, III, 18, pp. 440–442.

82. *Miracles de Notre-Dame par personnages*, ed. G. Paris and U. Robert, Paris, 8 vol., 1876–1893, t. 5, p. 178, the miracle of Berthe, v. 650 and sq.

83. P.-A. Sigal, *L'homme et le miracle dans la France médiévale (xie–xiie siècle)*, Paris, Cerf, 1985, chap. 5; from the same volume, La typologie des miracles dans la littérature hagiographique occidentale (xiie–xve s.), *Les saints et leurs miracles à travers l'hagiographie chrétienne et islamique (ive-xve s.)*, ed. D. Aigle, Turnhout, Brepols, 2000, pp. 543–556: no cure of poisoning appears in about thirty collections of miracles.

84. *Miracles de Thomas Becket*, in ed. J. C. Robertson, *Materials for the History of Saint Thomas Becket, Archbishop of Canterbury*, Londres, 2 vol., 1875–1876, t. 1, pp. 410, 478 and 496.

85. *Le livre des miracles de sainte Catherine de Fierbois*, ed. Y. Chauvin, *Arch. hist. du Poitou*, fasc. LX, Poitiers, 1976, n° 41, p. 17: à l'Assomption, 1396, a girl swallows a spider; Saint Catherine cures her.

86. *Miracles de Notre-Dame de Rocamadour au xiie siècle*, p. 276.

87. J. Berlioz, M.-A. Polo, *Les exempla médiévaux, nouvelles perspectives*, Paris, Champion, 1998, p. 408.

88. There are many sources that are totally lacking in such stories: for example, Arnold de Liège, *Alphabetum narrationum*, ed. C. Ribaucourt, Paris, 1992 (800 *exempla*).

89. Césaire de Heisterbach, *Dialogus miraculorum*, ed. J. Strange, 2 vol., Cologne, 1851, distinction XI.

90. Etienne de Bourbon, *Tractatus de diversis materiis praedicabilibus*, ed. Lecoy de la Marche, Paris, 1877, III, 3, n°174, pp. 153–154.

91. Jacques de Vitry, *Sermones vulgares*, ed. T. F. Crane, Londres, 1890, n CLXII and CLXIII, pp. 70–71.

92. Jean Gobi, *Scala coeli*, ed. M. Polo de Beaulieu, Paris, IRHT, 1991, n 390, p. 131/Grégoire le Grand, III, 5, t. 2 p. 274 and sq.

93. *Ci nous dit*, chap. 169, p. 164: some servants found a stone of gold. While two watched over their discovery, the other two went to get some bread because they were hungry. They slipped some poison into the loaf to give to the ones who stayed near the treasure that they coveted. But, anticipating treachery of some sort, the two intended victims killed the poisoners before eating the deadly bread, leaving then the gold without an owner.

94. *Speculum exemplorum*, Strasbourg, 1490, ed. of Douai, revised and expanded, 1618, pp. 474 and 140.

95. It must be noted, however, the punishment for the sin of gluttony can consist of the guilty parties being forced to eat poisonous creatures such as scorpions, spiders, toads, and snakes.

96. Jean Gobi, *Scala coeli*, n°LVII, p. 185.

97. E. Mitre Fernandez, Muerte, veneno y enfermedad, metaforas medievales de la herejia, *Heresis*, 1995, n°25, pp. 63–84. Les *Grandes chroniques de France*, t. 6, p. 317, speak of the poison of heresy.

98. *Speculum exemplorum*, p. 480.

99. It is a question of a "formal" infraction that does not need to have been carried out in order for it to be considered punishable. Nouveau Code pénal, art. 221-5, ed. Dalloz, 2002, p. 240. See A. Prothais, Plaidoyer pour le maintien de l'incrimination spéciale d'empoisonnement, *Recueil Dalloz, chronique*, 1982, pp. 107–110.

100. *Recueil des anciennes lois françaises*, ed. Isambert, XIX, n°1022, pp. 396–401.

101. *Constitutio criminalis carolina*, ed. J. Kohler et W. Scheel, *Die peinliche Gerichtsordnung Kaisers Karl's V.*, Halle, 1900, reprint, 1968, articles 37, 50, and 130.

102. K. J. Kesselring, A Draft of the 1531 "Acte for Poysoning," p. 898.

103. Isidore de Séville, *Etymologiarum libri XX*, ed. Migne, *PL* 82, Paris, 1850, V, 26.

104. J.-C. Genin, *La répression des actes de tentative en droit romain*, Thèse de droit, Lyon, 1968, pp. 107–115. However, the author seems to us to exaggerate the importance of the autonomy of the accusation.

105. *Code théodosien*, III, 16, 1; IX, 38, 1, 4, 7, 8; XI, 36, 1, and 7; *Digeste*, IV, 18; XXIX, 5, 1; XLVII, 11; XLVIII, 8, 9, and 19; L, 16; *Codex justinianus*, VII, 45, 2, and 65; IX, 16, 18, and 41.

106. *Fontes juris romani antiqui*, ed. C. G. Bruns, I, *Leges et negotia*, Fribourg-Leipzig, 1893, p. 93.

107. *Codex justinianus*, IX, 16, *Ad legem corneliam de sicariis*, t. 2, p. 379.

108. Quintilien, *Institution oratoire*, ed.-tr. J. Cousin, t. 3, Paris, 1976, V, 7, t. 3 p. 120; V, 10, pp. 132, 134.

109. *Digeste*, XXIX, 5, *Quorum testamenta ne aperiantur*, 1 (Ulpien), 17 and sq., p. 411.

110. *Codex justinianus*, IX, 18, t. 2, p. 379. This is how *maleficia* must be translated here.

111. *Corpus juris civilis, Institutiones*, IV, 18.

112. *Code théodosien*, IX, 38, 7 and XI, 36, 7 repeated by the *Codex justinianus*, VII, 65, 2: *Observare curabis ne qui homicidarum, veneficorum, maleficorum, adulterorum… audiatur appellans.*

113. *Lex Alammanorum*, ed. *MGH, Legum sectio I, leges nationum germanicarum*, t. 5 in two parts, Hanovre, 1888–1926, IV, 21 and 22, p. 330.

114. *Leges Langobardorum*, ed. F. Bluhme, *MGH, Leges*, t. 4, Hanovre, 1868, art. 138–141.

115. *Leges Wisigothorum*, ed. K. Zeumer, *MGH, Legum sectio I, leges nationum germanicarum*, t. 1, Hanovre-Leipzig, 1902, VI, 1, 2, and II, 5, 19: *aut gladio interimere, aut mortifera veneni potione decipere.*

116. *Lex salica*, ed. K. A. Eckhardt, *MGH, Legum sectio I, leges nationum germanicarum*, t. 4, Hanovre, 1962, art. XIX: *De maleficiis vel herbis: Si quis alteri maleficiis fecerit aut herbas dederit bibere ut moriatur…*

117. *Lex ribuaria*, ed. F. Beyerle and R. Buchner, *MGH, Legum sectio I, leges nationum germanicarum*, t. 3, part. 2, Hanovre, 1954, art. 86, p. 131.

118. *Leges Burgundionum*, ed. L. R. de Salis, *MGH, Legum sectio I, leges nationum germanicarum*, t. 2, part. 1, Hanovre, 1892, titre 21, p. 143.

119. *Lex salica*, XIX, 4, p. 82.

120. *Capitularia regum Francorum*, ed. A. Boretius and V. Krause, *MGH, Legum sectio II*, Hanovre, 2 vol., 1883–1897, n 22 (789), art. 82, t. 1, p. 61 where is repeated *Galat*. V: 20.

121. *Constitutiones regni Siciliae*, II, 33, 47, 69 to 72, p. 105 and sq. from t. 4 to 1.

122. *Statuta Augustae Pretoriae, Historiae patriae monumenta, Leges municipales*, t. 1, Turin, 1888, p. 37; *Statuto di Forli, dell'anno MCCCLIX con le modificazioni del MCCCLXXIII*, ed. E. Rinaldi, Rome, 1913, II, 46 and II, 85.

123. Statutes published in *RIS*, XXVIII-5, Livre IV, art. 6, 9, and 10. In Bologna, the statutes of 1288 seem to have made reference to poisoning and in Venice provisions targeting the *venefici* were put in place as early as the end of the twelfth century.

124. *Siete partidas*, partie 5, titre 5, loi 17, t. 3, p. 302 and partie 7, titre 8, loi 7, t. 4, p. 495.

125. Pointed out by D. Nirenberg, p. 119.

126. *Assises de Jérusalem. Assises de la cour des Bourgeois, RHC, Lois*, t. 2, ed. Beugnot, Paris, 1843, chap. 277, p. 209: *ex judicis officio pendet homicidas, maleficos et veneficos morti tradere…*

127. *De priscis legibus Anglorum libri*, Cambridge, 1644, Lois d'Edgar, art. 41, p. 81: *Si quis veneficio utatur in alterius amore comparando eique ideo pharmacum misceat aut philtrum aut edendum vel bibendum aut arte utatur necromantica…*

128. *Lois de Guillaume le Conquérant*, ed. J. Matzke, Paris, 1899, art. 36; *Ancient Laws and Institutes of England*, ed. B. Thorpe, Londres, 1840, p. 251.

129. Bracton, *De legibus et consuetudinibus Anglie,* ed. G. E. Woodbine, New Haven, 1942, pp. 363–364; *Britton,* ed. F. M. Nichols, Oxford, 1865, I, 6. *Fleta,* ed. H. G. Richardson and G. O. Sayles, London, 1953, I, 31.

130. Lewin, p. 59; see the *Sachsenspiegel,* II, 14, 7.

131. Those of Bamberg (1507) determine the treatment reserved for the purchasers of poison. (Lewin, p. 59).

132. *Li livre de jostice et de plet,* ed. P.-N. Rapetti, Paris, 1850, p. 83.

133. Jacques d'Ableiges, *Le Grand Coutumier de France,* ed. E. Laboulaye et R. Dareste, Paris, 1868, p. 649; Jean Boutillier, *La Somme rural,* ed. L. Charondas Le Caron, Paris, 1603, titres 28 and 29.

134. Pierre de Fontaine, *Conseil à un ami,* ed. A.-J. Marnier, Paris, 1846, XXII, 28, p. 308.

135. Philippe de Beaumanoir, *Coutumes de Beauvaisis,* ed. A. Salmon, Paris, 2 vol., 1899–1900, t. 1, p. 432.

136. *Poines de la duchié d'Orliens,* ed. F. Olivier-Martin, *RHDFE,* 1928, pp. 413–440, art. 84, p. 438.

137. *Coutumes et institutions de l'Anjou et du Maine,* ed. C.-J. Beautemps-Beaupré, Paris, 4 vol., 1877–1897, t. 1, respectively pp. 491–492 et p. 435: "if anyone... does anything to a man or to a woman either with witchcraft or with enchantments, or if he gives him or her poison to drink..., that person is considered as a murderer" (*si aucun... fait aucune chose a homme ou a femme soit par sorcerie ou charouz, ou il luy donne venin a boire..., celui est tenu pour omicide*).

138. See *Gal.,* 5, 20; *Apoc.,* 9, 21, 21, 8 et 22, 15. Augustin, *La Cité de Dieu,* ed.-tr. P. de Labriolle, Paris, 1941, 2 vol., XXI, 6: *magorum opera quos nostra scriptura veneficos et incantatores vocat.*

139. *Capitularia regum Francorum,* n°228, t. 2, p. 122; n 252, chap. 50, t. 2, p. 241: *et si quempiam veneno vel herbis aut diversi generis maleficiis perdiderit...*

140. Burchard de Worms, *Décret,* VI, col. 771.

141. Yves de Chartres, *Décret,* X, 37, col. 702 et XI, 26, col. 752; *Panormia,* chap. 65, col. 1317–1318. The *malefici* act *sine ullo veneni haustu,* without administering poison.

142. Reginon de Prüm, *Libri duo de synodalibus causis,* II, 82 p. 246; Burchard de Worms, *Décret,* VI, col. 771; Yves de Chartres, *Décret,* chap. 155, col. 737.

143. *Corpus juris canonici,* t. 1, *Décret de Gratien,* partie II, Causa III, Questio V, canon IX, p. 515; partie II, Causa VI, questio I, canon XVII, p. 558. Nothing interesting is found in the *Décrétales.*

144. Thomas d'Aquin, *Summa totius theologiae,* Rome, 4 vol., 1896, III, q. 64, art. 10 or q. 74, art. 2. Nevertheless, the author evokes separately *exhibitio veneni* (II-II, q. 61, art. 3).

145. *Statuts synodaux français du xiii*[e] *siècle,* IV: *Statuts synodaux de l'ancienne province de Reims,* ed. J. Avril, Paris, 1995, § 35, p. 34.

146. Ibid., respectively p. 102 et 327. The word *toxicatio* benefits from texts that wish to avoid the use of the word *veneficium.*

147. *Sacrorum conciliorum amplissima collectio,* ed. Mansi, t. 32: Freising, 1440, canon 24, col. 18. Statuts d'Amiens, 1454, *Actes de la province ecclésiastique de Reims,* ed. Th. Gousset, Reims, 1843, p. 700.

148. Thomas de Chobham, *Summa confessorum*, ed. F. Broomfield, Louvain-Paris, 1968, VII, 4, 9, 2, p. 451.

149. Pénitentiel de Théodore, ed. Wasserschleben, *Die Bussordnungen...*, I, 4, 7, p. 188, or Pénitentiel d'Egbert, VII, 7, p. 239. Pénitentiel de Cumes, p. 480, canon VII on the *maleficos, veneficos, sacrilegos, ariolos, aruspices divinos et vota reddentes..., matimaticos et emissores tempestatum.*

150. Reginon de Prüm, *Libri duo de synodalibus causis...*, II, 82, p. 246: *Si quis vero maleficio interfecerit alterum...*; Burchard de Worms, *Décret*, col. 771: *Si quis vero veneficio interfecerit alterum...*

151. Alain de Lille, *Liber poenitentialis*, ed. J. Longère, 2 vol., Louvain-Lille, 1965, t. 2, p. 66, II, 36–37 and 39. Les *venefici per amorem* reviennent sans cesse: Burchard de Worms, *Corrector*, chap. 104, col. 1004.

152. Barthélemy de Pise, *Summa de casibus conscientiae*, ed. of Trèves or Turin, 1472.

153. A decision made in the general chapter of Genoa in 1513 on the punishment reserved for those guilty of *crimen propinati (etiam effectu non subsecuto) veneni* (*Acta capitulorum generalium ordinis Praedicatorum*, ed. B. M. Reichert, Rome, t. 5, 1898, p. 104).

154. Jean Faber or Faure, *In justiniani codicem breviarium*, Lyon, 1550.

155. Example from the thirteenth century, Rogerius, *Summa codicis*, ed. A. Gaudenzi, *Scripta anecdota antiquissimorum glossatorum*, Bologne, t. 1, 1888, p. 166.

156. Rainierus Perusinus, *Ars notariae*, ed. L. Wahrmund, *Quellen zur Geschichte des römisch-katholischen Prozesses im Mittelalter*, Heidelberg, 5 vol., 1905–1931, t. 3, p. 175.

157. Accurse, *Commentaires*, ed. of Lyon, 1589, col. 2124 and col. 1796. Azon, *Summa codicis*, éd. de Pavie, 1506, p. 31; Balde, *Commentaria in Institutionibus*, ed. of Venice, 1599, f. 52 v.

158. Balde, *Commentaria*, ed. of Venice, 1599, p. 219. In the writings of Hippolite de Marsiliis of Bologna, *Commentaria super titulis ad legem Corneliam...*, scarcely 5 percent of the points of the *Lex Cornelia* examined by the attorney concern *veneficium.*

159. Balde, *Consilia, consilium* 221, p. 44: it is a question of a statute that implicates those who supply poison in the same way as the murderers themselves.

160. Bartole, *Commentaria in Digesti partes*, t. 2, pp. 177 v–178: in the *Lex Cornelia, habetur plus respectus ad animum quam ad actum*; Placentin, *In codicis libris IX summa*, Mayence, 1536, p. 433 and sq.; Angelus Gambiglione, dit Aretinus, *De maleficiis tractatus*, ed. of Venice, 1584, p. 165.

161. Jacoppo Butrigario, *Lectura super prima parte Codicis*, f. 6; Balde, *Commentaria in libro I codicis*, f. 10 et *Commentaria in libro VI codicis*, f. 124; Andrea Barbazza, *Consilia, consilium* n 70, f. 150 v et sq.; Hippolite de Marsiliis, *Commentaria super titulis...*, f. 2 v.

162. Balde, *Commentaria in libro VI codicis*, f. 124: *Nota quod venenatio est crimen occultum.*

163. Bernardus Papiensis, *Summa decretalium*, ed. E. A. T. Laspeyres, Regensburg, 1860, pp. 219–220.

164. Hostiensis, *Summa aurea*, ed. of Bâle, 1573, col. 1235–1236.

165. Rufin, *Summa decretorum*, ed. H. Singer, Paderborn, 1902.

166. Pietro d'Ancharano, *Commentaria in decretalium libros*, t. 5, p. 73.

167. Felino Sandeo, *Commentaria super toto quinto decretalium*, f. 194 v.

168. Johannes Nider, *Formicarius*, VII, ed. of Lyon, 1584, p. 502.

169. Claude Tholosan, *Ut magorum et maleficiorum errores*, art. 8 to 10. The *Lex de mathematicis* is cited in articles11, 16, and 28. Note that he does not use the term *veneficium*.

170. Jean Bodin, *Fléaux des démons et sorciers*, IVe partie, p. 186.

171. J. Chiffoleau, *Les justices du pape . . .*, p. 212.

172. Example: *Registres du trésor des Chartes*, JJ 84, f. 145, 8-VIII-1355.

173. C. Gauvard, "*De grace especial*" . . . , p. 123, calculates that 26 percent of the letters of Parlement that she studied leave the crime that has been committed unidentified.

174. In a witchcraft trial in 1477, the label of *homicidium* is given to the destruction by evil spell of a herd: E. Maier, *Trente ans avec le diable. Une nouvelle chasse aux sorcières sur la riviera lémanique (1477–1484)*, Lausanne, 1996, trial of Jaquet Panissière, 26-VIII / 19-IX-1477, p. 318.

175. *Registre criminel de Saint-Maur, xiiie siècle*, ed. A. Terroine, *Un abbé de Saint-Maur au xiiie siècle: Pierre de Chevry, 1256–1285*, Paris, 1968, p. 112, man detained *pro morte uxoris sue*.

176. Example: *Parlement criminel*, X2a 10, f. 90, *Jehan Rose prisonnier ou chastellet de Paris pour souspecon de la mort feu messire Jehan de Verruyes* (1378).

177. Albe, pp. 163–164, commission given for the directive of the trial of Hugues Géraud, 22 avril 1317: *potiones et venena mortifera preparari fecerunt ut . . . nos et aliquos ex eisdem fratribus nostris extinguerent*.

178. Ps Quintilien, *Declamationes XIX majores*, ed. L. Hakansan, Stuttgart, 1982, n 2, 14, 15, and17.

179. Guillaume de Drogheda, *Summa aurea*, in *Quellen zur Geschichte des römisch-katholischen Prozesses im Mittelalter*, t. 2, p. 237 of fascicule 2.

180. *Decisiones magistri Guidonis Pape*, Grenoble, 1729. The same observation can be made after reading the *Questiones* of Jean le Coq, ed. M. Boulet, Paris, 1945, in which only one case of evil spells is noted.

181. *Parlement criminel*, X2a 25, 15-VII-1449, in P. Champion, *Guillaume de Flavy, capitaine de Compiègne*, Paris, 1906, Slatkine reprints, Genève, 1975, PJ LXXXVII, p. 238.

182. *Parlement criminel*, X2a 6, f. 368 v - 369.

183. *Confessions et jugements*, p. 30.

184. *Registre criminel du Châtelet*, t. 1, p. 328.

185. G. Modestin, *Le diable chez l'évêque. Chasse aux sorciers dans le diocèse de Lausanne (vers 1460)*, Lausanne, *Cahiers lausannois d'histoire médiévale*, n°25, 1999, p. 276 and sq., actes du procès de Périssone Gapit, 11-I/4-II-1464.

186. L. Pfister, *L'enfer sur terre. Sorcellerie à Dommartin (1498)*, Lausanne, 1997, p. 190, trial of François Marguet, 25-X / 6-XI-1498.

187. *Quellen und Untersuchungen*, p. 542.

188. Jean de Salisbury, *Epistolae*, ed.-tr. Millor, Buttler, and Brooke, Oxford, 2 vol., 1979–1986, n°s 16 and 18.

189. Jacques Fournier, t. 2, p. 135. The use of the weapon to designate the crime is also found in French: "with regard to poison . . . , we make no judgement" (*au regard des poisons . . . , nous n'en faisons aucun jugement*) says the sentencing decree

of Jacques Cœur, in May 1453 (P. Clément, *Jacques Cœur et Charles VII*, Paris, 2e ed., 1863, PJ XII, p. 292).

190. *Parlement criminel*, X2a 6, f. 181 v, 13-IX-1354: *pro facto inherbacionum et pocionum*. The equivalent in French is often found in judicial documents: in magistrate's court in Reims appears Miles le Barbier dou Chayne, prosecuted "on the suspicion of having formerly drugged or poisoned his wife..." (*sur le souppecçon de avoir ennerbé ou empusonnée jadis sa fame...*) (*Archives administratives de la ville de Reims*, ed. P. Varin, Paris, 3 vol., 1839–1848, t. 2-2 p. 1186).

191. *Parlement criminel*, X2a 15, f. 224 v. The same choice was made in the texts of the Cistercian general chapters not for reasons of jurisdiction but for reasons of language.

192. Carbonelli, p. 224 then 227.

193. Pasolini, n 1096, t. 3, p. 406, 21 novembre 1499.

194. See C. Gauvard, *De la difficulté...*, p. 91 and *Les sources judiciaires...*, p. 479; D. M. Nicholas, Crime and punishment in fourteenth century Ghent, *Revue belge de philologie et d'histoire*, 1970, n 48-2 et 4, pp. 289–334 and 1141–1176, p. 314: only 10 percent of the crimes were settled before a judge.

195. A. Soman, La décriminalisation de la sorcellerie en France, *Histoire, économie et société*, 1985, n°4, pp. 179–203, p. 200.

196. In French, "*empoisonnement*" ("poisoning") and "*emprisonnement*" ("imprisonment"), "poison" and "prison" are easily confused when read. Alain Bouchart, t. 1 p. 400, gives *emprisonnerent* concerning the Normans opposed to Alain III de Bretagne whereas his source, Pierre le Baud, III, 48, gives *empoisonnerent*.

197. J. Lecuir, Criminalité et " moralité:" Montyon, statisticien du Parlement de Paris, *Revue d'Histoire moderne et contemporaine*, 1974, n 21, pp. 445–493: during the period 1775–1786, poisoning was a factor in an average of 0.5 percent of the accused in comparison with 5.3 percent for murder, 1.1 percent for l'infanticide, 0.1 for suicide, 1.9 for murder. F. Bonef-Bouillon, *L'empoisonnement criminel dans le Nord au xixe siècle*, thèse de droit, Lille, ANRT, 1986, annexes: one sees about forty cases per year in the first half of the nineteenth century and only about ten in the 1880s.

198. J.-C. Chesnay, *Les morts violentes en France depuis 1826*, Paris, 1976, Table 100, criminality by the type of weapon between 1950 and 1972: per year, the portion of murders by poison never surpasses 6.5 percent of the total.

199. A. Dimier, Violences, rixes et homicides chez les cisterciens, *Revue des sciences religieuses*, 1972, n 46, pp. 38–57.

200. *Statuts, chapitres généraux et visites de l'ordre de Cluny*, ed. G. Charvin, Paris, 9 vol., 1965–1973, t. 5, p. 28.

201. *Registre criminel de Saint-Martin-des-Champs au xive siècle*, ed. L. Tanon, Paris, 1877, p. 105, 9 novembre 1337.

202. According to the often incomplete indices kept by Varin, the editor of the town's archives.

203. J. Boca, *La justice criminelle de l'échevinage d'Abbeville au Moyen Âge, 1184–1516*, Paris, 1930.

204. M. Schüssler, Statistiche Untersuchung des Verbrechens in Nürnberg im Zeitraum von 1285 bis 1400, *Zeitschrift der Savigny Stiftung für Rechtsgeschichte*,

1991, n°108, pp. 117–193, p. 148 and sq. Same observation for Augsbourg between 1350 and 1400 (*Zeitschrift des historischen Vereins für Schwaben und Neuburg*, 1878, n 4, pp. 160–231).

205. E. Verga, Le sentenze criminali dei podesta milanesi, 1385–1429, *Archivio storico lombardo*, 1901, n 28, pp. 96–142, 111, 131. Sentence in 1385.

206. Gundersheimer, p. 111.

207. Gyger, PJ 27, trial of Guillaume Gerfa, pp. 270–272.

208. A. Soman, La justice criminelle aux xvie-xviie siècle: le Parlement de Paris et les sièges subalternes, *Actes du 107e Congrès national des Sociétés savantes (Brest, 1982)*, Paris, 1984, pp. 15–52, p. 44.

209. *Documents nouveaux sur les murs populaires et le droit de vengeance dans les Pays-Bas au xve siècle. Lettres de rémission de Philippe le Bon*, ed. and comm. Ch. Petit-Dutaillis, Paris, 1908.

210. M. Bourin, B. Chevalier, *Le comportement criminel*...

211. R. Des Godins de Souhesmes, *Études sur la criminalité en Lorraine d'après les lettres de rémissions*, Paris, 1903, letters from1473 to 1737.

212. B. A. Hanawalt, *Crime and Conflict in English Communities, 1300–1348*, Cambridge-Londres, 1979, p. 117 and The Female Felon in 14th century England, *Viator*, 1974, n°5, pp. 253–268, p. 259.

213. J. Chiffoleau, *Les justices du pape*..., only two cases, given p. 149.

214. *Registre de l'officialité de Cerisy*, ed. L. Delisle, Caen, 1880. Same observation in the *Recueil de lettres des officialités de Marseille et d'Aix (xive-xve s.)*, ed. R. Aubenas, Paris, 1937, where there appear some homicides.

215. Liber sententiarum *de l'officialité de Bruxelles, 1448–1459*, ed. C. Vleeschouwers and M. Van Melkebeek, 2 vol., Bruxelles, 1982–1983. *Registre des sentences de l'officialité de Cambrai, 1438–1453*, ed. C. Vleeschouwers and M. Van Melkebeek, Bruxelles, 1998.

216. According to the *Inventaire sommaire des archives de l'Aube, série G*, t. 2, pp. 266–311. The transcription of G 4170 (1389–1396), examined unsuccessfully, contains especially civil actions and letters.

217. Jacques Fournier, t. 2, pp. 135–144, 56 and t. 3, p. 882 of the translation. *Le livre des sentences de l'inquisiteur Bernard Gui, 1308–1323*, ed.-tr. A. Pales-Gobilliard, Paris, 2 vol., 2002, p. 1185.

218. G. A. Brucker, Sorcery in early Renaissance Florence, *Studies in the Renaissance*, 1963, pp. 7–24.

219. Calculations made based on the study of various trials edited by the Lausanne school.

220. A. Murray, *Suicide in the Middle Ages*, t. 1, Oxford and New York, 1998, p. 464. It is appropriate to add the case mentioned by Grégoire de Tours, *Historia Francorum*, III, 33, t. 1, p. 344 of Latouche's ed. In the ninth century, Halitchaire, *De vitiis et virtutibus et ordine poenitentium libri V, Liber pnitentialis*, ed. Migne, *PL* 105, Paris, 1831, IV, 6, col. 681, takes into account this method of suicide, used by the Cathares (*Le livre des sentences de l'inquisiteur Bernard Gui*, pp. 311, 459 and sq.).

221. Volumes published in Paris in 1744 and 1749.

222. With respectively for the sixth to tenth, eleventh to thirteenth, and fourteenth to fifteenth centuries, the following numbers: Gaguin, 3 + 2 + 9; Gilles, 3 + 3 + 7; Bouchart, 7 + 0 + 3; Vigneulles, 2 + 1 + 18.

223. Jacques Grevin, *Deux livres des venins, bestes venimeuses, thériaques, poisons et contre-poisons*, Anvers, 1568, p. 4.

224. Franciscus de Sienne, *De venenis*, f. 2. See the references for the other treatises in the list of sources.

225. A. Paravicini Bagliani, *Le corps du pape*, p. 12 et sq.; L. Thorndike, *An History of Magic…*, t. 3, chap. 31, p. 526, et N. Weill-Parot, *Les "images astrologiques" au Moyen Âge et à la Renaissance*, p. 571, relates the flowering of the second half of the fourteenth century to the plague. But the movement, clearly before 1348, has nothing to do with the epidemic. Even after this date, works can be found that are linked more closely to the fear of the crime than to the fear of the illness.

226. E. Paschetto, *Pietro d'Abano, medico e filosofo*, Florence, 1984, counted 44 manuscrits of the treatise produced before 1500; 16 printed editions appeared starting in 1472, mainly in Italy. The fact that the treatise was not completed when the author speaks of a part that was never written could give the impression that it was composed at the very end of Pietro's life, which corresponds to the beginning of the pontificate of Jean XXII. Note that the translation of 1402 indicates *A tressaint pere… pape Jehan.*

227. A. Paravicini Bagliani, *La cour des papes*, Paris, Hachette, 1995, p. 187.

228. One ms. at the BM of Metz, n° 282, summarized in Thorndike, *An History of Magic…*, t. 3, pp. 527–534.

229. Giacomo Albini di Moncalieri, *De sanitatis custodia*, ed. G. Carbonelli, Pignerole, 1906, pp. 131–133.

230. Ms. lat. 11230 of the BNF. R. H. Bowers, C. F. Bühler, A medical manuscript presented to Charles VIII of France, *Bulletin of the History of Medicine*, 1942, n 11, pp. 69–86: manuscript offered to the King of France by Franciscus Pamoleus of Genoa a short time before the trip to Naples.

231. Manuscrit 352 of the Biblioteca communale Ariostea de Ferrare, cited by W. L. Gundersheimer, Crime and Punishment in Ferrara…, p. 122.

232. Jean de Hocsem, *Chronique*, ed. G. Kurth, Bruxelles, 1927, I, 29, p. 116; Thomas Basin, *Historia Karoli septimi*, ed. Ch. Samaran, Paris, 2 vol., 1933–1944, V, 21, t. 2, pp. 277–279.

233. P. Pluchon, *Vaudou, sorciers empoisonneurs…*, p. 212: in the language of the slaves of the Antilles, *ouanga* means poison as well as enchantment. F. Obringer, *L'aconit et l'orpiment*, p. 227, on the double concept of *gu* in ancient China.

2

A Unique Weapon

The expressions used most often to mean "to poison," *occidere veneno* and *faire mourir par poison* (*to kill with poison*) emphasize the "weapon" that constitutes the essential ingredient for this type of homicide. However, other factors must also be considered: the source of the poison, the different types of poison, the effects attributed to them as well as the methods available for protection against them. Beyond these considerations, a more general question comes to mind: Is poison nothing else but a substance for killing?

THE POISON "MARKET"

In his important work on pharmacy and medicine in the western Mediterranean area, J.-P. Bénezet points out the enormous increase in the sales of medicinal plants between the early Middle Ages and the twelfth century. The spread of books and the circulation of merchandise engendered a quadrupling of the number of products, and this number increased again at the end of the Middle Ages.[1] Since they were linked in many ways to pharmacology, did the poisons that were available to criminals enjoy a similar evolution?

Areas of Production and Distribution Points

An examination of medieval geography indicates that the places most affected by poison were outside areas of major population. This fact demonstrates the perception that the impure is universally expelled to a place outside the community. In ancient tradition, regions such as the famous Colchide, the mountains of the Hellespont or Iberia (present-day Georgia) are famous for an abundance of poisons in their natural state and also for individuals skilled in preparing poisonous substances.[2] About 700, in the China of the Tangs, the southern and western fringes of the empire were reputed to be highly contaminated with poison.[3] During the Middle Ages, the distant Orient (Java, Borneo, or Sumatra) was described as the cradle of poisonous trees from which it was thought that the Jews intended to bring the deadly fruit to poison Christianity in 1348.[4] In these regions of high toxicity lived beasts whose mouths were always wide open and dripping with poison. The soil itself produced poison. According to Henry of Mondeville, it is from India, "a poisonous and malignant land" that comes **realgar**.[5] To nature's generosity in providing poisonous substances is added mastery of their use. The story of the poisonous Virgin, introduced into the Latin world in the thirteenth century,[6] inspired the belief that people from India or Persia could make someone become toxic without causing death. This mysterious Asia also worried Islamic geographers. In the tenth century, Masudi said that **aconite** could be gathered in the land of the Turks and also in Tibet before being sent on to Baghdad.[7]

The Muslim world suffered from a reputation for poison that was strongly fixed in Western minds based on products imported to the area as well as the natural poisons combined with human skill that existed there. Writers who went to the East in order to promote the Crusades are eloquent on the subject. Foucher de Chartres and Ernoul depict the appalling snakes of the land of the Saracens.[8] Reflecting the negative impression that he received upon his arrival in Acre in 1216 or 1217, Jacques de Vitry writes that the city is full of people who sell or produce terrible poisons made from the animals they raise.[9] Jeanne de Bourgogne's physician, Guido Vigevano from Pavia, emphasizes that the Saracen regions abound with **aconite.**[10] *Venefici* are also abundant in these eastern lands. The physician whom Charles the Bad (*le Mauvais*) puts in charge of poisoning the Valois princes and probably asked to make an appropriate substance was from Cyprus, whereas the presumed poisoner of the Comte de Savoie was a "physician from the Orient" (*phisicien d'Orient*) who claimed to use products from overseas.[11] A *velano venuto di Levante* and a product from Constantinople are involved in two cases in 1453 and 1490.[12]

Nevertheless, the East is not the only source of poison in Western eyes. Indeed, the very existence of the following expressions, "Spanish figs" and "Italian 'boucon' "[bite or mouthful] referring to poison[13] indicate that these countries were also associated with poison. Because Italy was in contact with Islam, and because it was at the end of trade routes, it enjoyed a special reputation. Around the tenth or eleventh century, its southern part, which had been Muslim for a while, was thought to shelter experts in the making of poison, such as the doctor from Salerno described by Richer de Saint-Remi.[14] The expression *eruditio veneficiorum* was used to characterize even a princess who was closely linked to doctors from Salerno.[15] At this point the geography of Italian poison switches to the north. **Realgar** and **orpiment** of excellent quality arrived in Venice.[16] The murderer of Henry of Breslau was aware of this fact since he went to the city of the doges to buy the deadly substance (1293).[17] A century later, the poison destined for Amédéé VIII de Savoie was acquired in Florence.[18] But Tuscany was subsequently largely supplanted by Lombardy. About 1450, the poison given to Gilles de Bretagne had been bought in that region.[19] Jehan Coustain sent an accomplice to Lombardy to acquire what was necessary to murder the Comte de Charolais.[20] In Bâle, in 1430, the authorities ordered professionals who used Italian poison to be extremely vigilant. It is clear that Italy's reputation dates back much earlier than the sixteenth century.

Famous as the headquarters of magic ("the art of Toledo") and alchemy,[21] the Iberian peninsula was also known for being a land of the production and supply of poison. The investigations that occurred in Savoie in 1348 showed that the powders that were supposed to kill Christians there had been produced in Toledo.[22] The interrogation of the accused poisoner of the Comte de Savoie in 1395 revealed that the powder used to kill the Count had been bought in Léon.[23] The presence of Jews and Infidels in those regions was strongly linked to their poisonous reputation. On the contrary, some regions were reputed to be totally lacking in poison of any kind. For reasons linked to nature or to the miracles of Saint Patrick, Ireland was not only thought to be venom free, but its air was also known for having a curative effect.[24]

There exists a certain distance between the location of production and the delivery point. The places where poison could be found largely coincided with places where toxic products were needed for medical, surgical, and pharmaceutical use. Apothecary shops were excellent sources of poison. Some apothecary inventories included products that were essentially mineral in nature such as quicksilver (mercury) or arsenic[25] and that were useful for many purposes. Criminals were aware of the presence of these substances in apothecary shops: Robert Wourdreton justified his purchase of a quarter of an ounce of what he thought to be mercuric chloride by saying the he needed it to heal his horse's wound; and Willemine la Barbière asked for arsenic to kill rats.[26] At the end of the Middle Ages, a wide network of dispensaries served to increase the sales of poison. As early as 1305, thinking they would have to go to Montpellier to acquire the poison to kill their bishop, the canons of Avignon realized they could find everything they needed nearby.[27] Charles the Bad (*le Mauvais*) guaranteed Robert Wourdreton that he would find what he needed "in apothecary shops in Pampelona, Bordeaux, and Bayonne and in all the cities [he would pass through]" (*Pampelune, Bordiaux, Bayonne et par toutes les bonnes villes [où il passera] es ostelz des apoticaires*).[28] Therefore, Michelet was right to talk about the democratization of poison at the end of the Middle Ages.[29] Thanks to the increase of both international and local trade—the most important method of getting supplies[30]—as well as the effect of the "medicalisation" of society, which led to the increase in number of apothecary pharmacies, the availability of poison increased and became more diverse, increasing its access to more modest people: a small amount of a toxic material cost only four sous in 1501.[31]

The easy availability of poison caused such products gradually to become regulated. As heir to the Arabic tradition, the Crown of Aragon put the distribution of toxic substances under strict control in the fourteenth century.[32] In 1326, the council of Avignon stipulated that the sale of poison would have to be reported to the common court (the bishop's?), so that the purchaser could be identified if necessary.[33] In 1384 France, one needed "approval and judicial authority" (*congié et auctorité de justice*) to market a particularly harmful form of arsenic.[34] Urban authorities controlled the possession and sale of poison by apothecaries. A text from Bordeaux dated 1414 quoted at the beginning of the sixteenth century predicts "that no owner will be allowed to have **realgar,** arsenic, quicksilver (mercury) or mercuric chloride in his shop if it is not under lock and key" (*qu'aucun maistre ne pourra tenir en sa boutique riarga, arsenic, argent vif ou sublimé si ce n'est sous la clef*).[35] In 1496, apothecaries in Nuremberg were required to keep a written record of their sales.[36] The 1492 arrest of a poisoner in Poitou while he was buying powder proves that the controls were effective.[37]

Another less perceptible source of supply, the sellers of ***thériaque*** sold dangerous substances wherever they went. Their trade implies, in fact, the possession of poison samples to be taken in small doses in order to demonstrate their efficacy to their customers, mainly as an antidote. In 1404, Jehan Guillerau's accusers blamed him for wanting to acquire **realgar** from a seller of ***thériaque***.[38] In 1482, a ***lettre de rémission*** presented a criminal who successively went to an apothecary and then to a seller of ***thériaque*** who provided him with poison for 20 sous but not without a warning.[39] Because of the potential danger such a job implied, the authorities reserved the making and selling of poison to people who were settled in one spot more or less under oath, who operated openly observing very strict regulations.[40]

At the end of the Middle Ages, the poison market followed a simple topography (in cities) and trade economy that the following expression from 1482 illustrates very well: "to make money from **realgar** and arsenic" (*faire finance de reagal et de arsenic*).[41] But these words ignore both the commerce in poison before the thirteenth century (which is hard to trace) and the most likely frequent avoidance of legitimate trade in poison in order to work in secret. In his account, Jacques Fournier mentions the case of a female poisoner who easily found some **hellebore** in the Pyrénées mountains while the purchase of **realgar** required a much more visible trip to an apothecary shop in a neighboring town.[42] There existed "commercial" poison, normally a mineral, and what can be called a "gathered poison," one that occurred naturally from plant sources and predominated in the early periods and in the country. **Aconite** could be gathered by the armfuls in the damp pastures of the Lombardian Alps where animals were not permitted to graze and Jews were not allowed to go for fear they would harvest the poison for criminal reasons.[43] Moreover, even when the supply was not so easily available, the sale of poison often escaped the open market. Street corners or private houses could be used as places where wrapped toxic products were distributed. A washerwoman who was suspected of providing a draper's widow with poison fits into that hidden poison trade.[44]

Producer and Provider: Separate Worlds?

In African societies there existed "masters of poison" who held very prestigious positions.[45] *Venenarii* or *venefici* from the ancient or Byzantine world had a similar status. Sometimes they were trained in schools and were known for producing and distributing poison. This is the narrow meaning that Isidore of Seville gives to the word *veneficus*.[46] One of their incarnations was the very skilled Locust whom Medea emulated.[47] Christine de Pizan describes the latter as capable of making poisoned brews since she possessed the knowledge of the qualities of plants.[48] Does that mean that Christine believed in the existence of such specialists in her time? Is the late example of Catherine Sforza, whose book entitled *Experimenti (1508)* contains one hundred and fifty recipes, widespread?

Expertise in poison was rarely limited only to the preparation of venom. In a fourteenth century novel entitled *Gaydon*, we read that Ganelon's brother had been informed by his uncle, who was trained in necromancy, how to get poison from a particular herb crushed in a mortar and then soaked in white wine.[49] From Félix Hermelin (about 1445) to Jean Bodin, experts on witchcraft point out that the making of poisonous substances is part of the activity of witches.[50] The three women who were burned on the Saturday before the Feast of Saint John in 1315 were accused of making the poisons given to the bishop of Châlons and, therefore, they were known as witches.[51] About 1400, Guillemette Blancpaine was solicited by a murderer who "knew her to be a witch who used enchantments or poisons" (*la savoit ester sorciere et user caraux ou poisons*).[52] During a trial in 1423, another Guillemette is mentioned. There she appears as a provider of powders, "a master of making poisons that work over an extended time" (*maistre de faire poison a long temps*), a title that endowed her with special knowledge.[53] The opposite sex also had this ability. Documents from a trial in 1448 mention a person who knew how to create *poncetum*, an evil powder the recipe for which was received from another man.[54] There is more! In the twelfth century, Hildegarde of Bingen, persuaded of the existence of special places where poisons were made, attributed the toxic effects of plants from the **Solanaceae** family to the devil.[55] During the fourteenth and fifteenth centuries, we go a step further. Without doubt, the designation of *venenator* attributed to the devil by Saint Augustine,[56] when taken literally, contributed to the idea that the Devil in person provided poison during the Sabbath.[57] As early as 1335, shepherds from the area of Carcassone were believed to have received deadly powder from the Fallen Angel.[58] During the Helvetian trials that took place during the second half of the fifteenth century, there were many references to powders and ointments made under inspiration from the devil[59] or given in small boxes by Satan himself.[60]

The Jews were also considered as *venefici* in the restricted sense. Hugues Géraud, the treasurer of the Bishop of Cahors solicited a Jew in order to obtain some wax (to bewitch) and also a poisonous substance.[61] An agent of Charles the Bad (*le Mauvais*) went to see a Jewess of Navare to buy some poison that she had made.[62] Trials in Parlement show in similar fashion murderers who went to Jews (both men and women), who were reputed to be able to provide them with what they needed to commit murder.[63] This fantastical vision of established providers of poison was widespread in the fourteenth and especially the fifteenth century. Yet, the majority of *venena* comes from more ordinary milieux.

An old historiographic tradition transformed practitioners corrupted by alchemy, the apothecary trade, or, to a lesser degree, medicine, into producers and sellers of poison. The increase in numbers of people involved in such activities would have led to the appearance of "black sheep" who used their knowledge for bad purposes because of the difficulty in finding decent jobs in a society in crisis.[64] In fact, the image of the specialist in pharmaceutics who provides poison dates back a long time: Cicero introduces it first in *Pro Cluentio*.[65] An 1192 text from London classifies the apothecary in the not very respectable group of magicians and witches.[66] During the second half of the fifteenth century, Saladin d'Ascali, the author of *Compendium aromatariorum*, warns against apothecaries who may be tempted to create deadly potions.[67] However, the gap between the theoretical and the historical cases is large. Less than 3 percent of extant cases record an accusation against an apothecary such as Cassien Petri, a Lombard by origin, who is the so-called provider of Guichard de Troyes, for his crime against Blanche de Navarre;[68] or such as Pierre Lompnes, the maker of dangerous potions that Jean de Grandville used against the Comte de Savoie Amédée VII.[69] A last example of this phenomenon is the poor apothecary from Clermont-en-Auvergne, who was literally diverted by Jean de Chalon in order to carry out a criminal project that targeted Louis XI.[70] Nevertheless, during the fourteenth and fifteenth centuries, the profession was more often reproached for its ignorance and negligence regarding medical procedures than for its criminal proclivity. French royal ordinances aimed above all at fighting against the nuisances triggered by the delivery of expired drugs which were adulterated, not correctly proportioned or harmful because of incompetence as the Parisian university of medicine declared in 1271.[71] Some members of the profession were even noted for their integrity. Jacques Fournier records that a targeted poison victim was saved by an apothecary who refused to deliver the deadly substance to her enemy.[72] An apothecary in Illiers sought to discover the purpose of powders that a lawyer had him make in 1482.[73] Strictly criminal suspicion was closely linked to the moral quality of those who practiced as apothecaries. Almost everywhere in the thirteenth century, Jews were forbidden to take up the trade of apothecary.[74] In 1312, authorities in Barcelona prohibited Jews from trading in **realgar**, but also strictly regulated the Christians who handled the poison.[75]

Scholarly doctors were another group suspected of producing dangerous substances. Guillaume Agasse, a leper questioned by Jacques Fournier, indicated that the powders put into the wells in 1321 had been made *de consilio medicorum*. The evil Robert depicted in 1350 in Ciperis de Vignevaux . . . "he had so much knowledge and was so well-educated / that it was not possible to find a better clerk wherever he may be assigned. / And there was no poison that he had not prepared" (*tant savoit clergié et tant fut doctrine / Ne toeuve si grant clerc ou il n'ait depute./Si n'estoit nul venin qu'il n'eust destrempé . . .*).[76] *A fortiori*, the therapists without "education" were considered as knowledgeable about poisons of a somewhat different nature. Skillful at making powders, Marguerite Daumas was initiated by a matron (*obstetrix*) into the making of evil spells, invocations, magical arts, and bewitchments.[77] As for alchemists, their place in extant documents is quite limited. Pietro d'Abano indicates that sublimate of mercury or arsenic were obtained *secundum alkimiam*, but it is a question here of practical alchemy (today we would call it chemistry)[78] and not speculative. Certain mineral or vegetable poisons were useful in alchemy experiments, reciprocally, one could obtain toxic products.[79] In the particular domain of the transmutation of metals, poison played a part as an agent of corrosion or alteration. But the idea of an explosion of the number of poisonings parallel to the development of alchemy activity is not soundly based.[80]

Overall, the use of poison as a weapon benefited from a better supply during the last medieval centuries. The knowledge of poison, not considered here because of little evidence of direct criminal use,[81] and actual availability expanded without causing the old ways of intuitive or natural access to disappear, and without abolishing the ancient idea of specialized producers. It is questionable to speak of the "banalisation" of toxic substances in the fourteenth century under the pretext that one could easily find rat poison.[82] A phantasmagorical geography of poisons subsists, doubled by an imaginary of the *veneficus* reinforced by the fantasy of witchcraft. The providers of poison were varied in relation to their trade. To make substances with an animal base, Guichard de Troyes is reputed to have asked a hermit for information whereas the poison that was to be given to Queen Blanche came from an apothecary capable of skillfully manipulating rarer materials.[83]

PRODUCTS THAT WERE USED AND THE INSTRUCTIONS

In a letter written from Orvieto, July 28, 1264, Urban IV warns Charles d'Anjou that a poisoner and assassins armed with fifty kinds of poison were preparing to kill him.[84] The treatise by Pietro d'Abano presents ninety-six poisons, mentions about thirty others and relates the instruction for obtaining a sublimated form (oxidized after heating) or lead oxide (**litharge**) or **realgar** from sulfur and lead.[85] A reflection of the rich choice available at the time to criminals, these two examples invite us to examine what kinds of products were used by criminals. Since the nature and the kind of poison used are mentioned in fewer than 15 percent of the cases, the data is rather scarce.

Simple Poisons

In an old study dedicated to poisonings that occurred in the sixteenth century, an author asserted that the medieval period only had poisons made from vegetable matter, uncomplicated products, unlike the poisons made from minerals that did not appear until the Renaissance.[86] The widespread use of the term "to give herbs" (*enherber*) to mean "to poison" implies indeed that a part of the criminal *venena* in the Middle Ages was vegetable in origin, particularly in the early period. However, "herbs" rarely appear in our collection of cases while the learned distribution of poisons attributes a large number to vegetable matter (almost half in the works of Pietro d'Abano). Nothing is said about those that were given to the Visigoth King Bamba nor about those that Jean de Jaux, the Provost of Compiègne, used (1354).[87] It may be that the pastel plant was used in the case of the poisoning of the waters in 1412.[88] **Aconite** is mentioned by the sources that wish to emphasize the cruelty of the enemies of Henry VII. Indeed, since the time of Ovid, Pliny, and Avicenna, this plant was considered as one of the strongest and irreparably toxic,[89] whose

Latin name *napellus* expresses its irresistible danger.[90] In addition, perhaps in contact with the mountainous areas where the Waldensian heresy was well-established, **aconite** was sometimes called *thora valdenis* or the Waldensian herb.[91] Another heretical herb, **hellebore** disappointed a female murderer pursued by Jacques Fournier. She chose to turn to a more reliable poison, **realgar**.[92] During the last medieval centuries, minerals appear much more often in the documents than vegetables as a source of poison.

Arsenic and **realgar** represent two-fifths of the poisons that are mentioned in the extant documents. Arsenic was known to the ancient world but mercuric chloride, which was much more toxic, a product known to the Arab world as early as the ninth century, appeared in the West at a date that is difficult to determine. Certain equipment and special manipulations (notably heating) were necessary to obtain a substance *ab arte procurata*.[93] On the advice of Charles the Bad (*le Mauvais*), obviously a connoisseur, Wordreton planned to use **sublimate** of arsenic (white arsenic) that was known for its effectiveness.[94]

The Arab name for what the ancients called "*sandaraque*," **realgar** is found at the top of the list of the poisons that are mentioned. Its frequent presence in criminal cases causes it to be suggested when the exact poison used in a murder is not clearly identified.

When Jacques de Rue had to determine what killed Seguin de Badefol, who was murdered at the King of Navarre's table, he said he did not know "what poisons were used but he thought it was *realgal*" (*quelles furent les poisons fors que il pense que ce fut par reagal*).[95] **Antimony** appears less often as does lead oxide (**litharge**) that was used about 1400 by a man from Palermo who was tired of his wife, or the magnet stone (iron oxide) that was suggested as the poison that killed Henry VII.[96]

In less than half of the cases for which data survives, toxic substances come from animal materials. The natural toxicity of certain beasts and decomposed organisms, pointed out by contemporary specialists, were put to use by poisoners. The fact that cats' brains are supposed to make people demented is found both in erudite treatises[97] and in the behavior of a nasty mother-in-law in 1469.[98] The flesh of corpses as well as hair and nails, which were considered impure superfluous substances rejected by the body to its extremities, were reputed to be toxic.[99] The armies of Frederick Barbarossa used corpses to poison the water supply of Pavia.[100] In 1390, the poisons placed in the fountains included among other substances the remains of hanged men. Indeed, materials useful for evil spells as well as for the making of poisons came from the gallows.[101] An act of Parlement in 1408 denounced "venomous" people who wandered around the gallows in order to acquire material for their trade.[102] These poisoners depended on the toxicity of putrefaction, which was thought to cause crawling animals to be poisonous since they came in contact with filthy and rotten substances in the earth.[103] Poisoners were less interested than witches in grilled and pulverized bones of young children.

Both dead flesh and menstrual blood were reputed to be toxic. It was considered as the body ridding itself of a harmful superfluous substance[104]: a variant of *The Secrets of Philosophers* (*Secrés as philosophes*) asserts that "menstrual blood is a worse and more dangerous poison than snake's venom" (*les fleurs est ung venin plus malvaiz et dangereuz que venin de sepent*).[105] Pietro d'Abano shares this opinion and also supports the idea that the blood and secretions of lepers are filled with venom.[106] This element was obviously of the utmost interest for the affair of 1321, even though, thanks to a strange paradox, the poison that was supposed to have been spread by the lepers in the fountains and the wells did not come from their bodies, although its purpose was to infect healthy people with the illness of the lepers.[107] As far as animals are concerned, the same species can be found from one case to another. A dismembered toad constituted the base of the substance given to the priest depicted by Guibert de Nogent. Spiders made up the gruel concocted by a woman taken to court in 1407. Four pieces of grass snake soaked in slurry were to be given to eat to a certain Jehan Chastellain (1408).[108] On the other hand, we hardly find any trace of **cantharadin** that was said to be the favorite poison of the Borgias.[109]

Compound Poisons

The documentation rarely indicates what poisonous substances are made of. Questioned on September 6, 1390, at the Châtelet, the suspect Jehan de Bloys said he did not know the composition of the poisons to be thrown into the wells and fountains.[110] Nevertheless, there are clues that indicate miscellaneous mixtures of substances clearly dominated by animal products.

Guichard de Troyes was accused of having poison made only from venomous animals (scorpions, toads, spiders), but often a combination of plant, animal, or mineral products are represented in the same mixture. The second poison produced for the Bishop of Cahors, Hugues Geraud, combined mineral and "learned" poisons (mercury, realgar, and arsenic) with powders made from lizards, toads, spiders, rats' and dogs' tails, pork bile, the leg of a hanged man, nails, and hair: a magnificent product of...cultural synthesis.[111] The substance thought to have been used by the lepers in 1321 and by the well poisoners in 1390 was composed of blood and bitter herbs among other substances.[112] In 1321, communion wafers were also listed among the ingredients because the sacrilegious mixture of the pure and the impure was supposed to increase tenfold the destructive power of the product.[113] Along the same lines of thought, incense was also used in combinations of some substances including urine and sperm.[114]

In some poisons, the immaterial was associated with the material. Present from the early periods and in hagiography,[115] magic words and gestures accompanied either the preparation of the poison or its administration in order to increase its effectiveness, in the same way that bewitching formulas were supposed to heighten the effect of a remedy. That is what a ***lettre de rémission*** from 1382 called "all the mystery" (*tout le mistere*) necessary for the effectiveness of a poison.[116] Le *vinum veneficatum* Guibert de Nogent talks about is more than a *vinum venenatum;* its preparation probably mixed words and substances, as does the priest when he consecrates the wine in the chalice.[117] At the end of the Middle Ages, the addition of new immaterial elements characterized the *materiae veneficae* of the witchcraft trials. In 1324, Alice Kyteler blended herbs and human and animal remains with incantations.[118] A case that exploded at the court of Henry IV of Lancaster mentions a toxic ointment made of magical art and "necromancy."[119] Thomas Basin describes the murderers of Charles of Guyenne as mixing poisons with enchantments.[120] The *venenis venefficis* (sic), mentioned by Tholosan, associate *res* (antimony) and *verba*.[121]

In 1466, Ysabeau de Combray is accused of having "compiled" (*compile*) poisons for her husband.[122] The term is suggestive but unfortunately, it does not give any clue about the composition of the poison. In his second justification of the murder of a tyrant (1409), Jehan Petit describes only briefly how the physician of the Orléans family, Mathieu Regnault, "had mixed in a mortar certain herbs with poisons" (*avoit broyé en un mortier chertaines herbes avec poisons*).[123] The confession of the hermit, who was also Guichard de Troyes' accomplice, gives a more concrete view on the preparation of a composed toxic substance. A grass snake, two toads, two worms, and two spiders are sliced or killed, and then boiled in the laundry water of the garments where they were found. The mixture has a consistency that resembles wine sediment and is left to settle until it is dry. Then, it is put into a container.[124] The Géraud affair indicates that poisonous animal remains were burned and then pulverized by an apothecary who was also in charge of blending together into a white substance **realgar,** mercury, and pork bile.[125] Soaking was often part of the preparation process: "softened" poisons, that is to say poisons that were plunged into a liquid were contrasted with powders that could be used immediately.[126] When poisoning and witchcraft are intermingled, technical indications reveal a formality with much more in common with the practice of magic than with chemistry. One of the rules for preparation that needed to be respected in the project to poison Henry VI of Lancaster (1440) was the use of human remains that had been buried for nine days and then blended with herbs.[127] The *Errores gazariorum* explains how to obtain a noxious ointment by grinding and reducing to powder the entrails of children, corpses of poisonous animals, fat from a hanged man, and a substance from the mouth of a red-headed man killed by a poisonous bite and hanged by his feet.[128] There is no need to say that the least divergence from these demanding requirements would decrease the *malicia veneni.*

Consistency, Media, and Methods of Administering Poison

One of the fundamental differences between poison and other weapons is that poison needs a go-between to reach its victim and that this go-between has to be concealed. This intermediary can be discerned in approximately half of the cases. The powder-drink-ingestion trilogy rather clearly predominated as a late fifteenth-century chronicler says: "to give a powder to drink" (*bailler une poudre a boire*).[129]

The words *pulveres* or *poudres* would have been sufficient to designate, by metonymy, the toxic weapon. As early as 810, Carolingian law designates poisoning by the expression *homicidiis factis (...) propter pulverem mortalem.*[130] Poisonous material appears with that expression in almost half of the cases because pulverization enabled poison to be hidden when the murderer transported it "wrapped in a paper or in little pieces of cloth" (*dedans ung papier envelope,* or *de petits drapiaulx*)[131] and when he added it, hidden under a fingernail, to the drink or the dish to be poisoned.[132] It also facilitated the spread of the poison into the organism, where it circulated like medication. It is a *venenum pulvereum* that Jean Delstein, an agent of Charles the Bad (*le Mauvais*), planned to use in 1385. "Take some of that and turn it into powder" (*Pren de cela et en fay de la poudre)* was the order that this same prince gave to another henchman.[133] The weapon designated to take the life of Geoffroi de Salagny is described as being a white powder whose name the jurist refused to say for fear that it could give ideas to other criminals.[134] Indeed, the color of the powders can either be white or verge on grey so that it can be mixed with pepper.[135] In 1245, the Infidels counted on just such a resemblance in the affair of the contaminated pepper.[136] In Bologna in 1379, the suspect powders found by the private tutor at the bottom of a dish served to the future Bishop of Mantua were shown to doctors and apothecaries who were unable to determine what it was even though it looked very much like arsenic.[137] With the same logic, a red powder (the color of **realgar**) was used to contaminate pomegranates and oranges about to be delivered to the Comte de Savoie, Amédée VIII.[138] The powder that Robert Wourdreton bought looked so much like a spice that he preferred to sew it in his doublet in order not to mix it up with other purchases made at the same time.[139] However, to link the growth of the crime of poisoning to the increase in consumption of spices that hid the fatal powders from sight and from taste is a dangerous leap.

Ointments and salves, both solid and liquid, were factors in about a third of the cases as early as the era of the Barbarian kingdoms.[140] Such is the poison that supposedly killed Otton III in 1002.[141] The Comte de Savoie blamed the creams and the plaster his doctor used on him as being the cause of the weakening of his health.[142] A substance that a doctor applied to the vagina of the daughter of King Lancelot of Naples in 1414 could have caused the king's death.[143] It is said that the persons who wanted to kill Guillaume de Flavy tried to put on his nose covered with warts a cream with "harmful salves" (*oignements contraires*).[144] In the Helvetian trials of the second half of the fifteenth century, "grease" was used both for night robberies (sticks and brooms were coated with it) and for poisoning.[145]

Poison itself was seldom found in liquid form even though it was often added to liquids. However, it is often difficult to distinguish between the medium used to carry the poison and the poisonous substance. Mathieu Paris reports that in 1258 locked vases containing a blue liquid were discovered.[146] In 1321, a certain poison consisted of a black, thick, and very putrid liquid that was impossible to burn, proof of its maximum potential to do harm.[147] Poison to be inhaled does not come to light very often either. One such example is the plot to kill François Sforza by throwing a product in his fireplace that was supposed to emit a toxic smoke[148] and another is the poisoned letter that Catherine Sforza was accused of sending to Alexander VI.[149] In the case (1425) of the prayer book of the former Bishop of Liège, Jean de Bavière, it is not certain that inhaling poison was the plan of the poisoner because it could also have been a poison transferred through touching as in Umberto Eco's novel.[150] Poisoning with gas was not as important as it was during the time of Catherine of Medicis with her Florentine perfumers who were omnipresent in the treatises on toxicity written by Ambroise Paré. On the other hand, air, which Avicenna already considered a carrier of disease,[151] played an important role. The days following the first plague epidemic in 1348, Alphonse of Cordoba warned that certain powders were present in earthenware vessels whose cracks enabled them to be spread by the wind from well-exposed places to inhabited places. Forty-two years later, the rector of the University of Prague, Henry of Brême, still referred to those *pulveres volantes in aere quae corrupunt aerem*.[152] Those accused of causing bad weather and cattle diseases in witchcraft trials used the same method.

During his interrogation, Robert Wourderton reports the advice given him by his master Charles de Navarre, who wanted him to poison King Charles VI and his relatives: "put this powder into the soup, the meat, or the wine of these lords" (*de celle poudre mets en potage, viands ou vins desditz seigneurs*).[153] This choice is representative of extant cases: the aim is to poison through food and beverage. The exact equivalent for *venenum* and "venom,"[154] and used more often, the words *potio* and "poison" do not designate the consistency of the toxic material as much as its primary medium: a liquid to be drunk (in more than half of the collected cases), and wine in particular. The carder Guillon Vassal from Carcassone drank "full cup" (*pleine tasse*) of wine to quench his thirst that resulted from the large amount of salt that had been added to his soup.[155] As emphasized in erudite treatises, wine has the advantage of spreading the poison quickly through an organism while, at the same time, concealing the taste.[156] Even sacred wine could serve as a vehicle for poison. Thomas of Chobham is eager to warn those who think that wine in a holy chalice is necessarily harmless[157] and Thomas Aquinas bases a question on this idea in his *Summa Theologica*.[158] Abélard claims that he almost died from a *poculum mortis* given instead of *poculum vitae*.[159] Wine used for cleansing was not less dangerous, such as Pope Victor III in 1086 or Archbishop William of York in 1154 are reputed to have taken, before Henry VII.[160] Water, less discreet but present everywhere, facilitated crimes on a large scale. In 1321, 1348, or 1390, water was the vehicle that the plotters planned to use in their grandiose toxic plots. In order to spread as much poison as possible into the water supply of Ariège, the lepers of 1321 were asked to put a linen bag containing poison under a stone or to attach it to something under the water in order to let it infuse.[161] The case of Ariège brings up the question of the nature of the infected waters. A letter designates the poisoners of 1321 as the source of the plot to poison cisterns, fountains, and streams, but it is particularly the wells that are targeted.[162] In 1390 also, it was again "the still waters" (*les eaux dormantes*) that were the focus of the poisoners.[163] Big and powerful rivers and streams were more difficult to poison. The physician of Ratisbonne, Konrad of Megenberg, doubts that the Danube could have been poisoned by a few bags of powder. Those who lived along rivers shared these doubts since they continued to use river water with no fear,[164] as the Parisians had done before them in 1321: "and they went every day to get water in barrels from the Seine and other rivers for the use of the king's court until the wells were safe again" (*et aloit-on tous les jours, jusques à tant que les puits fussent curés et nettyés, querres en tonniauls en Sainne ou en aultre rivieres l'iauve dont la court le roy usoit*).[165] Medication given *sub specie potionis* (potion or syrup) is another liquid vehicle linked to health that is particularly formidable.[166] Obviously, it is difficult to distinguish between an incorrect dosage that is accidentally fatal and a poison given deliberately disguised as medication. The difference is even more difficult considering that the vocabulary is ambiguous: Arnaud de Villeneuve asserts that "[a]ll poison is medication," while in the fifteenth century, Galeazzo Marzioda Narni notes that in Greek "medication" carries the ambiguous meaning of *pharmakoi* that also means "poison."[167]

Food or *le mangier* represents one-third of the identifiable media. Between solid and liquid nourishment, soup conceals poison very well.[168] Meat (in its present-day meaning) and fish (in fact spoiled)[169] represent media somewhat less common than fruits and vegetables. Unsurprisingly, the apple appears as the favorite fruit for poisoning. Robert Giroie died after taking a bite of one for fun; the son of the Orléans family died after stealing an apple that was rolling toward the Dauphin.[170] The poisoning of a foodstuff can be accomplished with a knife covered with poison that is used to cut the fruit, or more subtly, "by a little hole near the stem" (*par un petit pertuix ... emprés la queue*) where powder can be introduced.[171] Poisoning with an apple is a literary staple whose symbolism cannot be missed.[172] Convenient vehicles for poison thanks to their sweetness, pears, figs, and quince appear at the pope's table and at the very dangerous table of the King of Navarre.[173] Less commonly, pastry and bread can also be used to convey poison.[174] Like wine, bread can also be sacred. The poisoning of the communion wafer does not frighten the most resolute murderers who then transform the bread of life into the bread of death: *sic transit* the Bishop of Maguelone.[175] More elaborate preparation left to women's hands also served to conceal poison: pâté and sponge cake serve as examples as shown by cases in 1404 and 1484.[176]

Two strategies were thus available to the poisoner: the choice of a medium whose simplicity allays any suspicions (fruit, bread, wine), and the choice of complex dishes and beverages whose strong taste or sweetness efficiently conceals the poison. Pietro d'Abano thinks that poisoned foods and liquids have the sweetest and strongest flavors so that the bitter presence of the poison is masked.[177] The poisoned vinaigrette that Richer de Saint-Remi talks about,[178] absinthe mixed with honey wine given, according to Grégoire de Tours, to Romacharde de Coutances, illustrates the words of the doctor from Padua.[179]

The holy water in churches provides the treacherous target of the Sultan of Constantinople according to a rumor in 1478.[180] Next to consider are water to be drunk and water to be touched. Learned treatises suggest that readers should be careful of toxic baths,[181] a method that Jeanne de Bourgogne supposedly considered for killing Jean de Marigny, the Archbishop of Rouen.[182] If a bath that is too warm could cause suffocation and death, if the thirst that it causes could facilitate the *propinatio* of a poisoned cup—see the Lombard Helmigis who emptied in one gulp the fatal *poculum* upon leaving his bath,[183]—it is not clear what toxic method the wife of Philippe VI chose. Mathieu Paris mentions Pierre de la Vigne's intention to have poison mixed with Frederick II's bath water.[184] Without doubt this was also the queen's approach.

Medical objects (equipment for enemas,[185] a lancet used for bleeding a patient[186]) as well as clothing (the tunic and belt of the *Landgrave* [the title of certain German princes] of Thuringa in 1247[187]) can be added to a probably incomplete list. The plot of the Prince of Orange did not lack genius when he planned to "anoint the ground at the spot the king usually kisses after mass or at other times, when he does his devotions. And also to anoint the cloth on the altar that the king will probably kiss... and if the [agent] sees that there are traces of another color, such as green, black, red, and blue, he should use poisons that are of similar colors" (*oïndre la terre à l'endroit où le roy l'a acoustumé baiser après la messe ou autre heure, quant il fait ses devotions. Et aussi de oïndre la nappe de l'autel que le Roy va semblablement baiser... et que, si* [the agent] *veoit qu'il y eust parement d'autre couleur, et comme vert, noir, rouge et bleu, il mist de celles desdictes poisons qui seroit de couleur pareille*).[188] The method of poisoning through touch should not be underestimated.[189] The *apositio* may be a mode of operation that was less efficient because it was superficial,[190] but not less often used, particularly in cases of witchcraft where it constituted a sort of inversion of the sacraments.

During a trial in 1459 recorded by Hansen, a victim said he owed his redemption only to the fact that his enemy could not approach or touch him. Yet there are cases of poisoning where contact is not involved.[191] A "potion" made of a dismembered toad and other poisons can work by simply being present under the victim's table (1460), similar to the case in which *causas venenosas* were placed under the pillow and mattress of a man from Manosque (1300).[192] Operating at a greater distance, there was an attempt to symbolically poison the bewitched victim of the Visconti family (during the 1320s)[193] by setting on fire **aconite** sap and directing the smoke toward him. An addition to the *Manuel* of Bernard Gui describes the sorcerers filling up wax statuettes with a toxic mixture that was supposed to cause an intestinal disease.[194] We can add the poisoned look that both fascinates and kills. According to a theory about the expulsion of humors, *vetula* is supposed to make bad humors leave the body through the eyes, humors that *vetula* can no longer expel by the *ad hoc* path, and which concentrate to form an intense toxicity.[195] There is an account of a poison that kills by sight in a case totally foreign to this universe. Juvénal des Ursins tells, according to the Religieux de Saint-Denis, how an enemy of Louis d'Anjou got the idea to have him poisoned by a little poisoned spear whose effect could be fatal to whoever looked at it.[196]

During the last medieval centuries, it is tempting to separate on the one hand erudite poisons obtained by alchemy[197] and on the other hand, poisons made of common or base substances that were easy to collect and to transform by an individual "from the country and with little understanding" (*rural et de petit entendement*).[198] In truth, such a distinction is largely artificial because criminals purposefully took no chances by using a combination of diverse toxic materials that were easily accessible. There are no poisons for the elite that can be contrasted to popular poisons.

THE EFFECTS AND THE MARKS

During his interrogation in 1450, one of the murderers of Gilles de Bretagne revealed that three sachets of poison on which he had written "strong," "strong, strong," and "strong, strong, strong,"[199] were destined for the brother of the Duc de Bretagne. The question about the effect and marks of *venenum* was the subject of much medical attention beginning in the thirteenth century.[200] This question was also of much concern to those who were interested in the crime of poisoning, both those who wished to commit it and those who wished to combat it. Indeed, it was a key element to determining the cause of death, and therefore, the signature of the homicide. It was also a fundamental factor in determining the causes of death and then the signs of murder. It was also a fundamental piece of data concerning the approach of the murderers who counted on discretion in the act of poisoning or on its lack of connection with the death in order to remain unnoticed. The reactions of some poisons were related also to the sphere of occult forces in nature.[201] These phenomena cannot be ignored in an attempt to understand the perception of *veneficium*.

The Effects

In 90 percent of the cases in this study, the outcome of the crime, near to or far from its execution, is death. The weapon is then considered as formidable. Yet, it is not absolutely fatal for various reasons: insufficient strength of the *malicia veneni*, a victim's unexpectedly strong constitution, or the victim's particular temperament (a warm temperament facilitates the venom's work), effective remedies (we will come to that later), the skill of the therapist, or simply the poisoner's plan not to kill the victim. In a certain number of cases, the mental and physical disruption, which becomes a sort of possession, is limited to emotional relationships. Powders that cause people to fall out of love have as a goal to destroy affection and sexual powers, or more rarely, to direct the affection. The drama arises when substances go beyond this objective to globally harm the organism. Then, they really deserve the name of *venenum*, defined in the learned treatises as a force opposed to the principle of life, by assimilating the organism into its toxic nature.[202] What some theoreticians call "absolute poisons" invade the body with all their force, laying siege on it mainly through the veins.[203] They have a corrosive, putrefying, burning, cooling, warming, or stupefying effect.[204]

"It happened that they brought him a dish that he ate and soon afterwards he was completely dead" (*Si advint que on lui aporta ung mes de quoi il menga et tantos apres il quei toulx mors*). This is how the *Chronicle of Flanders and of France* (*Chronique de Flandres et de France*) describes the effects of poison administered in 1280.[205] One could think that this quick death is the norm, and one of the parties in a trial at the Parlement in December 1404 begins with this assumption when he declares, in order to invalidate the hypothesis of the poisoning of someone who had survived four months after the alleged murder attempt: "for as soon as one takes the poison, one feels sick and has pain in the heart and shivers" (*car incontinent que on a pris poisons, on sent mal et douleur au cuer et frissons*). But the other side replies that "among poisonous substances, some are cold and corrosive and kill immediately, others are warm and act a while after being administered" (*des choses venneneuses, les unes sont froides et corrosives, et mortifient incontinent, les autres sont chaudes et commectent plus après leur operation*).[206]

A small number (5 percent) of criminal poisons encountered during this research have an immediate effect. Grégoire de Tours reports that Francillon died as soon as he had drunk the poisoned beverage and that Romacharde de Coutances collapsed before taking three steps. Hugues d'Amboise fell down immediately after swallowing poison (1152).[207] After riding ten leagues on horseback King Henry IV of England "died suddenly sitting up straight on his saddle" (*subitement mort seant droitement en soun selle*) covered with poison.[208] There was even a way to accelerate the lethal process. At the end of the fifth century, the Breton King Aurelius had been put in a warm place on purpose by his murderer so that the poison would work more quickly.[209] For narrative drama, literature favors this kind of rapid effect. Gaheris de Karaheu dies immediately after eating the poisoned fruit innocently offered by Guinevere.[210] The slave charged with the poisoning of a woman's stepson asks for a *veneno subitano* in a short story from the *Pecorone*.[211]

Some poisons (approximately 10 percent of the cases collected) kill more slowly and provoke a slow deterioration of the state of health until death strikes. Murderers take advantage of this fact. A ***lettre de rémission*** from 1469 reveals someone who wanted to administer "such poisons so that the victim would not die immediately but that he would continue to live and would languish two years in order that it would not be known that he had been poisoned" (*telles poisons . . . qu'il* [the poisoned person] *ne mourroit pas icontinent mais qu'il viroit et languiroit bien deux ans affin que on ne cogneust qu'ils eust esté empoisonné*).[212] Thietmar of Mersebourg tells us about a bishop who died after ten years of excruciating suffering.[213] Apart from this eleventh-century example, very long delays attributed to the action of a poison are found more often at the end of the Middle Ages. The nine years of suffering of the Black Prince, who was supposed to have been poisoned at Najera, and the twenty-three years for Charles V, who was poisoned even before his accession to the throne (1357), and in only one attempt, constitute some kind of record.[214] In the area of ordinary criminality, a certain slowness of effect can also be seen: eleven months for the victim of Pierre Menetrey who was convicted in 1498.[215] No other weapon permits such a separation between the criminal act and its result, all the more so since there existed some substances even more subtle than slow poisons.

The question about the existence of slow working poisons is not only a scholarly argument.[216] Their use also preoccupied the imagination of fiction writers: for example, in the *Roman d'Alexandre*, there is a poison that does not have any effect on the victim for eight days but kills him in ten.[217] Far from a literary whim, the jurist Geoffroy de Salagny, speaking from an almost fatal experience, observes that a *venenum temporale* that postpones the poison's effect for ten years poses judicial problems in finding the responsible party.[218] Nevertheless, there are very few examples of this crime. It is very difficult to distinguish between poisons that work slowly and those with a delayed effect. Guichardin claims that such a poison was used in 1495 against Djem, the brother of the Sultan Bajazet.[219] Catherine Sforza gives a recipe for such a poison in her *Experimenti*.[220] In fact, this kind of poison presumes a mastery possessed only by those who have made a pact with the devil, such as the relapsed converted Jewish doctor, Nicolas of Bari, the source of a poison that took seven days to act.[221] In any case, it is clear that the effects of some of the poisons, the diabolic powders and the ones that operate with "all their substance" or by "specific shape" work outside the realm of reason and act by means of an "occult and indescribable power" (*occulte et indicible cause*).[222] The hidden crime makes use of a weapon with occult power. Yet, it leaves marks, closely linked to its effects.

The Marks

The very logic of an allegation of poisoning assumes that it leaves marks. Chevrier's adversaries, brought before the Parlement of Paris in 1404, maintained that the appearance alone of the supposed victim sufficed to prove poisoning.[223] In 1430, the doctors who examined the body of the Duc de Brabant were looking for *signa certa intoxicationis* mentioned in scholarly books.[224] Indeed, Pietro d'Abano distinguishes seventy-six different signs that permitted the recognition of a poisoning and especially its origin. What are they?

In the *Tristan* written by Thomas (mid-twelfth century), we read: "Poison spreads throughout the body, / It causes it to swell inside and out; / Turn black and change color, and lose its strength, / The bones are completely uncovered" (*li venims espans par tut le cors, / Emfler le fait dedenz e dehors; / Nercist e teint, sa force pert, / Li os sunt ja mult descovert*).[225] Now, let us listen to Gui de Chauliac, in his *Grande chirurgie* of 1363: "One finds the signs of a man who has died from poison that has been given to him in the writings of Galen in the sixth of the Internes where he says: 'As for someone who has become pale or black, or another color, or limp, or rotten, suddenly stinking, that means that he has taken poison. But if he has a different appearance, he has died from natural causes'" (*Les signes d'un homme mort de poison qu'on luy a donné, on les a de Galen, au sixiesme des* Internes *où il dit: 'Quant à aucun ... devient livide, ou noir, ou de diverse couleur, ou lasche, ou pourrissant, soudain est fait puant, cela signifie qu'il a prins poison. Mais s'il est autrement, il est mort selon les corruptions qui procedent du corps'*).[226] The poet, like the surgeon puts together a certain number of symptoms encountered in specific cases, not including the vague mention of pain and suffering.[227]

The physical transformations of Jean de Touraine, "with cheeks, tongue, lips and throat extremely swollen and eyes bulging" (*tout enflé parmi les joues, la langue, les baulevres et la gorge et les yeux exorbités et saillants*), recorded in April 1417, are considered as being characteristic of poisoning.[228] Rather frequently mentioned (about 12 percent of the cases), the swelling sometimes makes the body burst into pieces: this is what happened to Boleslaw of Masowie, the victim of the Ruthènes.[229] A frightening growth under the skin caused by wet poisons pierced the ventral wall of Frederick of Austria (1330).[230] Pietro d'Abano considers bulging eyes as a sign of poisoning by **aconite**.[231] There is no proof that the Greeks from Andrinopoulos used this product to poison the wine given to the crusaders led by Frederick Barbarossa, but the unfortunate guinea pig forced by the German soldiers to sample it, had his eyes come out of his head, as if they were ejected by the poison's power.[232] Literature seized this image: the author of the *Gaydon* repeats over and over "his eyes flew out of his head" (*li volerent li bel oil de son chief*) to describe a character's reaction to poison.[233] Sight in general is also affected by poison, as much in hagiographical texts as in historiographical ones.[234]

In 1402, during a trial in Parlement, the accusing party observed that "from certain poisons, the toenails and fingernails fall out providing a sound proof of poison" (*des dictes poisons, les ongles des piez et des mains lui cheirent, qui fu grant demonstrance de poison*).[235] The loss of nails and hair are as common as swelling; Guillaume le Breton, the author of the *Chronique de Rains*, detected in the sudden baldness of Philippe Auguste, the effect of a poison given to him in the Holy Land.[236] In 1258, the complex poison plot organized against the English barons was supposed to have the same effect.[237] In 1390, the poisoners of the wells confessed that their act was supposed to cause within a year the loss of hair and baldness among those who drank from the infected fountains.[238] *A contrario*, those who denied poisoning Henry VII used the absence of such marks as evidence in their defense.[239] The loss of hair can be explained by the fact that the characteristic of warm poisons (that is, the fourth degree of the prime quality that is heat) is the destruction of the humidity necessary for all life.[240] Drying afflicted Perette Andiguelle during her sickness and then after her death, she swelled up (1423).[241] Skinniness, languor, and feverishness resulting from the internal consumption of poison overcame many victims such as the Duc de Guyenne.[242] Burning causes corrosion. Jacques du Clerq talks about the wounds and the holes that tortured the body of the Doyen d'Arras, Jacques Dubois, the victim of a poison from the Valdensians.[243] An insatiable thirst seized some poison victims: according to Edmund of Dynter, that could explain the drunkenness of Wenceslas, who was poisoned twice.[244] Robert Wourderton reveals that the people he wanted to poison would have felt as if their bodies were being burned from the inside by a hot iron.[245] "The body cooks inside and burns" (*Le cors li frist dedenz e art*) wrote the author of *Yder* at the beginning of the thirteenth century, about his hero, who drank from a poisoned fountain.[246] The only advantage, somewhat absurd, is that the heat of the poison that kills also dries out the humors, so that the corpses of certain victims do not smell.[247]

"He who was as white as a flower is now completely black" (*Lui qui étoit blanc comme fleur, le voilà maintenant tout noir*). Thus, a poem depicts the end of Henry VII, an account inspired by Alexander's death.[248] The change of the color of the skin is commonly attributed to the absorption of poison. The skin of the poison victim cured by Saint Benedict was covered with spots.[249] Orderic Vital assumed that the persistent pallor of Louis the Fat (*le Gros*) and Bohemond was due to their being poisoned.[250] This paleness indicates the exhaustion of the vital forces resulting from the fight against poison. On the other hand, the blackening of the body of Hugues de Grammont was explained by the indubitable effect of poisoning.[251] Questioned after the death of Amédée VII (1391), the practitioner Homebon referred to Galien (*De interioribus*) when he said that the greening or the blackening of a corpse proves *toxicatio*.[252] The blackening of teeth—signs of **ceruse** according to Pietro d'Abano—makes some people insist that the archbishop of York was poisoned in 1154.[253] The hideous black face of Alexander VI caused the same reaction.[254]

Another sign of the destruction of the vital force is the paralysis that strikes the victims. Joinville tells how a sultan became paralyzed on one side after a wound came in contact with a poisoned mat.[255] In 1402, a trial in Parlement describes a paralysis on the right side that was fatal after six months.[256] Finally, let us talk about psychological and neurological effects, pointed out by medical and judicial tradition,[257] but seldom appearing in our cases. Paul Diacre mentions two Lombard potentates rendered unable to reign because of a powerful poison,[258] and other cases can be found, among which one of the most interesting is that of Charles VI, even if the *veneficias* responsible for his madness can be explained more easily by "curses" than by "poisonings."[259]

Confusing Symptoms

For the perpetrators, poison had the advantage that its effects and marks could be confused with other pathological symptoms. The weapon of poison was redoubtable because it could imitate nature to the point of making a criminal action seem natural. Favorable to *venefici*, this confusion existed also for the accusers since genuine illness could be mistaken for *toxicatio*.

Medical tradition made "poisonous humours" issuing from the organism responsible for some diseases[260]; along the same lines, poisons were considered similar to some illnesses that destroy health.[261] In 1380, prestigious doctors were solicited to determine, by seeing or rather by reading about the symptoms of the victim, whether the Sire de Grammont had been poisoned. Refering to Galien (*De morbo*, VI), the eminent Raymond Chalmel and Jean de Tournemire replied that the victim could very well have died from a poison created by his own body. Other doctors, less famous (is there a connection?) supported that, on the contrary, all the signs presented by the Sire de Grammont matched those of an "administered" poisoning.[262] Conceptually and literally, poison can therefore be hidden by disease and some of its symptoms. "Pestilence," a rather vague word that can cover many things, is one of these. According to Chastellain, Lancelot of Hungary ingested a poison "of such composition that it could make the body appear that death resulted from pestilence" (*de telle composition qu'elle pouvoit mettre le corps en telle semblance comme si mort fust de pestilence*).[263] This similarity found in all the treatises, was not insignificant in the accusations of 1348 against the Jews who distributed poison containing the plague.[264]

Concerning the death of Charles, son of Charles the Bad (*le Mauvais*), the author of the *Chronicle of the Four First Valois Kings* (*Chronique des quatre premiers Valois*) writes: "My Lord Charles of Navarre was poisoned by a poison that caused severe diarrhea" (*fut empoisonné le dit monseigneur Charles de Navarre de une poison telle de flux de ventre*).[265] Dysentery has been believed for a long time to cause symptoms identical to those caused by poison,[266] to the extent that the Frankish Queen Austrigilde believed that poisoning was the real cause of her illness.[267] Jehan Petit answered Valentine Visconti's lawyer who claimed that one of the victims of the Orléans couple had, in fact, died from dysentery and that this symptom is precisely the sign of the crime.[268] Sometimes linked to dysentery, the abdominal swelling mentioned above, presents the same ambiguity: the effect of poison or of nature, the answer depends on the party to be defended. Shortly after 1400, the litigant in a trial in Parlement stated that "many people die swollen up who have not been poisoned" (*maintes gens meurent enflez qui ne sont pas empoisonnez*). Twenty years later, another man of law said the opposite in front of the same court: "when she died, she suddenly became very swollen, which is the sign of poisoning according to the doctrine given us by physicians" (*quant fu morte, subito devint tres enflée, qui sont signes d'empoisonnement selon la doctrine que avoient baillée les medecins*).[269] Another disturbance of the organism that is difficult to distinguish from the effects of a violent poison is apoplexy, which can be the result of criminal poisoning or natural affliction. Jean de Viktring hesitated to speak his mind when he dealt with the death of Frederick of Austria (1330), and Jean de Roye mentioned the alternative concerning the death of Edward IV of England.[270]

Another confusing theme, certainly less important since it does not question the criminal origin of the death, is the similarity between the effects of poison and evil spells. Petrus Cararius indicates that those who fade away, victims of a poison with delayed effect, can appear to have been bewitched.[271] During the fourteenth and the fifteenth centuries, distinguishing between these two ways of killing was difficult. It can be chroniclers or witnesses who hesitate between the two methods, as in the case of Jacques Dubois, or the victim, such as the supplicant of a ***lettre de rémission*** in 1481. But it can also be physicians who are unable to say, for example, whether in 1308, Eléonore de Trie died from poisoning or bewitchment, or if, in 1323, Beatrice Galian poisoned her husband.[272] The jurist Hippolite de Marsiliis writes that some poisons are more like evil spells.[273] The result is the same, whether possessed by a curse or having ingested a poison, the organism succumbs without a blow being struck.

The action of poison and its *modus operandi* offer a wide diversity and cannot be easily verified. Even if a Mondeville ridicules the notion of "specific form," designed, according to him, to mask the ignorance and incomprehension of his colleagues,[274] it certainly plays a role in the image of the weapon of poison that is complex, ambiguous, and somewhat mysterious like a dagger made of an unknown metal that can kill without ever leaving its case. The lack of visibility of the weapon is partly compensated for by the marks it is supposed to leave, to make up for the blood that never flows.

AN INVINCIBLE WEAPON? HOW TO PREVENT AND TO RECOVER FROM POISONING

In a small minority of the cases (less than 10 percent), the poisoned person survived the crime. In a certain number of the others (a maximum of 13 percent), the weapon was discovered before it was used. This fact proves that poison can be foreseen or contained. The main justification for the existence of Western toxicological literature is to introduce the two main ways to fight against poisons: *defensio cum cautela, destructio cum virtute*.[275] Let us look at one and then the other.

Prevention

In the writings of Pietro d'Abano, prevention represents approximately 6 percent of the measures indicated against poisoning. This low number can be explained by the fact that the interest of the Italian doctor lies more with remedies, which is part of his specialty, whereas protection against poison exists as a less erudite dimension. Yet, every treatise on poison emphasizes the precautions to be taken by those who fear being poisoned. What are these precautions?

Sante Ardoini de Pesaro suggests six lines of preventive action: the choice of good servants, the interception of poisoners, the detection of the presence of poison, suspicion of food with unusual appearance or taste, restraint with food and beverage, and finally the ingestion of preventive drugs.[276] In addition, it is vital that dishes and cups located in the kitchen or on the tables be guarded because that is where *toxicatores* lurk, like the ones of the Comtesse de La Marche in 1242, the ones of Charles the Bad (*le Mauvais*) whose strategy consisted in infiltrating the "kitchen, sick room and wine cellar" (*cuisine, dispense et bouteillerie*) of his enemies.[277] It is wise to cover the pots into which poisonous animals could fall by accident, risking the appearance of a crime.[278] *A fortiori*, one should avoid exposing dishes and *pocula* to a poisoner's threat. The *leges palatinae* of the King of Majorca, Jacques II (1337) recommend that royal meals be prepared in a safe place, or even in secret, by people above all suspicion. It is necessary to employ servants whom one can trust completely and whose loyalty has been thoroughly tested.[279] Generosity and good treatment also enable the master to ensure the total loyalty of those who serve him, so that poisoning the *dominus* would result in self-poisoning since the demise of the prince would also mean their own end.[280] Examples of powerful personalities saved by members of their entourage are plentiful. The exemplary fidelity of Louis XI's kitchen staff prevented the crime that the Duc de Bourgogne planned in 1473.[281]

A healthy life that favors moderation and self-control also helps to escape the crime of poison. Before eating, it is advisable to rinse the mouth so that the tongue and the palate are capable of reacting to any suspicious taste.[282] Gluttony is dangerous because *voracitas impedit judicium*, as the humanist Bonifazio Simonetta wrote in 1492.[283] The appetite opens wide the veins through which toxic material can easily rush,[284] hence the necessity to eat without excessive hunger. Chestnuts, nuts, and dry figs are perfect for moderating the craving for food. It is because he did not follow these instructions that Pope Benedict XI, craving figs, swallowed poison without noticing. Matteo Visconti's excessive love for pork kidneys led him to a death that could have been avoided.[285] It would be an exaggeration to say that the recommendations in the treatises contributed to the movement toward "the civilization of mores" by lessening the importance of food and by restraining gluttony; the theories of N. Elias have somewhat caricatured the uncouthness of the people of the Middle Ages. On the other hand, in the evolution of table manners, there is an undeniable meeting point between cultural and preventive factors. Some additional clues will enable us to say more on this subject.

Most treatises state that on dining tables there should be some items that can indicate the presence of poison.[286] Jean d'Arezzo asserts that the cunning fraud of poisoners is revealed by the horn of a snake, men's diligence, and the help of Providence.[287] It comes from a beast called a "cerastes" (from the Greek *ceros* meaning horn), described by many authors.[288] Snakes tongues are obtained from the solid mass located in a reptile's head[289] and are assembled by silversmiths on "trees" or "***languiers***," which require the close presence of salt in order to maintain the humidity necessary for the good "functioning" of that kind of detector. The snake tongues belonging to the King of France always accompanied the saltcellars in the inventory of the crown jewels done in 1418.[290] Beyond the erudite arguments that are devoted to them,[291] testimonies of the use of similar detectors do exist, perhaps originating in the East. Thomas de Cantimpré indicates that in the first decades of the thirteenth century, (Byzantine) emperors put knives whose handles were made of such materials on their table.[292] Robert Guiscard's son, who was knowledgeable about Eastern customs, had a knife whose handle revealed the presence of a poison by sweating.[293] It is the sweating of the ***languier*** that was acquired overseas, that revealed to Robert de Béthune the presence of poison in his meat.[294] The inventories of the Popes are filled with ***languiers*** that look like metallic or coral trees whose weight can reach more than six pounds. The pontiffs sometimes borrowed them, promising in writing to return them, or received them as Christmas gifts.[295] In 1295, the inventory ordered by Boniface VIII at the time of his accession included fifteen such items. The inventory made at the time of the accession of Clement VI (1343), included twelve *arbores pro proba*, that is to say, the test to try on all dishes.[296] Not long after his election, Benedict XIII, wanting to inspect all the items in the pontifical treasure noted seven of them, which he ordered to be placed in the small chapel of the palace where the jewels were kept.[297] Such overzealousness indicates that these objects were extremely precious to him. The practical and aesthetic value attributed to them did not decrease during the fifteenth century: a tree-shaped ***languier*** was found at the death of Pious II in 1464. The princes of Europe were not to be outdone, from Mahaut d'Artois to the Comte de Savoie in 1380 including the court at Naples (1316)[298] and that of Charles V.[299] In an inventory done in 1395 of the precious things stolen from the Marquis Nicolo d'Este, there is a ***languier*** mounted with seventeen snake tongues.[300] A "coral tree with several snake tongues" (*arbre de corail a plusieurs langues de serpens*) is listed among the belongings of the Duchesse d'Orléans in 1408.[301] In 1453, the prosperous King René spent a large amount of money to have a snake tongue mounted in silver.[302] However, according to a tradition dating back to Avicenna, a snake's horn is known for sweating only in the presence of specific poisons.[303] During the thirteenth century, Albert the Great stated that the effectiveness of this detector with all poisons was not proved.[304] Christoforus de Honestis observed that it remained dry when placed in front of a scorpion.[305] Guido da Vigevano showed his scepticism founded on experience, but he thought it was useful to put it on the table in order to dissuade the criminal. What counts is that the criminals believe in it.[306]

An object more precious and universal than the snake horn that caught the fancy of powerful men is the horn of the unicorn, a mythic animal belonging to the Christian bestiary and reputed to have purified the water of a poisoned pond.[307] For a longer time than can be measured,[308] the unicorn horn was believed to be able to make poison effervescent if it possessed a warm nature, or make it smoke if it had a cold nature.[309] In reality, the horn of the unicorn came from the tooth of a narwhal, the horn of an oryx or a rhinoceros, or was taken from even more common animals not likely to be identified by those who wanted to get the best price for their merchandise. Boniface VIII found four unicorn horns in the treasury of the papacy, and his successor had three. Benedict XIII possessed pieces of unicorn horn that were of a good size and weight.[310] The one in the inventory of Gregory XII (1416) was complete.[311] The 1421 inventory of the jewels located in different castles of the kings of France reveals an incense box and its lid within which there is gold stick where there is a piece of unicorn horn to be used to test food, as well as a gold pot containing a "chain where hangs a piece of unicorn horn" (*chayenne où pend de la lycorne*).[312] In the inventory of the Abbey of Saint- Denis done in 1505, there is a huge horn weighing 25 marks and 6 1/2 feet long.[313] Along with other precious objects in the treasury of the kings of France, the unicorn horn of Saint-Denis illustrates the sumptuous dimension of the object: a big unicorn for an important monarch. And very likely, princes of doubtful pedigree or recently promoted princes knew how to acquire such objects: Pierre de Medicis and his son Laurent possessed horns that cost 1,500 and 6,000 florins.[314] During the sixteenth century, even if doubts increased concerning their effectiveness based on ideas very close to necromancy, Charles IX still cherished the ones he had, to the despair of Ambroise Paré who was convinced of the fabulous character of their reputation.[315]

Some metals were known for revealing the presence of poison. Nicolas of Florence mentions a pair of copper scissors that changed color, a phenomenon also found in Majorcan palatine laws.[316] In the rich lapidary tradition inherited from Antiquity, stones were also used as detectors by their change in color when they were close to poison. During the twelfth century, the blue topaz was highly valued by Hildegarde of Bingen.[317] Pietro d'Abano talks about quartz, prase (a variety of quartz), as well as the emerald with which he himself experimented.[318] Pulverized into a dish or a drink, some stones prevent the person who has poisoned food in his mouth from swallowing.[319] The popes obviously possessed such stones: the inventory of 1353 lists a leather case that contained seven.[320] In January 1390, Clement VII had gold rings endowed with small antivenom stones purchased from an artisan from Compiègne.[321] The saltcellar in the French royal inventory of 1418 is provided with sapphires, emeralds, and **cassidoines.**[322] From belief in the properties of stones to faith in the amulets, the step is very small. The detection powers of **hematite** were increased when the ring hewed inside was engraved with the astrological face of the serpent-eater: the taming of this poisonous animal provided the ring with the power to overcome poison.[323] That kind of object automatically found its place in literature. The author of *Ciperis de Vignevaux* (after 1350) portrays a young woman whose ring suddenly became wet when close to poison.[324]

Other detectors were abstract. According to the apostolic tradition (Mark 16:18), some gestures revealed poison hidden by a murderer. The sign of the cross caused a cup handed to Saint Benedict to break.[325] It could also neutralize the *malicia veneni*, or make it leave a poisoned beverage, so that it could be drunk safely: following the example of Saints John and George, Bishop Sabin escaped a poisonous trap thanks to this very real exorcism.[326] His contemporary Samson exemplarily added the two virtues of the sign of the cross.[327]

Those objects are used according to a prophylactic ritual in rapid development in the courts at the end of the Middle Ages.[328] At the dangerous court of the Visconti family, no fewer than twenty people tasted the dishes destined for Galeas, who always ate by himself to avoid any kind of attempt to poison him.[329] The test of dishes before a meal is a tradition well attested in the Roman world: Claudius had a *praegustor* who was suspected of doing his job so badly that he would have facilitated the poisoning of the emperor.[330] The tradition is repeated in Byzantium: during the tenth century, Liutprand of Cremona tells us that to harass him, the "***curopalate***" obliged him to taste dishes with the slaves instead of sitting at the imperial table.[331] But it is hard to follow the evolution before the thirteenth century. No attempts were made at the table of the Sire d'Amboise in the middle of the twelfth century, but was it because of his rank, which was quite modest, or because of the time period that was less mistrustful than later ones? Yet, at the beginning of the thirteenth century, the Duc de Lorraine Thibaud, received by the emperor Frederick, did not taste any dish before his chamberlain had tried it.[332] Not long before 1300, a simple archdeacon of the Albi diocese had a taster who lost all his hair for having done his dangerous duty.[333] As early as the beginning of the fourteenth century (1305–1307), protocol at the pontifical court determined that *supracoqui* and *buticularii* should taste the food before the Pope. The *Avvisamenta pro regimine et dispositione officiorum in* *palatio domini papae* of 1409 confirmed the luxury of the precautions that were taken.[334] The *proba*, a word that designates both the action of the tasting and the method by which it is done, is obviously performed on all dishes passed on to cardinals in conclave.[335] If the plan for the organization of the dwelling of Philippe V gives few details, the reflections of a criminal wanting to get rid of Louis X and his brother prove the existence of rigorous measures at the French court: "You would never succeed with poisons, for they are too well guarded" (*Par poisonz vous n'en vendriez jamais a chief, quar il sont trop gardez*).[336] The Majorcan palatine laws enacted in 1337 and partly adopted by Pierre III of Aragon in 1344 provide for several tests: first of all, in the kitchens, by the cooks and the providers, then by the butler or the head waiter, and finally by the ***camerlingue*** or finance minister or the one who holds that position. The wine steward tastes the wines and prevents any stranger from approaching the table.[337] The *Voeux de l'épervier* written on the day following the death of Henry VII illustrates spectacularly the expansion of food tasting. The herald of Flanders Gui de Namur gave a magnificent sermon and then paid with his life for his zeal as a taster, a rather particular feat of chivalry.[338] It goes without saying that potions and medications were tasted in the same way, usually by those who prescribed them. The palatine laws of Jacques of Majorca provide for a test of **electuaries** as well as lotions for the hair by the royal apothecary.[339] The test ensured by the doctor of the Comte de Nassau proves the use of this practice around the middle of the fourteenth century.[340] It probably occurred with less ostentation than the tasting of dishes.

During the fifteenth century, suspicion justified an important display of gestures integrated to the ceremonies associated with eating. Olivier de la Marche makes several such references in his *Etats de la maison de Bourgogne* (1473). A "meat" test was first done in the kitchens by the first headwaiter, then, with the help of a unicorn horn in a sideroom, salt and napkins were tested as well as sauces, fruits, and trenchers. The headwaiter did "two tests for each dish" (*deux assays pour chascuns mets*) always keeping an eye on the dishes. Besides, "the dish of the prince could be recognized by a piece of unicorn horn hanging from it by a chain" (*doit estre le pot du prince recongneu à une pièce de lycorne pendant à iceluy pot à une chaisne*).[341] An important part of the "ceremony" was delegated to the trencher squire, as Olivier de la Marche significantly calls him, and which indicates the political and ostentatious dimension: "he takes the bread ... then tests it with the unicorn horn in the small sideroom touches the bread all over, and then cuts it in front of the prince ... And when he has put each dish in front of the prince, he must uncover it and test it with the unicorn horn and afterwards taste it before the prince eats it" (*il prent le pain ... puis prend l'espreuve de la licorne en la petite nef et touché le pain tout à l'entour, et puis trenche devant le prince ... Et quant il a mis chascun plat devant le prince, il le doibt descouvrir et puis faire l'espreuve de la lycorne et après faire son essay avant que le prince en mange.*)[342] The addition of two kinds of testing, one with a tool and the other one with a human taster, was considered a way to preserve the lives of servants. Another way to spare them was to use dogs, in courts or in more humble places where no other kind of taster existed. A man persecuted by a bad woman told Jacques Fournier that he systematically gave a portion of his food to his pet before eating it himself.[343]

Sometimes the test took place far from banquets and sick rooms. The alleged poisoning of the Eucharist inspired locally, even if not as part of the ritual, a test on the host and wine. After the death of a bishop from Maguelone in 1249, it was decided, perhaps by the chapter, that two clerks would taste the host and the wine before the Holy Mass.[344] The Majorcan palatine laws made provision for the same test, including the ablution wine before the Prince's communion.[345] Secular objects underwent the same tests. Antonio Guainerie believed it to be desirable that a naked servant enter his master's bed in order to make sure that there was nothing harmful in the bed, and at the same time, to warm it up. He expanded these precautions to the clothes and even to the horse that would be ridden by a valet an hour before a departure, probably a response to stories of the poisoning of saddles.[346]

Tests were not always feasible: captivity rendered the high-born prisoner extremely vulnerable since any testing of his food was forbidden.[347] The safety of the food and drink could not be guaranteed, and the eating customs as well as the rules of hospitality required that they be shared. Jean d'Outremeuse explains that the poison destined for Henry VII was badly distributed in the imperial bowl, so that the test did not touch the dangerous part of the poisoned dish that was swallowed by the empress.[348] Even though it is only speculation, this scenario is not unlikely. Franciscus of Siena claims that the conditions of a trustworthy *praegutatio* were rarely met and that in reality, the test of the food had a double function: honorific (*ad honorem domini*) and deterrent—once again we find an ideological dimension.[349] Besides, the vigilance was not constant, even in the most important courts. The trial that occurred after the death of Amédée VII indicated that his doctor was giving him medicine without taking any precautions.[350] About 1460, Jehan Coustain experienced the negligence of the Burgundian ducal household: in Brussels, he managed to have the Comte de Charolais drink wine with no *proba*, which encouraged him in his murderous schemes.[351]

Remedies

Suffering from the poison administered by Bertrade de Montfort, Prince Louis owed his life to a magician who came from pagan lands (**al-Andalous**: Andalusia) where he had learned the deep secrets of physics.

On the contrary, lack of care caused the death of Ernaud d'Echauffour.[352] Those two stories told by Orderic Vital demonstrate that the salvation of poisoned victims could come from various kinds of remedies. What were these remedies and how were they used?

Numerous ways to counter poison are mentioned in theoretical sources, as early as the ninth century,[353] for example, in narrations, or even in manuscripts dealing with completely different subjects.[354] Surgery is hardly ever mentioned, even though it could sometimes be useful: the jealous man from Salerno poisoned by Déroud d'Amiens escaped death only because of help from his rival and an amputation. The Bishop-Count of Nantes died because he refused to have his arm amputated.[355] Even if the death of Mithridates Eupator (120–63 before our era) was well known among medieval men of letters,[356] the idea of an immunization with poison against poison was not promoted. The Hippocratic principle about habituation to poison occurs in the story of the poisonous Virgin, but this kind of prevention that worked too well for the King of Pont is not advised anywhere. It seemed too exotic to be reliable. Antonio Guaineri mentions it only in the case of a sultan.[357] Popular remedies were quite different.

Pietro d'Abano provides 135 remedies with the amounts of the ingredients and the duration of treatment. Knowledge of them does not imply any erudite readings. For Albert the Great, the antitoxic qualities of the streets can be inferred from the fact that weasels bitten by a snake instinctively eat the attacker.[358] The poisonous servant of Geoffroy de Salagny knew that the consumption of large quantities of onions could serve as an antidote to poison.[359] The same power is attributed to garlic, which is called "a common **thériaque**" (*thériaque à vilain*).[360] Oil, milk, tepid water, herbs, nuts, chestnuts, clay, and lemon seeds are all part of the advised remedies as well as **sigillated** soil taken preventively every day by Oriental princes.[361] Most of the time, the effects of the remedies are emetic.

The expulsion of poison by vomiting permits the body to rid itself of the substance and, at the same time, in some cases, allows the substance to be identified. This approach was so common that it became an almost obligatory scene in literature: Alexander rushed to get a feather to induce vomiting as soon as he felt the first signs of poison. Alas! The feather was also poisoned.[362] There were other emetic methods: perhaps inspired by Pietro d'Abano, the physician of the Comte de Savoie, who tried hard to make his sick master sneeze.[363] Sweating, purging, and cleansing are other methods available to caregivers,[364] as well as drainage. Poisoned twenty-three years before his death, Charles V owed his survival solely to the talent of a doctor who was sent by his uncle the emperor, who had himself been saved from poison. The expert inserted a duct into the Valois that permitted the toxic substance to leave his body. Having become bald and dry as a stick, he was unable to recover his health, but at least, he was able to regrow his hair by this method. The drying up of bodily fluids announced the death of the king two weeks in advance, according to a medical logic that is hard to understand.[365]

It seems that "the drainage theory" (*le principe de l'écoulement*) played an important role in a strange and limited method belonging to the Germanic regions. Medicine as practiced by learned physicians ignored or advised against it.[366] This method consisted in hanging the victim by the feet so that the poison left the body by gravity, leaving through one of the orifices in the head, normally the eyes. This was the treatment given to Wenceslas II of Bohemia much to the surprise of a chronicler who discovered him hanging upside down when he arrived at his court in 1278.[367] Despite the strangeness of this approach, this therapy had its supporters. In 1295, the Duke of Austria Albert lost half of his sight but stayed alive thanks to this treatment that was also successful in the case of Sigismund, King of Hungary and future emperor (1404).[368] This remedy is said to have been suggested to the emperor Henry VII who rejected it, not because of the indecency of the position but because he was horrified by the possibility of vomiting up the Eucharist.[369]

"Under the sky, there is no medicine as effective against poison as treacle" (*Sus ciel n'ad si bone medcine encuntre venim fors triacle*). This sentence is found in an Anglo-Norman medical book from the thirteenth century that is incorrectly called "a letter from Hippocrates."[370] ***Thériaques*** were used as antidotes to poison, either against specific poisons or general poisonings. Three types of ***thériaques*** were distinguishable from each other: "***thériaque*** **diatessaron**," "Mithridates' *thériaque*" (*thériaque mithridate*), and a third called "Galien's *thériaque*" (*thériaque de Galien).* But it is the great **thériaque** (*la grande thériaque*), called that of Andromaque, that attracts the most attention because of its reputed universal effectiveness, even though its effectiveness as an antidote for **aconite** was disputed.[371] It contains flesh of a viper and works according to the adage *venenum veneno curare potest*.[372] Its use against criminal poison, attested during the Byzantine Empire,[373] occurs many times in the sources. Déroud d'Amiens recovered from the attempt on his life made by his rival from Salerno thanks to this remedy. This remedy also saved Frederick II in 1224.[374] Charles V always wore a *thriaclier* [perhaps based on the word *bouclier* or shield]; it is impossible to know whether this fact reflects his fear of poison or his constant hypochondria.[375] The exact nature of what the documents call ***thériaque*** is uncertain. The great ***thériaque*** (*la grande thériaque*), which is the most effective, is composed of tens of ingredients that were not easy to assemble. At the beginning of the fourteenth century, Henri de Mondeville believed that it was seldom used in the regions of northwest European where people preferred the more accessible "**tormentille**" root.[376] At the end of the fifteenth century, Jacoppo Manlio regrets that the Milanese apothecaries do not make *la grande* ***thériaque*** themselves but instead buy it from merchants in Genoa who sell a preparation that is ineffective.[377] Symphorien Champier indicates that Charles VIII and his sister had one of the ingredients necessary for the preparation of a remedy imported from Egypt since Westerners were unable to produce it for economical and intellectual reasons.[378]

Bezoars and precious stones are endowed with curative qualities that were also used. "In the Arabic language '*bethasar*' means saving from death" (*En langue arabique bethasar (…) est a entendre delivrant de mort)* states a treatise from the fifteenth century.[379] In his last chapter, Pietro d'Abano devotes special space to "**bezoar**," a word to which he first gives the meaning of a method of curing particular to each poison. He mentions seven universal vegetal "**bezoars**."[380] The stone itself, a solidification of limestone that can be found in the stomachs of herbivores[381] and was considered a universal antidote effective against all poisons. Stabbed with a dagger poisoned by an assassin in 1272, Edward I owed his life to this remedy.[382] Convinced of its superiority, alchemists believed that the philosopher's stone chased away the poison by repulsion whereas the ***thériaque*** expulsed it by attraction.[383] The pulverization of different materials into a beverage drunk right after a poisoning was considered life-saving. Powder made from the horn of a unicorn was believed to neutralize poison that had been absorbed; panic-stricken in face of the worsening of his patient's state, the physician of Amédée VII of Savoie's offered him this remedy.[384]

Sometimes, spiritual remedies were also helpful. Grégoire de Tours quotes Mark 16:18 concerning the apostles, such as Saint John, who were immunized against poison simply by the invocation of the Trinity.[385] The origin of these beliefs is related to the symbolism of poison as a metaphor of evil: Alexander Nequam compares the Christ to a ***thériaque*** that chases away sin spread by the devil.[386] To call upon Christ, to make his sign or to call upon the apostles who have vanquished poison destroys the power of poison.[387] In the same way, substances linked to saints have the same qualities, whether it be dust from the tomb of Saint Marcel, which was life-saving for the poisoned priest depicted by Guibert de Nogent, or Saint Maurice's ring, which proved useful for the troops of the Comte de Savoie, who were ambushed by the Milanese.[388]

The mobilization of ways to fight against poisoning, in existence from the end of the thirteenth century was not without success. In a certain number of cases, the poison was vanquished. Thanks to diverse ways that may seem sometimes strange to us and where the supernatural played an important role (see Pietro d'Abano's remarks about the ***thériaque***[389]), there was an attempt to combat poison and this struggle brought about other cultural and even ideological changes. With the development of eating rituals, the prince's position was regarded with more awe and he was distanced from those around him. The rituals enabled him to accumulate objects that were as precious for their value as for the services they were supposed to offer.

The crime of poison brings into play unique weapons, sometimes provided by nature, most of the time by men, when it is not by the devil. It is tempting to think that the poison "market" became more important during the last centuries of the Middle Ages, both materially and intellectually, with perhaps the key being a certain familiarization. Some rather elaborate and harmful substances were used in everyday life. Despite some creative criminals, the variety of poisons that were used is not great and their ways of administration were not very diverse. The effects of criminal poison normally caused the death of the victim, but such an end was not inevitable since there were ways to avoid or to counteract poisonings. The properties attributed to poison and to its antidotes reflect a philosophy about poison that was coming into its own at the end of the thirteenth century. The fact that it was founded on scholastic reasoning does not mean that knowledge other than that from the University was excluded. A dimension of mystery was included in *venenum* that affected the domain of its prevention. Indeed, such a reflection applied first and foremost to *sine culpa* poisonings, but it is not unreasonable to believe that it also responded to the increasing fear of criminal poison.

NOTES

1. J.-P. Bénezet, *Pharmacie et médicament en Méditerranée occidentale (xiii*[e]*–xvi*[e] *siècles)*, Paris, Champion, 1999, p. 55.

2. Jacoppo Manlio, *Luminare majus super descriptiones antidotarii et practice Johannis Mesue*, Venice edition, 1499, f. 58.

3. The saliva alone of people from Taiyang can kill the unfortunate officials sent into a region that is moreover rich in toxic plant and animals: F. Obringer, *L'aconit et l'orpiment*, pp. 246–248.

4. Jehan de Mandeville, *Voyages*, ed. M. Letts, Londres, 1953, t. 2, p. 337: "He speaks of trees that bear flour and other poisons ... The Jews had sent for some of this poison during this time in order to poison all Christendom." (*Li parle des arbres qui portent farine et les autres venins .... De ceste venin avoient envoié querre les Iuyfz un des ces ans pour empoisonner toute crestienté ...*)

5. Henri de Mondeville, *Chirurgie*, ed. trans. E. Nicaise, Paris, 1893, p. 803.

6. Cf. W. Hertz, Die Sage vom Giftmädchen, *Abhandlungen der königlischen bayerischen Akademie der Wissenchaften, I. Kl.* XX, Bd I, Abtheilungen, 1893, pp. 89–167 et A. Grinaschi, La diffusion du *Secretum secretorum (Sirr al'Asrar)* dans l'Europe occidentale, *Archives d'histoire doctrinale et littéraire du Moyen Âge*, 1980, n 47, pp. 7–70.

7. Masudi, *The Meadows of Gold*, ed. and trans. P. Lunde et C. Stone, London and New York, 1989, pp. 327–328 (poisoning of Mutamid, 892).

8. Foucher de Chartres, *Historia hierosolomytana, RHC; historiens occidentaux*, t. 3, Paris, 1866, pp. 311–487, chap. 49, p. 475; Ernoul, *Continuation de Guillaume de Tyr*, ed. P. Paris in *Descriptions et traditions légendaires de la Terre sainte*, Paris, 2 vol., 1879–1880, t. 2, p. 506.

9. Jacques de Vitry, *Lettres de la cinquième croisade*, ed. R. B. C. Huygens, tr. G. Duchet-Suchaux, Turnhout, Brepols, 1998, lettre II, nov. 1216–févr. 1217, p. 54.

10. Guido da Vigevano, *Texaurus*..., f. 39.

11. Secousse, p. 374 and Carbonelli, p. 238.

12. Neri di Gino Capponi, *Commentaires*, ed. Muratori, *RIS*, XVIII, Milan, 1731, col. 1211; Stefano Infessura, *Diaire*, ed. *RIS*, III-2, Citta di Castello, 1908, col. 1231.

13. A. Le Roux de Lincy, *Le livre des proverbes français*, Paris, 2 vol., 1859, p. 288.

14. Richer de Saint-Remi, *Historia Francorum*, ed. R. Latouche, Paris, 1930, ii, 59.

15. Orderic Vital, VII, t. 3, pp. 181–182.

16. Sante Ardoini de Pesaro, *Opus de venenis*, p. 99.

17. Ottokar, *Österreichische Reimchronik*, éd. *MGH Scriptorum qui vernacula lingua usi sunt*, V-1, Hanovre, 1890, pp. 287–288.

18. Carbonelli, PJ XXXIV, p. 332.

19. Bouchart, iv, 218, t. 2, p. 349.

20. Du Clercq, p. 636.

21. Martin le Franc, *Le champion des dames*, t. 4, str. 2270.

22. C. Ginzburg, *Le sabbat* ..., p. 74.

23. Carbonelli, PJ XXXIV, p. 351.

24. Ranulf Higden, *Polychronicon*, I, 32, t. 1, p. 338; Johann de Saxe, *Compendium de epidemia*, beginning of the fifteenth century, in *Pestschriften*, 1924, n 16, p. 24.

25. As an example see the inventory of Guillaume Lefort, 1439, dans *Inventaires d'anciennes pharmacies dijonnaises*, ed. P. Dorveaux, Dijon, 1892: **orpiment** (n 57), arsenic, and **réalgar** (n°102), etc.

26. Secousse, p. 500; *Documents nouveaux*, pièce X, pp. 29–31, 20-II-1459.

27. Labande, pp. 137–144.

28. Secousse, p. 499.

29. J. Michelet, *La sorcière*, chap. IX. An idea pursued by R. W. Ireland, Chaucer's toxicology, p. 78.

30. J.-P. Bénezet, 30. *Pharmacie et médicament*..., estimates that 16 percent of the simple plants and 20 percent of the minerals used in pharmacology at the end of the Middle Ages were imported from afar (p. 505 and sq.).

31. *Registres du trésor des Chartes*, JJ 234, f. 107 v–108.

32. J.-P. Bénezet, p. 169 and sq.

33. *Sacrorum conciliorum... collectio*, concile d'Avignon, 18 juin 1326, canon 17, t. 25, col. 754. Contrary to other resolutions that are based on decisions of earlier councils, this resolution appears to be new.

34. Secousse, p. 502.

35. An edict of the parlement of Bordeaux edited in *Les statuts et règlements des apothicaires*, ed. F. Prévet, Paris, 15 vol., 1950, t. 6, p. 1174.

36. Lewin, p. 163 and sq.

37. *Registres du trésor des Chartes*, JJ 226 b, f. 2.

38. *Parlement criminel*, X2a 14, f. 154 v.

39. *Registres du trésor des Chartes*, JJ 209, f. 119 v: "in order to test the ***thériaque***, he had **realgar** and arsenic" (*pour bien l'*[la thériaque] *esprouver, il avoit du reagal et arcenic*).

40. Valence employed as early as1329 a *magister in arte conficiendi triagam* (M. McVaugh, p. 157).
41. *Registres du trésor des Chartes,* JJ 209, f. 119 v.
42. Jacques Fournier, t. 2, p. 56.
43. Henri Reibnitz de Breslau, *Tractatus de praeservationibus et remediis pestilenciarum,* in *Pestschriften...,* 1911, n 4, p. 215.
44. *Parlement criminel,* X2a 14, f. 93 v.
45. A. Retel-Laurentin, *Sorcellerie et ordalies,* p. 64.
46. Isidore de Séville, *Etymologiarum libri XX,* XI, col. 382.
47. Sur Locuste, Suétone, *Vie des XII Césars,* ed. trans. H. Ailloud, Paris, 3 vol., 1964–1967, Néron, 33, t. 2, p. 177. Sur Byzance, voir S. N. Troianos, Zauberei und Giftmischerei..., p. 48: according to *Digeste* XLVIII, 19, 28, l'*Isagogê* considers the *Giftmischer* as such, without confusing them with the *Giftmörder.*
48. Christine de Pizan, *Le livre de la Cité des dames,* p. 98.
49. *Gaydon,* p. 3.
50. Félix Hemmerlin, *Dialogus de nobilitate et rusticitate,* in *Quellen und Untersuchungen,* p. 110. Jean Bodin, *Fléaux des démons et sorciers,* p. 199: "He also notes that all witches normally make poisons" (*Encores faict il à noter que tous sorciers font ordinairement des poisons*).
51. *Grandes chroniques,* p. 696 du t. XXI du *RHGF.*
52. *Registres du trésor des Chartes,* JJ 120, f. 85–85 v and *Parlement criminel,* X2a 14, f. 173 and sq.
53. *Parlement criminel,* X2a 18, f. 13.
54. M. Ostorero, *Folâtrer avec les démons. Sabbat et chasse aux sorciers à Vevey (1448),* Lausanne, 1995, actes du procès, p. 204.
55. Hildegarde de Bingen, *Le livre des subtilités des créatures divines,* t. 1: *Plantes, pierres, métaux, éléments,* t. 2: *Arbres, poissons, oiseaux, animaux,* Paris, tr. P. Monat, Paris, Atopia, 1989, t. 1, p. 43.
56. Augustin, *Sermons,* ed. Migne, *PL* 38, col. 944 (sermon CLXXIII, chap. VIII): *universam massam generis humani in homine primo venenator ille percussit.*
57. Claude Tholosan, *Ut magorum...,* p. 357.
58. Voir J. Russel, p. 181. A case of a document of doubtful authenticity.
59. *Quellen und Untersuchungen,* p. 542: *ministerio dyabolorum fiunt venena.*
60. Maier, p. 188
61. Albe, p. 59.
62. Secousse, p. 379.
63. *Registres du trésor des Chartes,* JJ 106, f. 191 v–192.
64. Leleux, chap. 5.
65. Ciceron, *Pro Cluentio,* ed.-trans. P. Boyancé, Paris, 1953 (discours de Cicéron, t. 8), XIV, 40, p. 83.
66. Trachtenberg, p. 98, n. 6.
67. Saladin d'Ascoli, *Compendium aromatariorum,* ed. L. Zimermann, Leipzig, 1919, p. 83.
68. Rigault, p. 95 and sq., 22e article in the second series.
69. Carbonelli, p. 274.
70. *Lettres de Louis XI,* n 1164.
71. *Chartularium universitatis parisiensis,* ed. Denifle and Châtelain, Paris, 3 vol., 1889–1897, t. 1, pp. 488–490.
72. Jacques Fournier, t. 2, p. 56.

73. *Registres du trésor des Chartes*, JJ 209, f. 119 v.

74. J.-P. Bénezet, p. 75. A complete reversal in comparison with the period preceding 1200: in his charters concerning the Jews of Spire and of Worms, about 1090, Henry IV authorizes them to sell to Christians *vinum et pigmenta et antidota* (B. Blumenkranz, *Juifs et chrétiens . . .* , p. 345).

75. M. McVaugh, p. 60, n 87 and p. 158, n 104.

76. *Ciperis de Vignevaux*, v. 2911 and sq., p. 82.

77. Marx, pp. 132–133.

78. Pietro d'Abano, *De venenis*, chap. 2.

79. Ibid., BNF ms. lat. 11230, f. 6, concerning sublimated poisons.

80. G. Minois, p. 21.

81. In the affair of Benedict XI, the supposed supplier of the poison is not the learned Arnaud de Villeneuve, the accomplice de Bernard Délicieux, who was well-versed in toxicology, but Bernard himself (*Processus Bernardi Delitiosi*, p. 62 and sq.).

82. R. W. Ireland, Chaucer's toxicology, p. 78.

83. Rigault, p. 95 and sq. and Provost, *passim*.

84. *Novus thesaurus anecdotorum*, éd. U. Martène, t. 2, Paris, 1717, p. 86, lettre LVII.

85. Pietro d'Abano, *Tractatus de venenis*, BNF, ms lat. 11230, f. 6.

86. M. Robert, *Les empoisonnements criminels au xvi*^e^ *siècle*, Paris-Lyon, 1903, conclusion. Same reasoning concerning poisons in African societies. See A. Retel-Laurentin, *Sorcellerie et ordalies . . .* , pp. 73, 78, and 81.

87. Rodrigo Jimenez de Rada, III, 12, p. 92; *Parlement criminel*, X2a 6, f. 178–181.

88. Monstrelet, t. 2, p. 273. He gives the Latin (*gesdo*) and Greek (*ysatis*) names of the plant in question.

89. *Chronica di Pisa*, ed. Muratori, *RIS*, XV, Milan, 1729, col. 986. See Pietro d'Abano, *De venenis*, chap. 4; Galeazzo Marzio da Narni, *De doctrina promiscua*, ed. from Lyon, 1552, p. 116; Guido Da Vigevano, *Texaurus . . .* , f. 39 v–40, protests this statute and criticizes Avicenna.

90. *Placides et Timeo ou li secrés as philosophes*, ed. C. Thomasset, Genève-Paris, 1980, p. 113: " 'anapellis' comes from 'ana' which means 'retro' or 'behind,' and from 'pello' which means 'to push,' for it possesses a nature that is pushed back and changeable . . . , or because poison must be pushed away from all things because it is too cruel" (*"anapellis" si est dit de "ana" qui vaut a dire "retro" c'est a dire "deriere", et de " pello " qui vaut a dire "bouter", car c'est nature deboutee ariere et muee . . . , ou pour ce que ce venin doit estre arriere boutés de toutes coses, pour ce que il est trop crueulx*).

91. Ostorero, p. 205.

92. Jacques Fournier, t. 2 p. 56.

93. Pietro d'Abano, *De venenis*, chap. 2, p. 10 of the 1537 edition.

94. Secousse, p. 499: "if a man ate some the size of a pea, he would not live" (*se un homme en mangoit aussi gros que un poiz, jamais ne vivroit*).

95. Ibid., p. 388.

96. J. Marx, *L'inquisition en Dauphiné. Étude sur le développement et la répression de la sorcellerie du xiv*^e^ *siècle au début du règne de François I*^er^, Paris, 1914, PJ XI, pp. 226–227; A. Giuffrida, *La giustizia nel medioevo siciliano*, Palerme, 1975, p. 89; Jean de Saint-Victor, p. 657.

97. Pietro d'Abano, *De venenis*, chap. 68; Sante Ardoini de Pesaro, *Opus de venenis*, f. 250, is, however, skeptical.

98. *Registres du trésor des Chartes*, JJ 196, f. 72.

99. Sante Ardoini de Pesaro, *Opus de venenis*, p. 435. See the reflections of M. Mauss, *Sociologie et anthropologie*, p. 37 on the items used in the fabrication of objects used in witchcraft.

100. Lewin, p. 341.

101. *Chronique du Religieux de Saint-Denis*, XI, 5, t. 1, pp. 682–686.

102. Juvénal des Ursins, p. 143 of the 1653 edition.

103. Hildegarde de Bingen, *Causae et curae*, p. 50 of the tr.

104. See D. Jacquart, C. Thomasset, *Sexualité et savoir médical au Moyen Âge*, Paris, 1985, pp. 98–109; J. L. Canet, *La mujer venenosa en la época medieval*, Lemir, 1996, n 1.

105. *Placides et Timeo*, p. 264.

106. Pietro d'Abano, *De venenis*, chap. 2 and 71.

107. According to the confession of a leper from Périgord; cf. D. Nirenberg, p. 54.

108. Guibert de Nogent, *De vita sua*, III, 18, pp. 440–442; *Parlement criminel*, X2a 14, f. 384, et f. 411 v; *Registres du trésor des Chartes*, JJ 162, f. 76 v.

109. I. Cloulas, *Les Borgia*, Paris, Fayard, 1987, p. 317 and Guichardin, VI, 4.

110. *Registre criminel du Châtelet*, p. 442.

111. Albe, pp. 59–60.

112. Jacques Fournier, t. 2, pp. 135–144; *Registre criminel du Châtelet*, t. 1, pp. 311–322 et 409–480. This stereotype probably plays a role in the connection between the two cases.

113. Nangis, t. 2, pp. 31–36.

114. For example, Godefroy Ménilglaise, article X brought against Mahaut d'Artois.

115. Jacques de Voragine, *Légende dorée*, LVIII, Saint George.

116. *Registres du trésor des Chartes*, JJ 120, f. 85–85 v.

117. Guibert de Nogent, *De vita sua*, III, 18, pp. 440–442.

118. *Contemporary Narrative*, p. 2 and sq.: *pulveres cum variis incantationibus*.

119. *Select Cases in the Court of King's Bench. Richard II, Henry IV and Henry V*, ed. M. S. Arnold, London, 3 vol., 1985 1987, p. 113.

120. Basin, t. 2, pp. 116 and 132. The commentator on the journal of Jean de Roye, p. 285 of volume 2 of Mandrot's edition, indicates that the partisans of the Duc de Guyenne maintained that he "had been poisoned and cursed" (*avoit esté empoisonné et maleficié*).

121. Marx, PJ XI, p. 226. Jacques Grevin, *Deux livres des venins*, p. 31: "poisons mixed with words" (*venins meslés avec paroles*).

122. Jean de Roye, p. 275 of the Michaud-Poujoulat edition.

123. Coville, p. 330.

124. Provost, p. 286 and p. 535 and sq. (transcript of the confession).

125. Albe, p. 59.

126. *Mémoires pour servir de preuves à l'histoire de la Bretagne*, ed. Dom Morice, Paris, 3 vol, 1742–1746, t. 2, col. 1550–1554; in this case, poison put to soak only one day before its use is reputed to be less strong than those that can be mixed directly with meat or soup, but the literary sources, on the contrary, imply that

poison that has been mixed with water is all the more powerful the longer that it has been left to soak.

127. M. Aston, A Kent Approver of 1440, *Bulletin of the Institute of Historical Research*, 1963, n°36, pp. 82–90, p. 86.

128. J. Russel, p. 240, according to the text of the *Errores*.

129. Nicole Gilles, t. 1, f. 66 v.

130. *Capitularia regum Francorum*, n°54, t. 1 p. 153. In a judicial text from the fifteenth century, the two words are used as synonyms. (Marx, p. 133: *de dicto pulvere et veneno*).

131. Geoffroy de Salagny, t. 1, f. 113 et t. 3, f. 107 v. *Registre criminel du Châtelet*, p. 438.

132. Mathias von Neuenburg, p. 93 then 354.

133. *Chronique du Religieux de Saint-Denis*, VI, 4, t. 1, pp. 355–357. Secousse, p. 499.

134. Geoffroy de Salagny, t. 3, f. 107 v, col. b.

135. *Registre criminel du Châtelet*, p. 420: powder "approaching the color of ground pepper" (*trayant sur la couleur de poudre de poivre*).

136. Matthieu Paris, t. 4, p. 490.

137. Monfrin, p. 231 and sq. Among them is found Christoforus de Honestis, the author of a treatise on poisons.

138. Carbonelli, PJ XXXIV.

139. Secousse p. 500.

140. Frédégaire, *Chronique*, ed. B. Krusch, *MGH Ss rr mer.*, II, Hanovre, 1888, IV, 49, p. 145: salve applied after a bath.

141. Landolphe, *Mediolanenses historiae libri IV*, ed. Muratori, *RIS*, IV, Milan, 1723, II, 19, pp. 81–82. G. Althoff, *Otto III*, Darmstadt, 1997, pp. 186–187, denies the reality of this poisoning. The emperor would have succumbed instead to a mysterious *morbus italicus*.

142. Carbonelli, p. 225 puis 230.

143. Monstrelet, t. 3, pp. 44–46.

144. Matthieu d'Escouchy, *Chronique*, ed. Du Fresne de Beaucourt, Paris, 3 vol., 1863–1864, t. 3, pp. 346 and 352.

145. Modestin, n°25, p. 252 and sq., acts from the trial of Jeannette Anyo.

146. Matthieu Paris, t. 5, p. 702 and sq.

147. Nangis, t. 2, pp. 31–36. The inability to burn of poisoned organs is another well known sign in the Middle Ages of the power of poison: John of Salisbury mentions it when speaking of the emperor Tiberius. (*Policraticus*, tr. de D. Foulechat (1372), VIII, 19, p. 100).

148. Neri di Gino Capponi, col. 121; Nicolas Falcucci, *De dispositionibus venenorum*, f. 83 v gives the example of a captain of Forli who was poisoned when he approached a fire where a noxious substance was burning.

149. Burchard, *Diarium*, ed. L. Thuasne, Paris, 3 vol., 1883–1885, t. 2 p. 579.

150. Zantfliet, col. 417.

151. D. Jacquart, Influence de la médecine arabe en Occident médiéval, *Histoire des sciences arabes*, 3, *Technologies, alchimie et sciences de la vie*, sd. R. Rashed, Paris, Le Seuil, 1997, pp. 213–232, p. 221. Malaria has this reputation as a consequence, and it probably gave to central Italy its poisonous reputation. See J. Nelson, La mort de Charles le Chauve.

152. *Epistola et regimen Alphontii Cordubensis de pestilentia*, in *Pestschriften . . .*, 1910, n°3, p. 225. Henri de Brême, *Causae, signa et remedia contra pestilentiam*, in *Pestschriften . . .*, 1914, n°7, p. 85.

153. Secousse, p. 499.

154. In the act that clears Mahaut d'Artois in 1317, one reads that Louis X died *non ex causa veneni seu potionum*. Acte publié par Godefroy Ménilglaise, pp. 195–218.

155. *Registres du trésor des Chartes*, JJ 196, f. 104–105.

156. Maïmonide, *Traité des poisons*, p. 51.

157. Thomas de Chobham, *Summa confessorum*, IV, 2, 6, 4, *Si aranea incidat*, pp. 138–139, certainly this concerns an accidental poisoning.

158. Thomas d'Aquin, *Somme théologique*, Pars III, Q. 73, art. 6, p. 294: *cognoscit sacerdos calici venenum esse immissum ab aliquo malevolo causa occidendi ipsum*; what must the priest do? To drink from the chalice is suicide, not to drink is a sin against the laws of the Church: it is necessary to commit a sin; it is better to empty the chalice and to reconsecrate other wine, *ne calix vite vertatur in mortem*. On earlier reflections by Thomas Aquinas, P. Browe, Die angebliche Vergiftung Kaiser Heinrichs VII, *Historisches Jahrbuch*, 1929, n°49, pp. 479–488.

159. Abélard, *Historia calamitatum*, ed. J. Monfrin, Paris, Vrin, 1967, pp. 106–107.

160. Guillaume de Malmesbury, t. 2, p. 326 and Guillaume de Newburgh, t. 1, p. 71 and sq.; Mathias von Neuenburg, p. 93 then 354.

161. Jacques Fournier, t. 2, p. 14; *Grandes chroniques de France*, t. 8, p. 358: "and when the packet breaks, the poison is released" (*et quant le sachet rompoit, si espandoit le venin*).

162. Letter published by M. Freher, *Scriptores rerum bohemicarum*, Hanovre, 1602, pp. 35–36.

163. *Chronique des premiers Valois*, p. 315.

164. Konrad de Megenberg, p. 867. L'*Epistola et regimen Alphontii Cordubensis*, p. 224, limits poisonous action to *aquis praaecipue non fluentibus*.

165. *Istore et croniques de Flandres*, ed. Kervyn de Lettenhove, Bruxelles, 2 vol., 1879–1880, p. 325.

166. Pietro d'Abano, *De venenis*, I, p. 5.

167. Arnaud de Villeneuve, *Epistola de dosi tyrialicium medicinarum*, in *Opera omnia medica*, ed. L. Garcia-Ballester, J. A. Paniagua et M. McVaugh, Barcelone, 1975–1990, t. 3, p. 87. Galeotto Marzio da Narni, *De doctrina promiscua*, p. 47: *venenum ergo et medicina sive medicamen eiusdem naturae sunt . . . Est igitur apud nos medicina et venenum quod apud Graecos pharmacon*.

168. Escouchy, t. 3, p. 346 and sq.

169. Grégoire de Tours, V, 36, t. 1, p. 300 from the trans. of R. Latouche: Marachaire poisoned by a fish head.

170. Orderic Vital, III, t. 2, p. 28 then 73, and Froissart, t. 3, p. 243 from the Buchon edition.

171. Commynes, VI, 12 p. 495, writes more exactly that it was in the handle of the knife that the poison was concealed; Carbonelli, PJ XXXIV, p. 349: the fruit to be poisoned was a pomegranate.

172. Example in *Gaydon*, v. 90; *Parise la Duchesse*, pp. 1–5; on the theme of poisoned fruit in literature, see J. Frappier, *Étude sur la mort le roi Artu*, Genève, 3e éd., 1972, pp. 196–198.

173. Ferretus Vicentinus, *Historia*, ed. Muratori, *RIS*, IX, Milan, 1726, col. 1013; Secousse, p. 381. Pears have the reputation of easily absorbing contaminated air and causing pestilence according to Konrad de Megenberg.

174. *Parlement criminel*, X2a 14, f. 214 v–217 v: "pastry full of garbage" [meaning foreign material or poison] (*bugnes pleins d'ordures*).

175. Arnaud de Verdale, *Catalogus episcoporum magalonensium*, ed. A. Germain, Montpellier, 1881, p. 133.

176. *Parlement criminel*, X2a 14, f. 214 v–217 v, and *Registres du trésor des Chartes*, JJ 215, f. 75 v.

177. Pietro d'Abano, *De venenis*, I, p. 28 from the edition of 1537.

178. Richer, II, 59.

179. Grégoire de Tours, t. 2, p. 206 from the Büchner edition.

180. P. Preto, *Epidemia, paura e politica nell'Italia moderna*, Bari, 1987, p. 24.

181. See, for example, Nicolas Falcucci, *De dispositionibus venenorum*, f. 83 v.

182. Pierre Cochon, *Chronique normande*, ed. C. de Robillard de Beaurepaire, Rouen, 1870, pp. 62–63.

183. Matthieu Paris, t. 6, p. 464 from the translated edition; Paul Diacre, *Historia Langobardorum*, ed. L. Bethmann and G. Waitz, Hanovre, 1881, II, 29. Numerous learned treatises mention the danger of drinking upon leaving a bath, whatever the content of the drink.

184. Matthieu Paris, t. 5, pp. 68–69.

185. Domenico da Gravina, *Chronicon*, ed. A. Sorbelli, *RIS*, XII-3, Milan, 1903, col. 559.

186. *Chronique du Religieux de Saint-Denis*, t. 1, p. 166.

187. *Gesta abbatum Horti sanctae Mariae*, ed. *MGH SS*, XXIII, Hanover, 1874, p. 595.

188. *Lettres de Louis XI*, t. 7, PJ VI, p. 311.

189. Froissart, t. 12, pp. 81–88 from the ed. SHF, concerning the poison destined for Gaston Phoebus: "powder of such a kind that there was no living thing that could touch or eat it without being killed" (*pouldre de telle condition que il n'estoit chose vivant que se de la poudre atouchoit ne mengoit que tantost ne le convenist morir sans nul remede*).

190. Coville, p. 328, second justification: in response to the argument according to which the chaplain who had touched the powder of the Duc d'Orléans at Neauphle had not died until six years later (Monstrelet, *Chronique*, t. 1, p. 326), the theologian in the pay of Jean sans Peur answers that the individual did not die right away because he had only touched the poisoned food.

191. *Quellen und Untersuchungen*, pp. 571–575.

192. Du Clercq, p. 668 from Buchon and Shatzmiller's edition, pp. 88–89.

193. See R. Michel, Le procès de Matteo et Galeazo Visconti, *MAHEFR*, 1909, pp. 277–327.

194. Bernard Gui, *Manuel de l'inquisiteur*, ed.-transl. G. Mollat, Paris, 2 vol., reedited, 1964, p. 22, n 1.

195. See J. Agrimi, C. Crisciani, Savoir médical et anthropologie religieuse...

196. Juvénal des Ursins, p. 27 from the 1614 edition. The idea of a poisonous glance was invoked against the nobles to explain the epidemic of 1348.

197. Secousse, p. 502.

198. *Registres du trésor des Chartes*, JJ 234, f. 107 v–108.

199. *Mémoires pour servir de preuves à l'histoire de la Bretagne*, col. 1550–1554.

200. Jean de Saint-Amand, *Concordanciae*, ed. J. Pagel, Berlin, 1894, p. 498, wrote an article of impressive length on *venenum*.

201. Thorndike, *An History of Magic . . .*, t. 3, p. 525.

202. Pietro d'Abano, *De venenis*, chap. 1: *venenum oppositum est cibo nostri corporis*. On the difficulty of distinguishing philtre/poison, see Ps. Quintilien, *Declamationes*, p. 292 and sq.: *venenum negat esse nisi tantum quod occidit* claims an accused woman.

203. Avicenne, *Liber canonis*, p. 69; Isidore de Séville, *Etymologiarum libri XX*, XII, 4, col. 447, rapproche *venenum* de *venae*. The larger the veins, the more quickly poison works.

204. Avicenne, *Liber canonis*, ed. from Bâle, 1566, f. 912.

205. *Chronique de France et de Flandre de saint Louis à 1383*, BNF, ms. fr. 12272, f. 11 v–12.

206. *Parlement criminel*, X2a 14, f. 217. See the same argument in X2a 18, f. 12 v, defended by Jouvenel: "it is not possible to keep the poisons such a long time . . . For if they were realgar or arsenic, the lady could have lived only two days at the most" (*n'eust pu garder les poisons si longtemps . . . Car s'ils furent de reagas ou d'arsenic, la dame n'eust pu vivre que deux jours au plus*).

207. Grégoire de Tours, t. 1, p. 162 from Latouche's edition, et t. 2, p. 206 from Büchner's edition; *Chronique des comtes d'Anjou et des seigneurs d'Amboise*, ed. L. Halphen, R. Poupardin, Paris, 1913, p. 124.

208. *Select case; Richard II, etc.*, p. 113.

209. Pierre le Baud, t. 2, p. 56.

210. *La mort le roi Artu*, p. 76: "And as soon as it had passed his throat, he fell dead immediately (*Et si tost comme il en ot le col passé, il chaï morz erranment*).

211. Ser Giovanni Fiorentino, *Il pecorone*, 23e journée, p. 215.

212. *Registres du trésor des Chartes*, JJ 196, f. 104–105.

213. Thietmar de Mersebourg, *Gesta Saxonum*, ed. R. Holtzmann, Berlin, 1955, VI, 36, p. 319.

214. *Chronicon Angliae, 1328–1388*, ed. Edward. M. Thompson, Londres, 1874, p. 60. Froissart, t. 2, p. 110 of Buchon's edition. Petrus Cararius claims that a poison can wait thirty years before killing a victim. (*Questio de venenis ad terminum*, f. 270).

215. Pfister, actes du procès, p. 254.

216. Avicenne, *Liber canonis*, ed. of Bâle, 1566, f. 912; Petrus Cararius, *Questio de venenis ad terminum*, f. 268–271: certain words can hasten a cure, others can very well determine the moment of the poison's acting.

217. *Roman d'Alexandre*, p. 740, v. 7824–7833.

218. Geoffroy de Salagny, t.1, f. 113, col. B.

219. Guichardin, II, 3, p. 156.

220. P. D. Pasolini, *Catherina Sforza*, t. 3, p. 775.

221. Marx, p. 224.

222. Ambroise Paré, *Traité des venins . . .*, chap. 45 and p. 339. An entire tradition maintains that certain poisons have properties that are not affected by pharmacology and can be influenced by stallar emanations. (See Galeotto Marzio da Narni, *De doctrina promiscua*, p. 126 or Jean Martin de Ferrare, *De venenis evitandis*, f. 6).

223. *Parlement criminel*, X2a 14, f. 215: "she was found with her abdomen swollen up, shiny, and red, signs of poisoning" (*fut trouvee enflee et reluisant et rouge par le ventre qui sont signes d'empoisonnements*).

224. Dynter, t. 3, pp. 497–499.

225. *Les fragments du Roman de Tristan . . .*, p. 128.

226. Gui de Chauliac, *La grande chirurgie*, traité VI, doctrine I, chap. 8, p. 434.

227. Grégoire de Tours, t. 2, p. 206 of Büchner's edition; *Chronique des comtes d'Anjou . . .*, p. 124; Basin, t. 2, p. 118.

228. Y. Grandeau, Le dauphin Jean de Touraine (1398–1417), *Bulletin philologique et historique*, 1968, n 2, pp. 665–722, p. 721.

229. Jean de Winterthur, *Chronica*, ed. F. Baethgen, *MGH, ss rr g in us. sch.*, n. série (3), Berlin, 1923, p. 184.

230. Henri Stero, *Chronique*, ed. M. Freher, *Scriptores rerum germanicarum*, Strasbourg, 1717, p. 596.

231. Pietro d'Abano, *De venenis*, chap. 30.

232. *Historia de expeditione Friderici imperatoris*, ed. A. Chroust, Berlin, 1928, *MGH, ss rr g. in us. sc.*, n. s. 5, pp. 1–115, pp. 54–55.

233. *Gaydon*, v. 214, 243, perhaps inspired by *Parise la Duchesse*, v. 109: "Both eyes immediately flew out of his forehead" (*Andui li oil li volent tot maintenant del front*) or p. 9: "He gave him the apple that poisoned him, / As a result, his eyes flew out of his head" (*La pome li dona dont il fu enherbez, / Par coi li fist les ieuz de la teste voler*).

234. Cf. Jacques de Voragine, *Legenda aurea*, chap. 45, Saint Matthias: he cured in Macedonia more than 250 persons who had been blinded by poison. Jean de Winterthur, p. 85: the wife of the Duke of Austria who became blind in 1327.

235. *Parlement criminel*, X2a 14, f. 174.

236. *Chronique de Rains*, ed. P. Paris, Paris, 1837, p. 42 puis 49: "the nails fell from the feet and the hands and all became bald" (*li ongle li cheirent des pies et des mains et pela tous*).

237. Matthieu Paris, t. 5, p. 702 and sq., and *Annales de Burton*, in *Annales monastici*, ed. R. Luard, t. 1, Londres, 1864, p. 460: The count of Gloucester came out of it *semi-vivus, tonsis capillis et ungulis cadentibus.*

238. *Chronique du Religieux de Saint-Denis*, t. 1, p. 682. The balding effect is also found in the beliefs of African peoples. See E. E. Evans-Pritchard, *Sorcellerie, oracle et magie chez les Azandé*, p. 327.

239. *Brevis historia ordinis Fratrum Praedicatorum*, ed. Martène and Durand, in *Veterum scriptorum et monumentorum historicorum, dogmaticorum, moralium amplissima collectio*, t. 6, Paris, 1729, col. 377.

240. Guillaume de Saliceto, *Cirurgia*, p. 18. In the case of poisons that act on the first quality, it is the excess of one of these qualities (heat, cold, dryness, humidity) that causes the destruction of life. Mercury is thus hot and dry to the 4th degree.

241. *Parlement criminel*, X2a 18, f. 11 v–14.

242. Basin, III, 16 and IV, 2.

243. Du Clercq, p. 632 of Michaud and Poujoulat's edition.

244. Dynter, t. 3, p. 73.

245. Secousse, p. 503.

246. *Yder*, v. 5752.

247. Orderic Vital, III, t. 2, p. 73, concerning the corpse of Robert Giroie. One finds in Pliny's *Histoire naturelle*, ed.-trans. Littré, Paris, 2 vol., 1848–1850, XXIV, 5, 11, the idea that a poisoned corpse does not rot.

248. Simon de Marville, *Vœux de l'Épervier*, v. 504; *Roman d'Alexandre*, p. 754, v. 157 and sq.

249. Grégoire le Grand, *Dialogues, Vita Benedicti*, 27, 3.
250. Orderic Vital, t. 3, pp. 181–182 and t. 4, pp. 196–197.
251. C. G. Carbonelli, *Come vissero i primi conti di Savoia*, Milan, 1931, p. 208.
252. Carbonelli, p. 243.
253. Guillaume de Newburgh, t. 1, p. 71 and sq. Pietro d'Abano, *De venenis*, chap. 13.
254. Guichardin, *Storia d'Italia*, VI, 4.
255. Jean de Joinville, *Histoire de saint Louis*, ed. N. de Wailly, Paris, 1881, p. 51.
256. *Parlement criminel*, X2a 14, f. 174 v.
257. About one-fifth of the effects of poisons inventoried by Pietro d'Abano are of this type. The *Theodosian Code* (IX, 38, 6) mentions the *mentis et corporis venena*, the *Liber augustalis* (II, 69, p. 166) puts in the same category *mala et noxia medicamenta ad alienandos animos seu venena*.
258. Frédégaire, p. 145, and Paul Diacre, IV, 45. See also in the Visigoth world, Isidore de Séville, *Historia Gothorum*, ed. Mommsen, *MGH AA*, XI, Berlin, 1894, pp. 291–292.
259. Froissart, t. 3, p. 279 from the edition by Buchon and Thomas Basin, *Historia Karoli septimi*, I, 2, t. 1, p. 10. Jean d'Outremeuse explains the Flagellant movement by the absorption of poison from the Jews (Trachtenberg, p. 105).
260. Guillaume de Brescia, *Questiones de tyriaca*, ed. M. McVaugh, *Sudhoffs Archiv*, 1972, n 56, pp. 130–143, compares a sick body to an organism filled with poison (*simili veneno repleto*). Since the sixteenth century, the "virus" has been described as a pathogenic agent as noticed by C. Boujot, *Le venin*, p. 139.
261. Cf. Thomas de Bologne, *Questio an lapis philosophicus valeat contra pestem*, published in *Theatrum chimicum*, ed. L. Zetzner, Starsbourg, 4 vol., 1659, t. 3, p. 182: *febris sive dysenteria sive hydrops sive lepra sive quecunque alia infirmitas ducens vel apta nata ducere ad mortem potest vocari venenum.*
262. Carbonelli, p. 206 then p. 208.
263. Chastellain, t. 3, p. 386.
264. In a *Regimen preservativum* of Breslau (about 1350), one can read a recipe pro *preservacione a veneno tempore pestilenciae et propter timorem intoxicationis (Pestschriften . . . ,* 1914, n 9, p. 164).
265. *Chronique des premiers Valois*, p. 274.
266. Pietro d'Abano, *De venenis*, chap. 11: he gives the symptoms of seven poisons including arsenic.
267. Grégoire de Tours, V, 35, t. 1, p. 298 of R. Latouche's tr.
268. See Coville, p. 330.
269. *Parlement criminel*, X2a 14, f. 215, et *Parlement criminel*, X2a 18, f. 11 v. This controversy is not at all surprising since Quintilian wrote earlier in his *Institution oratoire* (V, 9, p. 125) that swelling was an argument equally useful for the defense and the prosectution in a case in which *veneficium* was suspected. The text was rediscovered by le Pogge in 1417.
270. Jean de Viktring, *Liber certarum historiarum*, ed. F. Schneider, *MGH, ss rr gg in us. schap.* (36), t. 2, Hanovre et Leipzig, 1910, pp. 135–136, and Jean de Roye, t. 2, p. 131.
271. Petrus Cararius, *Questio de venenis ad terminum*, f. 270: *non est inconveniens aliquos esse venenatos qui continue exiccando procedant et tales appellantur apud vulgares herbati sive strigati.*

272. Du Clercq, p. 632 from the ed. Michaud and Poujoulat: "Some said that he had been poisoned or cursed by the Vaudois." (*Disoient aulcuns qu'il avoit esté empoisonné par les Vauldois ou ensorcelez*); *Registres du trésor des Chartes*, JJ 207, f. 148. Jean de Saint-Victor, p. 651; N. Gonthier, *Délinquance, justice et société dans le Lyonnais médiéval (fin xiiie—début xvie siècle)*, Paris, 1993, p. 231.

273. Hippolite de Marsiliis, *Commentaria . . .*, f. 26 v.

274. D. Jacquart, *La médecine . . .*, p. 322.

275. Formule de Gilbertus Anglicus, *Compendium medicine*, Lyon ed., 1510, f. 350. Sante Ardoini de Pesaro illustrates this double orientation by giving each of his items the headings *praeservatio et cura*.

276. Id., *Opus de venenis*, chap. 8.

277. Guillaume de Nangis, *Gesta Ludovici*, ed. *RHGF*, XX, Paris, 1840, p. 334. Secousse, t. 2, pp. 379 and 499.

278. Jean de Winterthur, p. 11.

279. *Leges palatinae regis Jacobi Majoricarum*, ed. in *Acta Sanctorum*, Junii, III, Anvers, 1701, p. xix et p. xv.

280. Franciscus de Sienne, *Liber de venenis*, f. 22 v.

281. Jean de Roye, p. 307 in the1837 edition.

282. Widespread advice; see, for example, Jean Martin de Ferrare, *De venenis evitandis*, f. 3.

283. Bonifazio Simonetta, *De christiane fidei et romanorum pontificum persecutione*, Bâle, 1509, f. 105.

284. Avicenna, *Liber canonis*, Bâle edition, 1566, f. 911–912.

285. Feretus Vicentinus, col. 1013; Froissart, t. 3, p. 241 of the Buchon edition.

286. Pietro d'Abano, *De venenis*, p. 26 of the1537 edition. Nicolas Falcucci, *De dispositionibus venenorum*, chap. 6 and 7.

287. Jean d'Arezzo, *De procuratione cordis*, III, 3, cited by L. Thorndike, *Science and Thought in the xvth Century*, New York, 1929, p. 115, n 18.

288. Texts cited by Pogatscher, p. 44.

289. Christoforus de Honestis, *Liber de venenis*, f. 89: *non est lingua serpentis ut vulgus eam appellat*.

290. *Choix de pièces inédites relatives au règne de Charles VI*, t. 2, pp. 281–360.

291. See, for example, *The Prose Salernitan Questions*, ed. B. Lawn, Londres, 1979, ms B, Oxford (xiiie–xve siècle), question 103, p. 48 and question 165, p. 84: *Queritur quare ex presentia toxici cornu serpentis sudet*.

292. Thomas de Cantimpré, *Liber de natura rerum*, ed. H. Boese, Berlin–New York, 1973, p. 44.

293. Guillaume de Malmesbury, t. 2, p. 455.

294. Jean d'Outremeuse, *Le myreur des histors*, ed. A. Borgnet and S. Bormans, Bruxelles, 6 vol., 1864–1886, t. 6, p. 253.

295. R. Lentsch, p. 158. A. Coulon, A gift from Philippe V, king of France, to Pope John XXII, *MHAEFR*, 1894, n° 14, pp. 611–614, cites the thank-you letter to Philippe V and describes the objects given as gifts between 1317 and 1320, perhaps following the affaire of Hugues Géraud.

296. *Inventaire du trésor du Saint-Siège sous Boniface VIII*. The heading is called *rami sive arbores cum linguis serpentinis*. *Die Inventare des papstlichen Schatzes in Avignon*, p. 52 and sq.

297. R. Lentsch, p. 158, n. 14, text cited by the author.

298. Pogatscher, p. 21 and chap. 3.

299. *Inventaire du mobilier de Charles V, roi de France*, ed. J. Labarte, Paris, 1879, n°324, 784, 1606 and 2160.

300. O. Mazzoni Toselli, *Racconti storici estratti dall'archivio criminale di Bologna*, Bologne, 3 vol., 1866–1870, t. 2, p. 451.

301. *Quelques pièces relatives à la vie de Louis I, duc d'Orléans, et de Valentine Visconti, sa femme*, ed. F. M. Graves, Paris, 1913, n°CXXXI, p. 233.

302. *Comptes du roi René*, ed. Arnaud d'Agnel, Paris, 3 vol., 1909, n°879, t. 1, p. 302.

303. For example, Nicolas Falcucci, *De dispositionibus venenorum*, f. 84.

304. Text cited by Pogatscher, p. 44.

305. Christoforus de Honestis, *Liber de venenis*, f. 87 v.

306. Guido da Vigevano, *Thesaurus*, f. 41.

307. Metaphor of the redemption of sins by Christ. Voir L. Réau, *Iconographie de l'art chrétien*, I, Paris, 1955, pp. 89–92; J. Voisenet, *Bestiaire chrétien. L'imagerie animale des auteurs du haut Moyen Âge (v^e^–xie siècle)*, Toulouse, 1994, p. 126.

308. Ambroise Paré, *Discours a scavoir . . .* , chap. 16, points out that neither Aristotle, Hippocrates, nor Galien speaks of the virtues of the unicorn horn.

309. Hildegarde de Bingen, *Le livre des subtilités des créatures divines*, t. 2, p. 197.

310. R. Lentsch, p. 158. Pogatscher, p. 15 and 20, believes that the *cornua unicornuum* of Boniface VIII were lost and that they do not reappear until the time of Benedict XIII.

311. Id., p. 27.

312. *Choix de pièces inédites relatives au règne de Charles VI*, n°39, 46, de la pièce 149, t. 2, pp. 370, 374.

313. Inventory of the treasury and precious objects kept in the church of the Abbey of Saint-Denis in 1505 and 1739, ed. H. Omont, *Mémoires de la société de l'histoire de Paris et de l'Île de France*, 1901, n°28, pp. 163–212, n°165.

314. Pogatscher, p. 33.

315. Ambroise Paré, *Discours a scavoir . . .* , p. 518. Jacques Grevin, *Deux livres des venins . . .* , p. 194, overwhelm Pietro d'Abano and Gilbert l'Anglais.

316. Nicolas Falcucci, *De dispositionibus venenorum*, f. 85; *Leges palatinae regis Jacobi Majoricarum*, p. x

317. Hildegarde de Bingen, *Le livre des subtilités des créatures divines*, t. 1, pp. 247–248.

318. Pietro d'Abano, *De venenis*, BNF, ms. lat. 11230, f. 11. See also Jean Martin de Ferrare, *De venenis evitandis . . .* , f. 3: *presentato veneno amittit viriditatem et ipso remoto recuperat*.

319. Nicolas Falcucci, *De dispositionibus venenorum*, f. 85.

320. *Die Inventare des papstlichen Schatzes . . .* , p. 264.

321. R. Lentsch, p. 159.

322. *Choix de pièces inédites relatives au règne de Charles VI*, t. 2, p. 303, n°120.

323. On this subject, see N. Weill-Parot, *Les "images astrologiques" . . .* , p. 530 and sq. Cf. Antonio Guaineri, *Opus praeclarum*, f. 231: *imago astri serpentarii alicui pretioso lapidi insculpta venena fugat omnia . . .*

324. *Ciperis de Vignevaux*, v. 2978 and sq.: "Then the beautiful Aragonde of Germany with blond hair, / Looks at one of her rings in a noble way. / As soon as

there is poison within ten feet / the stone that is in it becomes covered with water / She finds it damp and says in a loud voice, / ... / 'At this table there is poison.' " (*Adonc belle Aragonde d'Alemengne au crin blon, / Ung sien anel regarde de moult gente fachon. / Si tost qu'il a venin a X piés environ / La pierre qui est ens s'i rent yaue a foison. / Moullié le trouva, lors dit a hault ton, / ... / " A ceste table chi a venin ou poison"*).

325. Grégoire le Grand, *Dialogues*, II, *Vita Benedicti*, 3, t. 2, p. 140 and sq. In the *Vita patrum* de Grégoire de Tours, V, 2, ed. *MGH, SS rr mm*, I, p. 678, the abbot Pourçain from Auvergne († 540) breaks a poisoned cup with the sign of the cross.

326. Grégoire le Grand, *Dialogues*, III, 5, t. 2, p. 274 and sq.

327. *La vie ancienne de saint Samson de Dol*, I, 16 and 55.

328. Guido da Vigevano, *Texaurus* ..., f. 41.

329. *Chronique du Religieux de Saint-Denis*, t. 3, p. 134.

330. Suétone, *Vie des XII Césars*, Claude, 44, t. 2, p. 148.

331. Liutprand de Cremona, *Relatio de legatione Constantinopolitana*, in *Opera omnia*, ed. P. Chiesa, Turnhout, 1998, pp. 185–218, p. 196.

332. Richer de Sénones, *Gesta Senoniensis ecclesie*, ed. *MGH SS*, XXV, Hanover, 1880, Errard's French version, p. 300.

333. J. Théry, p. 42.

334. *Avvisamenta*, ed. *RIS*, III-2, col. 810-824, see col. 813; R. Lentsch, pp. 159–161, believes that at the end of the fourteenth century, the test was done only in the kitchens because the descriptions of the banquets never mention them; but this silence can also be explained by the habitual nature of the test.

335. See Burchard, *Diarium*, t. 1, p. 58 of the Thuasne edition (Conclave of 1484).

336. Ch.-V. Langlois, L'affaire du cardinal Francesco Caetani (avril 1316), *RH*, 1897, t. 63, pp. 56–71, p. 63, deposition of the cardinal's accuser, whose two henchmen are supposedly reflecting on the best way to kill the royal princes.

337. *Leges palatinae regis Jacobi Majoricarum*, p. x; p. xv on the wine steward and p. xxviii for the finance minister (le **camerlingue**).

338. See Simon de Marville, *Vœux de l'épervier*, v. 155–162.

339. *Leges palatinae regis Jacobi Majoricarum*, p. xxi et xxxi–xxxii.

340. Mathias von Neuenburg, pp. 276 and 431.

341. Olivier de la Marche, *Mémoires*, t. 4, pp. 1–94, text p. 46. See also Éléonore de Poitiers, *Les États de France (les honneurs de la cour)*, ed. J. Paviot, *ABSHF*, 1996, pp. 84–118. Composed in the 1480s, this treatise devotes a few lines to the belief and the test (p. 115).

342. Ibid.

343. Jacques Fournier, t. 3, p. 832 of the translation.

344. Arnaud de Verdale, p. 133.

345. *Leges palatinae regis Jacobi Majoricarum*, col. XLVI. Other examples concerning worldly princes like those of the Church in P. Browe, Die angebliche Vergiftung Kaiser Heinrichs VII, p. 488.

346. Antonio Guaineri, *Opus praeclarum*, f. 231. The test of linen also includes that used on dining tables.

347. Christoforus de Honestis, *Liber de venenis*, f. 87.

348. Jean d'Outremeuse, t. 6, p. 140.

349. Franciscus de Sienne, *Liber de venenis*, I, 2, f. 23: *ad timorem servitoribus inducendum*.

350. Carbonelli, p. 224; this observation often appears in trial records.

351. Chastellain, t. 4, p. 242.

352. Orderic Vital, t. 4, pp. 106–107, and t. 2, p. 107.

353. For example, BNF, ms. lat. 7021, f. 118 v.

354. An example of recipes, those that the future Pope Clement VI wrote in the margin of a manuscript made up of extracts from various works (Vat. Borghese 247, fol. 218 v); this reference was suggested by J.-P. Boudet whom we thank warmly. Another recipe copied in a manuscript in Munich and cited by K. Sudhoff dans *Pestschriften*, 1912, n°17, p. 138: a powder made for the king of England by a certain Jean Cesar.

355. Richer, II, 59, and Pierre le Baud, t. 3, p. 167.

356. See, for example, the *Philippide* of Guillaume le Breton, *Gesta Philippi Augusti*, ed. H.-F. Delaborde, Paris, 2 vol., 1882–1885, XII, v. 183–187, t. 2, p. 355.

357. Antonio Guaineri, *Opus praeclarum*, f. 234 v.

358. Albert le Grand, *Liber de mirabilibus mundi*, Anvers edition, 1555, without pagination.

359. Geoffroy de Salagny, t. 3, f. 107 v, col. b.

360. Platearius, *Le livre des simples médecines*, ed. P. Dorveaux, Paris, 1913, p. 7.

361. Pietro d'Abano, *De venenis*, p. 33.

362. *Roman d'Alexandre*, p. 754, v. 160.

363. Carbonelli, p. 278. This remedy appears in a number of treatises: Pietro d'Abano, *De venenis*, chap. 80; Jean Martin de Ferrara, *De venenis evitandis*, f. 5.

364. Pietro d'Abano, *De venenis*, chap. 15 et 80.

365. Froissart, t. 2, p. 110 of Buchon's edition: "he got rid of all or a part of the poison that he had taken and received; the king recovered his hair and nails for, little by little the poison flowed out by a small fistula in his arm" (*il amortit tout ou en partie le venin qu'il avoit pris et reçu*; le roi recouvre poils et ongles car, *petit à petit, le venin lui issoit et couloit par une petite fistule qu'il avoit dans le bras*). Is Antonio Guaineri making an allusion to this treatment, which he says was given to a king of France? (*Opus praeclarum*, f. 240 v).

366. See Thorndike, *An History of Magic . . .*, t. 3, p. 540. Christophorus de Honestis sees this method as emetic.

367. *Cronica de gestis principum*, p. 36.

368. Jean de Winterthur, p. 46; Thomas Ebendorfer, *Chronica pontificum romanorum*, ed. H. Zimmermann, *MGH, SS Rer. Ger.*, n. série (16), Munich, 1994, t. 2, p. 521.

369. Gilles li Muisit, *Chronique et annales*, ed. H. Lemaître, Paris, 1906, p. 81. Same account as Matthias von Neuenburg, p. 355: Henry is advised to return to Pisa, *ut per pedes suspensus et oculi amissione intoxicationem evaderet . . .*

370. Cited by T. Hunt, *Popular Medicine in Thirteenth Century England*, Cambridge, 1990, p. 117.

371. Pietro d'Abano, *De venenis*, chap. 4.

372. Id., chap. 3. The word "*thériaque*" is supposed to have come from the Greek word for "snake," but this is disputable.

373. Constantin Porphyrogénète, *Livre des cérémonies*, ed. J. Reiski, Bonn, 1829–1830, p. 467.

374. Richer, p. 226. *Chronicon turonense*, ed. *MGH SS*, XXVI, Hanover, 1882, p. 470.

375. *Inventaire du mobilier de Charles V*, n°342.

376. Henri de Mondeville, *Chirurgie*, pp. 692–693. Guillaume de Marra, *Sertum papale de venenis*, tells of having seen Maître Benoît de Mantoue experimenting with a pulverized herb called "tormentil" (Thorndike, *An history of Magic…*, t. 3, p. 530).

377. Jacoppo Manlio, *Luminare majus*, f. 35.

378. Symphorien Champier, *Le miroir des apothicaires*, ed. P. Dorveaux, Paris, 1894, pp. 27 and 33.

379. Anonymous fifteenth-century treatise, edited in *Pestschriften*, 1925, n°17, p. 98.

380. Pietro d'Abano, *De venenis*, last chapter.

381. Maïmonide, *Traité des poisons*, p. 54. Pietro d'Abano, *De venenis*, chap. 4 and chap. 80 for bezoar.

382. See *Chronographia regum Francorum*, ed. H. Moranvillé, Paris, 3 vol., 1891–1897, t. 1, p. 4.

383. *Questio* de Thomas de Bologne published in *Theatrum chimicum*, t. 3, p. 181 and sq.

384. Carbonelli, p. 227: *animalis dicti unicornu quod veneficatis et veneno infectis dari solitum est pro liberacione ipsorum.*

385. Grégoire de Tours, III, 31, p. 102 of Poupardin's edition. On Saint John persecuted by Domitien, *Renart le Contrefait*, t. 1, p. 347: "He crushed together toads and poison / And made him swallow them. / As soon as John made the sign of the cross / It could do him no harm" (*Boz et velin pesteler fist / Et ou cors avaler li fist. / Si tost com Jehans seigné l'avoit / Nul mal fere ne li pouoit*).

386. Alexandre Nequam, *De naturis rerum*, ed. T. Wright, Londres, 1863, II, 109, p. 190.

387. "By Saint John! You will not succeed! (*Par saint Jehan ! vous ne ferez jà bien*) Queen Blanche is supposed to have said to the Duc d'Orléans upon learning about his attempt to poison Charles VI. (Jehan Petit, *Apologie du tyrannicide*, in Monstrelet, t. 1, p. 234).

388. Guibert de Nogent, *De vita sua*, III, 18, pp. 440–442, and Jean Servion, *Gestez et croniques de la mayson de Savoye*, ed. F. Bollati, Turin, 1879, p. 196.

389. Pietro d'Abano, *De venenis…*, prologue: this type of product works *occulta virtute potius et divina quam genere vel natura.*

3

The Sociology of Poisoning

Because of trends in contemporary criminology, those who study the history of criminality show much interest in the social level of both victims and aggressors, as well as the factors that bring them together. Medieval documentation rarely offers sound information as a base for sociological statistics because it is randomly selected and fragmentary and because, in narrative sources, the authors' attention is directed mainly toward clerks and princes. Outside these two groups, it is most unlikely to find references to individuals who use poison or, more especially, who are the victims of poison. Besides, the fact that access of all levels of society to Parlement or to ***lettres de rémission*** was not guaranteed undermines the credibility of sociological use of judicial archives.[1] Finally, the sociology of *toxicatio* is totally subjective; it results from mental and cultural constructs, which are sometimes quite unrealistic. Therefore, this chapter will treat a social imaginary of criminal poison, which constructs the figures of the protagonists much more than it depicts them.

PROFILES OF THE VICTIMS OF POISONING

The social identity of the victims of criminal poison (supposed, alleged, anticipated, or real) is given in more than 80 percent of the cases. The overwhelming majority (more than 83 percent) of the crimes affect only one victim, a situation clearly less predominant than in cases of other homicides (between 60 percent and 70 percent) that occur in the majority of cases during brawls involving several individuals.[2] But, on the other hand, poison could also be used in massive crimes (5 percent of the total), which were impossible to commit with other weapons. Did victims exist who were likely to be poisoned, and what is it that propelled them toward this fate or did the crime occur randomly?

Gender and Age

Before treating the sociology of the crime, strictly speaking, of the victims of criminal poisoning, some general data must be examined, data that we will call "demographic" for the sake of convenience. First of all, did the sex of an individual increase the likelihood of being poisoned? The Comte du Mans, Gautier, and his wife Biote were indiscriminately poisoned in 1063.[3] Can it be said that the crime of poisoning touched men and women indifferently? Several factors could lead us to think not. In the thirteenth century, the *Dialogue de Placides et Timeo* supports the theory that women are naturally immunized against poison.[4] This idea could have diverted murderers of women who planned to use this method. Inversely, the adaptation of the *modus necandi* to the feminine sex is conceivable, for poison permits an economy of shameful physical aggression against a member of the weaker sex. This logic of avoiding violence is, however, highly doubtful. Membership in the feminine sex was not protection against blows or wounds. At high levels of Merovingian society, violence was not linked to the sex of the victims.[5] However, later periods abound in "beatings" and aggression against women.[6] Neither an inexistent "murderous sensitivity" nor the improbable reading of *Placide et Timeo* by poisoners protected women from poisoning or made them more vulnerable to this method of killing.

About 11 percent of the victims of poison were female while 89 percent were male. Is the disparity in these two percentages truly a reflection of criminal reality or is it due to the larger number of documents that concern men? Or is it the result of a cultural perception? If one considers only the cases known exclusively or notably from judicial sources, which are more likely to include women, the relationship between the percentages is 20 percent/80 percent. It is clear that men were the victims of poison much more often than women. But murder in general presented a much greater imbalance during the period 1380–1422: only 3 percent of the victims were women.[7] Women were more likely to die from poisoning than to be victims of street brawls or of fights in taverns, spaces more likely to be occupied by men. In any case, women were at less risk than men because there was less interest in the elimination of women, who were usually excluded from positions of power that invited rivalries and murder.

Were poisoners more likely to attack people who were weak or unimportant (because they were very young or very old), or people at their peak strength, who would be more difficult to kill with physical aggression? This question presents difficulties. On the one hand, documents rarely indicate the exact age of the victim of poison. On the other hand, age enters as much in the perception of the crime as in its execution, so that the statistics concerning the age of the victims muddles inextricably the criminal act and its perception. Of the total of countable victims of our corpus (somewhat less than 400), those who are oldest and youngest (under 15 and over 60) belong to the smallest group: about 1.5 percent each. The youngest, the dauphin of Charles VI, thought to have been poisoned in 1401 at the age of 9, and at the other end of the spectrum, a victim of advanced age (between 60 and 72) named Guiette Guillonne, are not typical.[8] Let us not believe in an anachronistic sensitivity that would spare children a bloody death from a knife in order for them to die more gently! A young age offered to the *toxicator* a chance to operate by seduction. In 1254 or 1255, Manfred intended to give to Conradin, the very young son of Conrad, poisoned candy, but the dangerous sweets did not succeed in killing him because the heir's mother Staufen, who was wise and followed the dress customs of the aristocracy, had had her child dressed just like the young nobles around him.[9] Those who wished to take the life of the 3-year-old Dauphin in 1395 counted on his childish quickness to seize an apple rolling toward him in order to kill him.[10]

Equally vulnerable to a fondness for food that can turn out to be fatal, advanced age presented other advantages. The calculation of Hugues Géraud with respect to the elderly John XXII was that a discreet poison could send him to the other world without arousing suspicion. Old age gave to impatient murderers many chances to act simply because of the frequent administration of medicines. However, we must not give too much importance to the relationship between age and the criminal act. Age was not really a factor in the choice of method.

On the other hand, age was certainly a factor in the accusation of poisoning, in particular when death or a sudden change in health afflicted people in the flower of life (this occurs in slightly less than 10 percent of the cases). Although an elevated rate of death also occurred with young adults, and especially those giving birth, many people were quick to conclude that poison had played a role in early deaths. The controversy associated with the exact age of Guiette Guillonne at her death is a good illustration of the articulation between the presumption of poisoning and the age of the victim. Those who maintained that she was poisoned insisted that she was not older than 60; those who disagreed claimed that she had reached 72, an age at which death would be expected.[11] Speaking of the death of the heir Louis de France (1276), the chronicler Guillaume Guiard generalizes: "he died from poisoning/which is often seen with those born healthy" (*fina per empoisonnement/C'on voit souvent sur les sains-nés*).[12] From Louis V to Gian Galeazzo Sforza and Charles VIII, there is a long list of princes who supposedly died from poison because they died between 20 and 30 years of age. Quick funerals increased the suspicion, as in the case of the Duchesse de Bourgogne, Michelle de France, who died in 1422. When Henry VII died at the peak of his strength at 35 years,[13] the "doctors" saw no other reason for his death than poison.[14] The illness and death at the age of 25 of the Duc de Brabant, *juvenis strenuus*, inspired loud rumors in 1430.[15] Without considering the unlikely basis of the statement in truth, the enemies of the late Louis XI, who wished to implicate him in the death of Charles de Guyenne, said that "all the doctors thought that he [Charles] would have a long life" (*extimé de tous médecins de longue vie*) implying that he had been killed by poison. These accusations seem to have had no basis in truth.[16] It is important to specify here that the conditions of age and health leading to death did not necessarily lead to the charge of poison. In 1382, the *mors subitanea* of the Count of Suffolk grieved everyone around him but instigated no investigation. This lack of inquiry concerning a sudden death is far from being the only one.[17] Nevertheless, the idea that a murderous hand is hidden behind many deaths was much more common at the end of the Middle Ages than in earlier periods when the will of God was considered a satisfactory explanation. This change in approach caused the reasons for death to be questioned much more often. Because of the lack of sufficient scientific knowledge to clear up the doubts about a given death, curious minds turned toward other sorts of explanation.

From the Emperor to the Beggar, from the Pope to the Vicar

According to a defendant in 1321, powder thrown into wells and fountains caused the death of everyone, *tam nobiles quam ignobiles*.[18] The lack of class distinction in the case of mass poisonings is obvious. But do the more common cases of poison concern uniformly all social classes or does poison cause death in only certain milieux?

After the account of the death of Benedict XI, Ferretus de Vicenza recalls incidents of great valiant princes who also were victims of poison. For him, the governing elite pay a high price to poison.[19] The literature of toxicology does not contradict this opinion. After Pietro d'Abano, Michele Savonarole observes in the fifteenth century that princes and magnates are consistently in danger of being poisoned.[20] Half of the victims of our corpus whose social class is known, including some whose class is unsure, were princes or princesses, to whom can be added nobles, knights, princely officers, the presence of whom raises the proportion of these upper classes to more than 70 percent of the individuals who suffered attempted poisoning. If the calculation is limited to the fourteenth and fifteenth centuries, a time when the sources cover the social spectrum more thoroughly, the result is even higher with more than 75 percent. Since the twelfth century, the powerful had been suffering from the weapon that was fatal to Alexander, the archetype of the powerful sovereign who was poisoned. A Bavarian chronicle from the fourteenth century emphasizes that all the kings of his time, in Bohemia as elsewhere, died by sword or by poison.[21] Out of the twenty-one kings who reigned in France from 987 to 1498, three-quarters are thought to have been exposed to poison, which permitted killing without laying a hand on "the anointed of the Lord" and thus avoiding the biblical prohibition. *L'Estoire de Eracles empereur* indicates that Richard the Lion-Hearted wanted to attack Philippe August "without laying a hand on him" (*sanz metre en lui main*).[22] But the goal of the expression may be simply to point out the cowardice of the King of England. It is doubtful that only the fact that Philippe was *rex Francorum* would lead a criminal to choose *venenatio*.[23]

It is possible that at the end of the Middle Ages, the opaqueness of the "affairs of State" was in part responsible for the increase in accusations of poison in courts and palaces.[24] Their high walls transformed them into incubators of rumors that resonated within because they did not permit those on the outside to see inside. Contemporary political reflections prefer, however, to emphasize another point. Jean Martin de Ferrara explained to the Master of Milan François Sforza that the threat of poison constituted one of the bondages that result from power.[25] Poggio suggests that the prospect of being poisoned caused, among other reasons, the "unhappiness of princes" because it kept them from enjoying the pleasures of life.[26] The example of Charles VII, reputed to have lost interest in eating out of fear of being poisoned, supports this suggestion.[27] And this fear extended to the entire princely entourage. Rhetoric that criticizes court life at the end of the fourteenth century does not exclude poison. The *Franc Gontier* by Philippe de Vitry maintains that it is more comfortable to live in the countryside than as a courtesan permanently exposed to poison served in a golden dish.[28]

A cultural construction as much as a criminal reality, the princely victim of poison prevails mostly in documents and in minds. About 1398, Honorat Bovet exclaims with exasperation: "Ignorant people claim that a prince has no illness that is not caused by treason, witchcraft, or poison" (*L'ygnorant gens prent tel propos/C'un prince n'aye maladie/... Si ce ne vient par traïson/Par sorcerie ou poison*).[29] "Foolish opinion from a simple imagination" (*Fole oppinion, simple ymagination*) from all eras,[30] certainly, but accentuated at a time when princely power took on such an importance that the prince's death created a vacuum filled only by discourse.

Dedicating his work to a pope, Pietro d'Abano naturally adds prelates to the number of frequent victims of criminal poisoning. The members of the high clergy supposedly poisoned are numerous through the twelfth century. One poisoned ecclesiastic out of two of our corpus belongs to the period 500–1200, when the documentation favors pontiffs and abbots. However, we must guard against optical illusions. Nearly half of the papal poison victims belong to the eleventh century, not after a renewed outbreak of *veneficium* against the head of the Church—Pierre Damien does not indicate any such situation in his minor work on the longevity of the successors of Saint Peter[31]—because anti-Gregorian propaganda attributes to Gregory VII the murder of many of his predecessors.

The Church lacks an archetypical figure of a poisoned pontiff. There is no Alexander wearing a tiara. This supposition applies less to abbots and even bishops. Victims from the Church account for nearly 11 percent of the total of the countable victims, spread equally on both sides of the year 1200, which makes the poisoned prelate a figure of the early Middle Ages. The story of Saint Benedict facing the persecutions of his monks and of a jealous priest plays an important role in the allegation of the poisoning of abbots during later centuries. The *Vita* of Saint Samson composed in the middle of the eighth century is much influenced by this model in its report of the misfortunes of the future bishop of Dol.[32] Without linking everything to common places and to archetypes, it can be assumed that the unexpected or early death of the head of a monastic community or diocese[33] recalled to the recording clerk or the historians the memory of Benoît de Nursie, whom Alvaro Pelayo uses, at the beginning of the fourteenth century, as the best example of an abbot exposed to the malice of his monks.[34] When poison appears, the founder of Western monasticism sometimes follows in its wake.[35] Somewhat distant from the hagiographic model, the prelate who dies brutally gives rise to the evocation of poison. The Patriarch Etienne of Jerusalem in 1130, the Archbishop of York in 1154, or the Bishop of Valence in 1239 all died from a *mors inopinata* that led to allegations of poisoning.[36] Such allegations were sometimes made because of a similarity to a preceding death or to a general narrative pattern. Guillaume de Tyr was declared to have died from poison by an author who was thinking about the fate of the Patriarch Raoul of Antioch, who died in 1141.[37] Guillaume de Nangis wrote that the Archbishop of Tours Geoffroi de Lande died from poison after two years of prelacy because he (Guillaume) read the *Chronique de Tours* too quickly and interpreted it to say that the prelate was poisoned, when in fact the chronicle speaks of poison only in a figurative sense, the poison of counselors with bad intentions.[38]

Legal texts were certainly little influenced by literary reminiscences. The Bishop of Amiens seems to have really been the target of poisoners (1281),[39] just like the Cistercian abbots and priors whose documents from the general chapters have conserved a record. From 1150 to 1200 on, what exposed the prelate was no longer so much his spiritual intransigence, which condemned ungodliness, or the laxity of his enemies but the possession of worldly goods, even if an Italian canon reflected that in 1379 people like him were particularly exposed to malicious traps because of the fact that their role was so little supported by the guardians of morality.[40] Ambroise Paré makes the following observation at the end of the sixteenth century, but his comment can be applied perfectly to earlier centuries: "prelates and the privileged are often poisoned by those who desire their wealth" ([poison] *souvent advient aux prelats et beneficiers pour avoir leur despoüille*).[41]

However, this theme does not take into account the use of poison as a weapon of death. Could one think that prelates would be more protected from bloody and violent crimes because of the proximity of their entourage, and therefore more vulnerable to murder committed without blood and blows? The story of the life of John VIII, ending with massive blows after his being given too little poison to be effective (at the end of the ninth century) makes us sceptical.[42] In any case, at the time of the Gregorian reform, the poisoning of a priest of the Beauvais region related by Guibert de Nogent resulted from a possible disgust with the use of open violence against a man of the Church.[43] Nevertheless, even if illicit, brutality is not reduced during the successive centuries. The canons of the councils consider an attempt against the life of a clerk only in respect to physical blows. Nothing suggests that a clerk might fall victim to poison.

Contrary to what he believes, Franc Gontier secluded in his forest is not safer than the King of France in his palaces. Outside the world of clerks and courts, poison also found victims. Even if the majority of individuals with no historical identity in the written sources remain anonymous because of their modest social rank, the number of ordinary people affected by poison increased by a little more than 17 percent and this kind of victim is seen especially in the fourteenth and fifteenth centuries. The judicial sources of this era focus on humble victims of modest social rank, peasants, artisans, or even bourgeois. In four cases out of seven, trials or ***lettres de rémission*** mention cases of poisoning or attempted poisoning that involve the common people of both town and country.

Sociological consensus concerning victims of poison (real or alleged) informs as much about the sociological perception as about the victims themselves. Legal documents correct this perspective and show that individuals targeted for poisoning came from all levels of society.[44] Vulnerability was general. When victims are considered without reference to their social rank, it is clear that the weapon of poison equalized social levels and its capacity to kill masses of people pushed this observation to its limit. John XXII wrote in 1317 that the exposure of the highest ranked Christian prelate to the danger of poison proves that no one can escape.[45] Probably in all social milieux, certain criminal strategies selected the weapon according to the targeted individual. But, far from being the decision of the murderers, this selection occurred often through the accounts that tell about the crime, even in some cases creating the crime. Is this also the case for poisoners?

THE FACES OF THE POISONERS

As is the case with the victims, the faces of those who murder with poison are hard to picture. Nearly 10 percent of them are totally unknown. Often, rumors leave only the vaguest notion of the murderer. The sociological coverage of the sources and the interweaving of facts and ramblings considerably blur the face of the presumed guilty party. It is more productive to consult the sociology of criminal descriptions than criminal sociology to look for the perpetrators of this crime.

A Shared Crime

Because of Latin classical literature or the novels of Alexandre Dumas, one of the accepted ideas about the crime of poisoning is that it is committed in the "warm greenhouse atmosphere" of the courts.[46] Poison would be an aristocratic weapon, elegant and muffled, the opposite of the uncalculated brutality of the peasants.[47] This perception, which is that of *Franc Gontier*, espouses the statements of Bernard de la Roche, the man implicated in a nasty affair in which he tried to exonerate himself by arguing precisely that the fact that he was a simple, country fellow made him incapable of such an act (1395).[48] Let us look at this subject more closely.

Princes and monarchs are implicated in 40 percent of the cases in our collection, and half of them occurred during the last two centuries of the Middle Ages. Of course, the poisoners of high social rank were almost exclusively the plotters. Fewer than 2 percent of those who carried out the plan came from their rank, such as the son of Gaston Phoebus.[49] Some figures stand out because of their reputation with poison, from William the Conqueror to Louis XI, with Charles the Bad (*le Mauvais*) at the head of the class. The status of the most highly placed must not, however, plunge the more ordinary players into the shadow. Norman chivalry, as depicted by Orderic Vital, indulged enthusiastically in poisoning. The chronicles like the judicial texts of the end of the Middle Ages identify many knights or squires as poisoners such as Lord D'Ormoy (1308),[50] Squire Regnaut de Fissericourt (in the 1340s),[51] and the knight Robert Gui (1358).[52] In 1404, the defenders of Pierre de Cuisel also known as Chevrier claimed that his status as squire proved that he was incapable of the murder of Guiette Guillonne.[53] But the argument is not linked as much to *modus necandi* as it is to murder as such, which is considered unthinkable for a soldier in service to the king.

High-level servers to powerful figures were implicated in many cases of poisoning during the last centuries of the Middle Ages, from the chamberlain Pierre de la Broce under Philippe III, to the president of the **Chambre des Comptes** in Savoie (1354), Pierre Gerbais, or to this Jehan Coustain, chamberlain of Philippe the Good accused in 1462. Poison is not a surprising weapon for these upstarts because of its horrible connotation, so foreign to the values that the aristocrats prided themselves on possessing exclusively.[54] A vile weapon for a vile person. Membership in the world of government, high or low, did not impede the use of poison, even when the functions carried out should have instructed the murderer on the consequences of the act. A Provost of Compiègne becomes involved in a case of poisoning (1354);[55] Juvénal des Ursins reports an unusually sensational case of a prosecutor of the king, executed in 1402 for having poisoned one of his colleagues.[56]

Well before Molière, doctors had a reputation for poisoning their patients, accidentally or deliberately.[57] In 1415, Antoine Didmaire asked for an inquest concerning the illness of his mistress, the Duchesse de Brabant, in order that he not be held responsible in any way.[58] This example of taking such an initiative demonstrates the overexposure of the medical profession to implication in the crime of poison. A relatively high number of accusations were made against princes as the instigator or the one who carried out *venenationes*. The Patriarch of Jerusalem appointed a special "doctor" to attend Guillaume de Tyr, so that he could kill him with the cover of caring for him (1187).[59] Charles the Bad (*le Mauvais*) counted on the interest in medicine of Charles V, who was ill but maintained his intellectual curiosity, to ease the acceptance of the "doctor" Angel, "a very great and subtile clerk [who] spoke Latin beautifully and enjoyed a good discussion" (*tres grant clerc et subtil* [qui] *parloit bel latin, estoit moult argumentatif*).[60] The avid search by the powerful for better health opened the door to dangerous healers, who promised the princes less suffering, better-looking hair, and many heirs.[61] A failure in treatment of the sick was probably perceived more frequently at the end of the Middle Ages as the result of a deliberate criminal act. This suspicion was nourished by jealousies among the noble houses. Richer de Saint-Remi tells about two specialists who were probably rivals in the service of the Carolingian King Louis IV about 940 and who poisoned each other.[62] In the fourteenth and fifteenth centuries, if the favor of the prince was inversely proportional to the academic baggage of the healer, the least misstep led to accusations and slander. Thus, the doctors of the house of Savoie unleashed their fury against Jean de Grandville, who found favor too quickly with Amédée VII de Savoie, when because of his unknown origins and suspicious degrees, he had been forbidden to practice in Montpelier.[63] If one continues to descend the social ladder, while staying within the courts, the cases of poisoning do not become rarer. Charles the Bad (*le Mauvais*) understood quickly how he could turn to his advantage the role of Robert Wourdreton, the valet of one of his courtiers who was often present in the chateaux and their kitchens.[64]

Less important people are, of course, well represented among the poisoners. In about a quarter of the crimes committed by individuals whose social class can be determined, the act of murder was or was supposed to be committed by recruits of humble origin with the promise that they would be able to escape their unhappy status. The well poisoners of 1390 correspond to this profile of men without land and "sitting and begging" (*seans a* [et] *querant leur vie*).[65] But poisoning did not occur only as a result of directions from higher up. About a quarter of the cases (a great majority of those in the fourteenth and fifteenth centuries) involved criminals from the common people. Guibert de Nogent points out the case of a poisoner whom he identifies as *rusticus*.[66] The criminal acts recorded by Parlement such as the ***lettres de rémission*** and the witchcraft trials involved numerous artisans, peasants, and other tradesmen who use poison as a weapon as much in town as in the country. The servant woman from Manosque, the peasant from Arras, the money changer from Toulouse, the wife of the barrel-maker in La Rochelle, the wife of a carder from Carcasonne, a chambermaid from Agen, a lawyer from Illiers, a cobbler from Freiburg, a ladykiller from the area of Lake Geneva, a wine grower from Lorraine, the wife of a pastry maker in Roye—all used poison. A surprising case, but not unique, is presented by an executioner, who was accused of having put poisonous powder in drinking water in Normandy.[67] To these individuals must be added the bonesetters or the healers whose talents and powers raised many suspicions after 1300 because of their lack of academic training.[68] Poison was not foreign to the common people; it was a weapon shared by many.

A Favorite Activity of Clerks?

In his treatise entitled *De Planctu ecclesie*, the Portuguese prelate Alvaro Pelayo (who died in 1349) mentions rapidly the giving of poison to someone else among the crimes that prevent their perpetrators from taking orders.[69] In 1337, men "wearing religious clothing" (*en habit de religion*) and with poisonous intentions presented themselves at the court of Philippe VI.[70] In 1350, the inhabitants of Rostock were persuaded that individuals dressed like ecclesiastics were *seminatores venenorum*.[71] These examples raise the question whether a particular link existed between the clergy and the crime of poisoning.

The Church's horror of blood as well as the fact that the ecclesiastics were forbidden to carry arms could have made them prefer weapons that did not make blood flow. The clerks' knowledge of plants (monks who were herbalists and apothecaries) and more generally their information on "the properties of things" could have made them expert users of toxic substances. However, the correlation between the clergy and the use of poison is very uncertain. The impossibility of open violence and the aversion to blood did not prevent the documents of Cluny and Cistercians chapters from including numerous fights with knives that the secular clerks also knew how to use.[72] At the beginning of the fifteenth century, the canon who had taken charge of the Clunisian priory of Bellevaux-en-Bauges distributed more mortal blows than violent poisons.[73] Abélard's bad monks, at Saint-Gildas-de-Rhuys, did not hesitate to convert to the sword when their poisons failed.[74] Two centuries later, the religious of the priory of Saint-Michel-de-Cruilles resorted to the sword instead of **realgar**.[75] The reasons for a clerk to prefer poison are not so obvious. And is this a marked preference?

In about 17 percent of the cases, about which there is enough information to judge, poisoners were associated with the Church. For a small portion of the crimes (13 percent), they only carried out the deed. No category of the clergy is excluded. According to Franc Vouloir, the *Le Champion des dames*, and the theories of the councils invented by Martin le Franc, "several popes truly covered their poison with honey" (*plusieurs papes vraiement/Soubx miel ont couvert leur venin*).[76] At the very top of the Church, the use of *toxicatio* appears to be linked to the closed character of ecclesiastic affairs. At the time of the conclaves, the most closed off places in the Church, poison could remove from the ballot a candidate judged to be too dangerous. The Cardinal Robert de Sumercot certainly suffered from the jealousy of the other cardinals who were worried about his distinguished qualities (1241).[77] After the conclaves, poison served to hasten the reunion of another conclave. The unfounded rumor about the poisoning of Alexander V in 1410, after a reign of only one year, implicated his successor John XXIII.[78] About 1500, Alexander VI incarnated the symbolic figure of the scandalous pontiff who was a poisoner.[79]

Members of the high clergy were implicated in cases involving poison beginning in the twelfth century, and the beginning of the fourteenth century was marked by an accumulation of accusations against bishops who had the reputation of being poisoners and witches such as Guichard de Troyes, Pierre de Latilly, or Hugues Géraud. Abbots and priors were suspected less often.[80] In total numbers, the princes of the Church do not form a large group of poisoners, neither do the members of the low clergy. In 1460, a priest of the Soissonnais region financed a murder that was carried out with a combination of poison and magic.[81] But the crime of poison cannot be considered an ecclesiastical crime. If *ecclesia non abhorret a veneno*, the homicidal clergyman had many other weapons at his disposal and normally the clergy did not hesitate to use them.

An Affair of Women?

In Roman antiquity, poisoning was considered a crime greatly valued by women.[82] In 1595, Condrochi considers that for one *veneficus*, one finds fifty *veneficae*.[83] It would be surprising if there were a gap between these two eras. An idea popular with historians of poison and inspired by the criminology of the nineteenth and twentieth centuries links the claimed predominance of female poisoners to the *imbecillitas sexus*, judged unable to use force, and to feminine psychology that finds women to be underhanded, deceitful, and sensitive, in the tradition of a misogyny that has lasted for millennia and is almost universal.[84] But the historians of today do not believe in the existence of a criminality that is specifically feminine, in Merovingian times or in the fourteenth and fifteenth centuries.[85] Women did not shy away from violence: dozens of ***lettres de rémission*** as well as archives from the English courts demonstrate this fact clearly.[86] One must distinguish between factual data and representations of the facts.

An entire cultural heritage encouraged the male of the Middle Ages to attribute to women a proclivity for poisoning.[87] Roman history supplies examples known by Gautier Map or Boccacio.[88] The Bible associates the first woman with poison. Orderic Vital cannot keep from pointing out the parallel between the poison of Sichelgaïte and the malice of Eve,[89] whose error Hildegarde of Bingen considers the origin of the appearance of poison on the earth.[90] For the Norman monk, poisoning illustrates the *feminea fraus*, the opposite of chivalric virtue, by a male definition.[91] The claimed toxicity of menstrual blood is the natural translation of the poisonous essence of the woman whose seductive activity poisons man literally and figuratively: this is the moral lesson to learn from the story of the poisonous virgin.[92] Her knowledge of the secrets of nature as well as her fragility that exposes her more than man to the temptations of the "Enemy" appears to lead her fatally to the use of poison. The toxic malice of the feminine sex is a widespread theme, both literal and metaphorical. The clerks were obviously the first to exploit it. Burchard of Worms invited pastors to track especially the use of dangerous herbs[93] or harmful substances such as menstrual blood.[94] In his *Livre des manières*, certainly addressed to a woman, the Countess of Hereford, the Bishop of Rennes Etienne de Fougères condemns witches, abortionists, and poisoners (twelfth century)[95] and this misogyny continues into the fourteenth and fifteenth centuries in the writings of theoreticians and preachers such as Alvaro Pelayo, Antonin de Florence, Bernardin de Siena, or Jean Raulin.[96] The quarrel of the women that troubled Western culture beginning with the *Roman de la Rose* does not ignore feminine *venenositas*. Jean de Meun, the main instigator of the misogynous camp, affirms that the nature of woman commands it to do the worst, in particular to have recourse to poison, charms, and "enchantments" among other works of the devil (*granz deablies*).[97] This is their trade: lying, betraying, and poisoning people (*Ceo est lur mestier/Mentir, trahir et gent enpoisoner*) exclaims the author of *Blasme des fames* at approximately the same time.[98] In the *Champion des Dames* by Martin le Franc, Lourd Entendement (Heavy Intellect) criticizes the tendency of the weaker sex to use poison, eventually delivered on the Sabbath. "Beware her betrayals/Either from a hammer or from poison,"

(*Garde toy de ses trahisons/Ou de cuignie ou de poisons*) he hurls at the speaker before adding: "She has neither forgiveness nor mercy/For she can throw her black venom or bitter poison/here or there/like a spiteful snake" (*Elle n'a pardon ne mercy/Car se peut par là ou par cy/Comme une despiteuse wuivre/Jettera son venin noircy*...ou *le poison amere*).[99] By exalting Circe and Medea, even Christine de Pizan validates the link that exists between femininity and the knowledge of poisons, when she exalts the potential of feminine genius, which many authors had condemned.[100]

Produced by men and often clerks, the factual sources are obviously impregnated by the culture of misogyny. In our collection, murder by poison is exclusively feminine in slightly more than 18 percent of the cases, masculine in 75 percent, and shared in somewhat less than 7 percent. In one-fourth of the total cases, one or more women are participants in *toxicatio*. This figure is close to the 20 to 22 percent of the women implicated in English crime in the first half of the fourteenth century and in the crimes in Lyon of the fifteenth century (all crime mixed together)[101] but very far from the 1 percent calculated by C. Gauvard for crime in general.[102] Poisoning then seems to involve more women than other crimes. Killing with poison involves such creatures as Willemine la Barbière, "handicapped by her body" (*debilitée de son corps*), according to the ***lettre de remission*** written on her behalf (1459).[103] Qualitatively, some cases present a high degree of feminization. In 1382, a certain Gilette joined with two other women, Margueritte and Jehanette, to carry out her crime.[104] An act of Parlement of 1382 unites three women in a somber case of the same sort: a witch, Jeanne Sauverelle, gave a potion to a woman through an intermediary named Arzent.[105] A ***lettre de rémission*** of 1469 puts a mother and daughter together in a poisonous plot.[106] Telling her troubles to an unknown woman whom she met on the steps of a church where she was crying, Gillon Honoré received good advice on improving her lot (1501).[107] *Toxicatio* was firmly grounded in the networks of feminine sociability and solidarity.

The implication of women in cases of poisoning must be viewed with the understanding that they are not necessarily acting alone. In the France of Charles VI or in England in the fourteenth century, a male accomplice usually helped the woman in the crime, in a society where women usually didn't take the initiative.[108] The services of a woman were necessary when the plot involved the seduction of an enemy. A *venefica* acted for the Robert, a Norman cadet, against Richard III;[109] Frederick II sent a *meretrix* to the Duke of Lorraine (1220), who was poisoned by wine "by means of her flirtatious words and flattery" (*en ses cajoleries et blandicies*).[110] Innocent or pious appearances often facilitated the execution of a criminal deed. The death of Benedict XI is sometimes attributed to a woman disguised as a nun who was working for unknown plotters; a beguine from

Metz lent her services to the enemies of Charles de Valois.[111] The statistics that we have, however, indicate that the majority of female poisoners worked alone. They were four times less likely to work in collaboration with a man than alone, and they sometimes used someone else to execute a crime that they had conceived. In 1493, Jenette tried twice to kill someone by herself, before asking her nailsmith lover to get her a third poison that she hoped would be more effective.[112] Masculine intervention occurred when the murderess did not have all that she needed to commit the act: thus Hawis Brunet sent her brother to get poison at Saint-Nicolas-du-Port (1491).[113] Still it would be erroneous to think that a man had to purchase the arsenic or **realgar**.[114]

In the imaginary world of chivalry, Queen Guinevere incarnates the poisonous princess. Guinevere is the "*wuivre*," or *vouivre*, a name taken from "*vipère*" (snake).[115] This figure certainly deserves special attention because she crops up frequently, from the famous Rosamund to Valentine Visconti and Jacqueline de Brabant. She is found in about 10 percent of the cases, of which a third occur before the year 1000. From the early Middle Ages, the figure of the princess accused of poisoning appears with a certain regularity in the Breton or Lombard courts.[116] From the ninth to the fourteenth century, there was no scarcity of royal women accused of poisoning others or causing others to be poisoned. Considering only the kingdom of France, from Emma, Lothaire's wife, to Jeanne de Bourgogne, Philippe VI's spouse, at least one queen per century left rumors of poison in her wake. In the Germanic empire, the Duchess of Austria was wrongfully accused of having killed Louis de Bavaria. Her flight on horseback after an encounter with the sovereign confirmed her guilt.[117] The weapon associated with banquets and steam rooms, poison played a role in the atmosphere of the palace where the princess was part of the entourage before the appearance of separate quarters for the royal couple. With responsibility for the meals and the physical comforts of the court, the queen had every chance to utilize this nourishing role as a means to cause harm.[118] And this negative power was attributed to her all the more when she was a foreigner. Rosamund was the daughter of the King of Gépides. Brunehaut came from the Visigoths of Spain. Eadburh, the Queen of Wessex, was the daughter of the King of Mercia. Sichelguaïte was from Apulia while the first wife of Robert Guiscard was Norman. The Belgian origin (she came from Brabant) of the second wife of Philippe III was enough to cause her to be accused of the death of Louis de France in 1276. Of Hungarian origin, Queen Cunégonde of Bohemia suffered the same outrage at the time of the illness of Wenceslas II.[119] Because she was from an unknown culture and spoke an incomprehensible language, the presence of a foreign queen nourished suspicion that increased as national monarchies were formed.[120]

Comparatively, as crimes are divided according to the sex of the perpetrator, the feminine presence among those accused of poisoning is noticeable. Nevertheless, it remains in the minority. More than witchcraft, *venenatio* is mostly a masculine crime. It is difficult to correlate the practice of poisoning with the sex of the perpetrator. What is certain is that the tasks normally assigned to women in medieval society put them in contact with food, clothing, or bodies, thus giving them the perfect opportunities and access to the targets of poison. At the same time, domestic functions facilitated the poisoner's act; the implication of women was founded on a long-term cultural tradition. Inversely, men, who were not involved with these activities, in theory, had nothing to do with poison. One of the protagonists of a story in the *Heptameron* of Marguerite of Navarre is surprised that the president of the Parlement of Grenoble poisoned his unfaithful wife: that was not supposed to be a male crime.[121]

A Crime of the Other

Still less than for any other crime, it is hard to relegate poisoning to the fringes of society. The role of the miserable wretches of the criminal register of the Châtelet, who are only the underlings, must not be exaggerated, neither must the role of the shepherds implicated in 1335 and on whom a solitary way of life favorable to sin and the knowledge of the secrets of nature easily cast suspicion.[122] Perfectly integrated into society, the poisoner was not an individual at odds with his culture who awaited his victim in the dark of the woods. In any case, in particular, starting with the twelfth century, documents attribute the use of *venenum* to individuals more or less foreign to the community. Without considering objective reality, the dominant discourse draws the face of the poisoner with the traits of the other, those of the pagan, the Infidel, the foreigner, and those on the fringes.

J. Chiffoleau observes: "Those guilty of crimes against nature, such as heretics, always come from the East."[123] The same profile exists for poisoning. As the depositaries of *scientia venenorum*, the Infidels were reputed to apply it without restraint. Pietro d'Abano clearly locates *in partibus orientalibus et meridionalibus* the historic and geographical origin of the crime of poison.[124] Eustache Deschamps repeats in the *envoi* of his *Ballade des empoisonneurs*: "Such beverages are served in the Orient" (*En Orient servent tels beuvrages*). The women of Acre who eliminated their husbands according to a long tradition, the sultans who poisoned each other maliciously[125] are examples of the criminal toxicity of Islam to which corresponds, of course, the pernicious character of its doctrine. It is not surprising that the Christians who had lived in contact with the Muslims were reputed to having adopted their poisonous ways. Melisande, the Queen of Jerusalem, is reputed to have killed the Comte de Saint-Gilles with a poisoned drink in Caesarea in Palestine (1148).[126] The documents that report the affair involving Jean de Grandville, who was born in Bohemia, emphasize his stay *in patria Serrazenorum vel Grecie.*[127] But the poisonous enemy lurked also in the heart of the West. The Saracen population that had lived under the rule of the Christians conserved its poisonous heredity. The Muslim baker of the Calabrian monastery that Orderic Vital mentions belonged to the lineage of Ishmael, the persecutor of Isaac.[128] In Spain after the reconquest, the Moors were from time to time suspected of using poison.[129] Other Eastern peoples were afflicted with the same generic vice.

An anonymous story from the third crusade indicates that a city near Andrinople owed a tribute of poison to the *basileus.*[130] This detail places poison at the very heart of the Byzantine administrative system. As early as the tenth century, Greece inspired mistrust. In the story of his turbulent legation in Byzantium, where he thought he was going to die from the food and drinks, Liutprand de Cremona recalls the verses of Virgil on the traps of the "Danaäns" and depicts the Greek emperor as a man full of lies and tricks.[131] A century and a half later, Bohémond was aware of this reputation when he refused all food.[132] In his *Directorium ad passagium faciendum* written for Philippe VI in 1332, the German preacher Brocardus summarizes the "general character of all the nations of the East: you must avoid then, my lord king, all enemies in your breast and you do not nourish any scorpion or serpent in your bosom" (*generale proprieté de touttes les nations d'Orient: Sy vous gardé doncques, mon souverain seigneur . . . , que vous n'ayez nul ennemy en vostre pis et que vour ne nourrissiez nul escorpion ou serpent en vostre giron*). The metaphors of the bestiary speak for themselves.[133] Heretic or infidel, the Oriental is a born poisoner. Rome was already divided between fascination and suspicion with regard to a world personified by Mithridates. In the medieval Occident, religious alterity and military confrontation came to emphasize the trait.

Geographic boundaries were not limited to the distant Orient. *La Ballade des empoisonneurs* mentions also neighboring Christian countries: "In Spain, Calabria and Aragon/Cyprus et Pouille, in Romania and Sezille they often serve/the good mouthful [poison]" (*En Espaigne, Calabre et Arragon,/Chippre et Puille, en Romayne font prendre,/En Sezille souvent le bon bouquon. . . .*) A little further on, Eustache Deschamps evokes the Lombards and their "doubtful drink."[134]

Long before the words of the poet from Champagne, this Italian association with poison demands an explanation. The reasons for it are notably the cultural presence of the Muslims in the south of the peninsula and the bad health conditions that caused deaths that could easily be blamed on poison. In the eleventh century, Italy had the reputation of being the location of the poisoned tombs of the emperors[135] and several episodes during the following centuries reinforced this idea in the minds of the Germanic people. The death of Henry VI, the destiny of Henry VII, who died *in terra latina*, the misadventures of Charles of Luxembourg on the other side of the Alps and of Sigismond illustrate the poisonous nature of the Italian inhabitants of the peninsulas.[136] The poisonings of Robert Guiscard and of his son at the instigation of a princess from Benevento, the death of French-born Robert de Bourgogne because of Adèle de Pouille, the crimes directed against Norman clerks by Roman and Florentine monks were reasons to believe along with Orderic Vital that the people on the other side of the mountains were dangerous.[137] In the thirteenth century, Italians from the south of the country continued to be considered frightening. Matthieu Paris explains that the English pretender to the throne of Sicily was very fearful that the people of the region would poison him as was their custom.[138] Starting with the beginning of the fourteenth century, perhaps because of the intrigues of the Visconti family whose coat-of-arms bore a serpent,[139] perhaps because of imperial misadventures in the north of Italy, perhaps even because of their predominance in the universe of the apothecary business, the "Lombards" appear to have had the reputation of being dangerous poisoners. Chroniclers from Savoie tell about traps set by the Lord of Milan for the troops of Amédée VI.[140] The Religious of Saint-Denis wrote that in Lombardy, poisons and enchantments were used more than elsewhere and that the use of poison was common.[141] Bernard de la Roche, who was tortured in 1395, heard the following suggested testimony from the torturer: "You come from Lombardie and the Comte de Vertux gave you these poisons to poison the king, my lord of Savoy and several other lords" (*Tu viens de Lombardie et t'a baillié ces poisons le conte de Vertux pour empoisonner le roy, monsegneur de Savoye et plusieurs aultres seigneurs*).[142] The scenario appears ordinary and serves as an alibi to cover other criminals. It is known that the fact that Valentine Visconti came from Milan served as reason enough for her to be accused of poisonings.[143] At the end of the fifteenth century, when the activity of the Lombards was still strong,[144] the Venetians and the Tuscans joined them. In a work that was certainly polemical, Jean Lemaire de Belges condemned Venice in particular.[145] On a more global level, the French people, cry out for the benefit of the Italian people, in the *Jeu du Prince des sots* by Pierre Gringore (1506): "Everyone has noticed your behavior/You give poison instead of good spices, against the law" (*Chascun a de ton cas notice:/Poison, en lieu de bonne espice,/Tu bailles, offensant la loy*).[146] Thus, it was not Cathérine de Médicis who was the source of the reputation of Italians as poisoners. One could say that she carried on an old tradition.

Other neighbors of France do not enjoy such a distinct reputation. Capetian Navarre cannot be considered foreign and the Iberian kingdoms, despite what Deschamps says about the people of Spain, cannot be taken as protectors of masses of poisoners, except for the Jewish and Infidel minorities. *Toxicatio* was not generically Iberian. Neither was it British. Although, about 1300, a farce presented the English *scorpionibus similes*,[147] the French sources did not point out any English propensity for poisoning. The German origin of the presumed poisoner of Michelle de France contributed to arousing the people in the streets of Ghent against her in 1422,[148] but she was not generically a synonym of poisoning. This form of murder was decidedly linked to the shores of the Mediterranean, there where the mores of the infidel propagated.

In the heart of the kingdoms and principalities of the West and also outside the normal social structure, there existed two groups reportedly given to the crime of poisoning because they carried inherently a spiritual or natural toxicity. One of these groups is known to have been involved in only one incident, but one with very serious consequences: these are the lepers. The second group, on the other hand, was the object of recurring accusations as early as the eleventh century and these accusations reached their highest point in 1348: the Jews.

Before 1321, lepers were already considered carriers of poison, the poison that caused their illness. According to the poet Gautier de Coincy, "Poison flows out of them/From every part below their face" (*Li venins li sort et degote/De tote part aval lou vis*).[149] Leprosy acts in them like a poison that corrupts the flesh and it gives to their breath an "evil aroma" (*fumet malin*) caused by the fearful power of contagion, explaining their necessary separation from the world. In the thirteenth century, the wells in Amiens were forbidden to lepers because of the strong belief that they could contaminate the water.[150] The perceived malice of the lepers has already been mentioned: the traitor Béranger of *Parise la Duchesse* (about 1225) is said to have learned the art of poison from an old leper who had withdrawn into a monastery in Ravenna.[151] The episode of 1321 transformed this natural toxicity into criminal toxicity. According to the late translation (end of the fifteenth century) of a chronicle from Rouen contemporary to the incident, the drama stemmed from the frequenting of the common wells by the lepers, who were suspected of wanting to contaminate them with their illness.[152] This incident remained inscribed in the memories of the people in 1348 when an act of Philippe VI refers to it,[153] and its reverberations carried on much longer. Certain chroniclers at the end of the fifteenth century still call lepers the poisoners of 1390 in whom they incorrectly see the offenders of 1321.[154] The strong relationship established between the mass poisoning of water and lepers caused a long-lived misconception. At the same time, another misconception was in full bloom.

In 1422, Martin V forbad that Jews be called well-poisoners, an attribution in the process of being substituted for the long-term label of godkillers.[155] This act says much about the deep-seated reputation of the Elected People as poisoners. This act came at the beginning of a terrible century. In mid-June 1321, a leper being interrogated in Parthenay had denounced Jews as being the source of the plot.[156] Thought to be immune to leprosy, or to the contrary, being accused of the illness's introduction into the West,[157] the Jews appear in a certain number of documents as the intermediaries between the Muslim sources and the lepers who carried out the plot.[158] In 1348, the same charge was reiterated, but the lepers were not in the foreground. Globally, the Black Death appears to be the supreme manifestation of the harmfulness of the Jews. However, the treatises on the plague invalidate their guilt and numerous chroniclers express serious doubts about their involvement.[159] But the accusation persisted. The Jews who were dependent on the crown of Aragon asked the pope in 1354 for an official exoneration.[160]

The accusation against the Jews as the cause of the plague was linked to the toxicity attributed to the *filii venenati judaei* (Matthew, chapter 3) by a long Christian tradition.[161] Spiritual poison, denounced by Burchard of Worms[162] and numerous other preachers, ended up becoming a natural and criminal poisonous reputation shared with the Muslims, whose status, let us remember, was clarified at the same time as that of the Jews at the Council of Lateran IV. The Jews' poison, sometimes associated with the scorpion,[163] had at its origin a metaphorical meaning[164] that went back to Judas's betrayal of Christ. A poem by Walter de Wimborne from the middle of the thirteenth century relates how the poison that was emitted from the traitor's hanged corpse infected all of Judea.[165] The moral impurity, sometimes compared to an interior leprosy,[166] contaminated Jews' bodies, which were also impure, because they were nourished and watered by things not consumed by Christians. Starting in the twelfth century, canonical texts warn the faithful against naturally harmful contact with Jews.[167] Baths and steam rooms for the two groups were separate.[168] And this segregation only increased in the following centuries, as shown by numerous documents from Provence and Languedoc.[169] This segregation served to increase the fantasy, according to a well-known mental mechanism.[170] The exclusion of the Jews from the world of fighters probably supported the idea that they could use only disloyal weapons.[171] The Jews of Nuremberg were accused of poisoning Christians already in 1096.[172] Canon 18 of the Council of Vienna (Austria) of 1267 forbids the faithful to have any interaction with Jews for fear of poisoning.[173] Conversion did not make the danger disappear. A poisonous hatred based on the reputation of the Jews surrounded the relapsed Jean de Bari brought to court in 1443; a converted Jew of Halle was suspected of having poisoned citizens of the city (1515).[174] Exclusion went well with poison. It is noteworthy that if the Muslim culture also considered Jews as fearful poisoners responsible for a trap set for the Prophet and for the death of the first Caliph,[175] it never implied that all relationships with the sons of Isaac exposed the descendents of Ishmael to their poison.

Between criminal reality and social imagination, the poisoner thus possessed a dual profile. From the village yokel to the king, from the pontiff to the subdeacon, poisoning covered the whole social spectrum. This crime could unite in a criminal alliance individuals at the top and at the bottom of society.[176] But the discourse and the representations attribute the use of poison to a few groups characterized in one way or another by alterity: of sex, of religion, of body, or of country. The weight of these parameters varied according to the locality. In the Aragon of 1321, the threat of poisoning was more clearly directed toward foreigners (Gênois of Barcelona, for example) than toward Jews or Muslims, who benefited, at least in theory, from the protection of authorities.[177] The imaginary poisoner is quite different from the banal person revealed by the extant sources. This is indeed a sign that this crime is not trivial.

THE CRIME OF POISONING IN THE WORLD OF RELATIONSHIPS

Up to this point, the poisoned and the poisoners have been considered separately. Now, the two groups will be put together in order to see how the crime of poison operates in social relationships. It is not our purpose to outline here the motives of the criminals but to understand what sorts of social links criminal poisoning involved. Burchard of Worms recommends that a priest ask a parishioner if he made a fatal potion to poison "another."[178] The relationship of this "other" to the poisoner is the issue to now explore.

Murder within the Family

A recent study on China in the eighteenth and nineteenth centuries entitled "Murder within the Family" has a large section on poisoning.[179] A ***lettre de rémission*** from 1501 presents a husband (the victim), his wife, and her parents[180] and illustrates the fact that for the medieval period, family ties are those most likely to be affected by *toxicatio*.

Relatively untouched by crime in general,[181] the conjugal relationship was an important setting for the crime of poison. Certainly, the crime between spouses was not limited to poisoning.[182] Mortal blows exceeded murderous drinks in fourteenth century England.[183] However, in more than 15 percent of the cases where the link between the murderer and his victim is known, the crime of poison involved spouses. This scenario was common enough that individuals brought to justice tried to use it to their advantage. In 1349, the supplicant of a ***lettre de rémission*** succeeded in convincing the authorities that his adversary died as a result of being poisoned by his wife, not from the benign blows that he gave him.[184] The original conjugal relationship was seen to be affected by poison, and Geoffroi de Vendôme compares Eve's sin to the poisoning of her companion.[185] Ancient stories of the poisoning of spouses are added to the Biblical model[186] including that of the famous Rosamund, the literary incarnation of matrimonial perfidy.[187] Certain barbaric codes of law and the **penitentials** treat the crime of poisoning starting essentially with the poisoning of spouses.[188] In two-thirds of the cases, the female poisoner is the spouse, *deceptrix* or *insidiatrix uxor*. The examples of wives reputed to be poisoners are spread all during the period and in all milieux, from the wife of Robert Guiscard[189] to that of Pierre Pinchepré, the pastry maker in Roye in 1501,[190] including Jeanne, the widow of Michel Lefort, who tried, in a classic scenario, to substitute poison for a powder that was supposed to lead to reconciliation and love (1355).[191] Christine de Pizan attempts to promote Xantippe who tried to snatch the cup of fatal hemlock from the hands of her husband Socrates, a marvelous inversed scene of the wife taking away the *poculum mortis* instead of offering it. Christine denies the use of poison by brutalized and submissive women whose patience she celebrates.[192] But the figure of the *venenosa conjux* does not fade one little bit. Eustache Deschamps observes, in his *Mirouer de mariage*, that as soon as a wife is annoyed by her husband, she considers using "toxins and charms/enchantments, poisons, tricks" (*illec venins et charays,/Enchantemens, poisons, agays*).[193] In a small number of cases (less that one out of three) that is the opposite of the statistics of conjugal crimes proposed by C. Gauvard,[194] it was the wife who undertook the poisoning. The *Lex romana* of the Burgundians observes that the numbers in the early Middle Ages are parallel to those of the *veneficae* wives.[195] Boson, marquis of Provence, who poisoned his wife in 876, is an isolated case of a poisoning husband in this period.[196] Poisoning husbands are more likely to have lived in the last centuries of the Middle Ages, and in all social ranks: princes (Albert of Austria), knights (le Sire d'Ormoy), bourgeois, or artisans (a cobbler from Freiburg in 1483). Proximity and intimate situations greatly influenced the choice of weapon, that of the common table and common roof.

Little affected by medieval criminality in general,[197] the family setting was the context for the crime of homicide by poison in 18 percent of the cases examined. We will consider here the relationships that led to contact between the participants in a homicide. The fratricides involving Robert de Normandie, the Staufens, the Viscontis, or Louis XI had more to do with power plays than family relationships.

The family relationship affected by the crime of poisoning is represented differently in different cases, but the relationship between the family link and the method of killing is quite close. Etienne de Bourbon poisoned both his father and his mother.[198] This situation is part of a criminal reality that was far from rare. Victims of poisoning and the accused poisoners were linked by a family relationship in somewhat less than 10 percent of the victims indexed, and four times more that was observed in the ***lettres de rémission***.[199] There were fathers or mothers poisoned by their sons or daughters—a type of murder treated specifically by Roman law and those who commented on it[200]—and infanticides, which, in one case out of three, involved children put in the care of a stepmother.

Not considering abortions brought about sometimes with powders that Alvaro Pelayo calls *venena sterilitatis*,[201] the poisoning of children was practiced on older victims—the murder of very young children was accomplished by very different means[202]—and can be categorized with the murder of husbands. Such a double homicide was attributed in 1363 to the Countess of Tyrol by Filippo Villani, who, of course, evoked the figure of Medea.[203] It can be observed that, with some exceptions, women were more often guilty of the poisoning of children—which is the reverse of their function as nurturer—than men, who are not considered nurturers. This situation is illustrated by the fate that the heretic Mersende provided for her daughter.[204]

The image of the stepmother as poisoner does not exist only in the imagination of moralists, poets, and storytellers.[205] It corresponds to a situation found in documents starting in the early Middle Ages. Marcatrude poisoned the young son of the King of Burgundy, Gontran, who was her husband (about 560).[206] Sichelgaïte faced with Bohémond and Bertrade de Montfort with Prince Louis[207] are examples of this Ovidian figure of *noverca*, a perception so general that when Philippe III's heir died, in 1276, popular Parisian opinion assumed that the king's second wife was responsible.[208] The event of 1280 that involved Yolande de Nevers and her stepson follows the same pattern. From a first marriage, the future Count of Flanders Robert de Béthune had a son, Charlot; from the second, with Yolande, he had four children: "her stepmother caused his death unfairly" (*sa marastre l'a fait mourir faulcement*), cried the father of the victim, whereas the distraught princess was persuaded that her husband's suspicions would be the cause of her own death, since the criminal scenario was so fixed in the culture.[209] This type of situation is also found in other milieux. Not content with attacking her husband, Philippe, the wife of Adam Bargon, sought to kill the daughter that he had had in a first marriage (1375). Convinced of her bad intentions Jordan Molard did not permit his stepmother Perrisonne Gapit to prepare his food (1462). It must not be believed, however, that stepmothers used only poison to carry out their plans. William of Malmesbury reports an episode that occurred in 975 to the son that King Edgar had in a first marriage. The second wife of the Saxon monarch was so jealous of this child that with vicious cunning (*dolum viperum*) she hired assassins to kill him, even though it was a situation where poison was usually used.[210] Adèle de Pouille got rid of her son-in-law Robert de Bourgogne, who was in charge of the government of Sicily during the minority of the future Roger II (1113).[211] René Colinet experienced the poisonous evil of the mother of his wife (1469).[212] Stepmothers and mothers-in-law detested any foreigners present in the family circle.

The poisoning of parents was also a factor in the Ostrogoth court in the sixth century, where the daughter of Theodoric Amalasuntha was accused of killing her mother Audofleda with poison.[213] An example of parricide, this time paternal, committed in ordinary milieux, can be found in the registers of Parlement in 1318: Bertranne de Noisilliez was strongly suspected of having killed her father Pierre Hubert.[214] Concerning children poisoned by their parents, the sources indicate or suggest a few such as that of the Duchesse de Bar who died brutally in 1404[215] or that of Bianca Maria Visconti whom some thought was poisoned (1468).[216] Finally, the most serious act, parricide committed or attempted by a son against his father takes on a dimension particularly dramatic at the court of Foix (1379).[217] It is possible that Froissart, who was well acquainted with chivalric literature, had in mind the similar story of the *Bastard de Bouillon* when he retold that terrible event.[218]

Outside of marriage and family relationships, kinship links about 8 percent of the victims to their aggressors. But, except when the accused is in the position of heir,[219] a situation that obviously arouses suspicion, lesser degrees of kinship are more difficult to link to poison since there is less contact between the poisoned and the poisoner. They confirm simply that poisoning is indeed a typical method of murder within a family that scorns bloodlines while avoiding the spilling of any blood.

Spiritual kinship that brings together members of a religious community must be considered briefly. Monastic or canonical groups provide a context in which crimes of poisoning were not frequent, but certainly not unknown. Umberto Eco's heroes existed, and well before the fourteenth century. The air in the cloister could be toxic; confinement tended to exacerbate conflicts. However, one cannot say that the crime of poisoning particularly affected monastic or cloistered relationships. The number of such cases noted amounts to less than 8 percent of the total. Poison given in the guise of brotherly charity is similar to fratricide, in fact less common in our sources than parricide to which Bartole compares logically the murder by poisoning of the Father Abbot.[220] Despite the assumptions that one can make on the reason for existence of certain works by the Abbess Hildegarde of Bingen, we have not encountered a convent that was the location of *veneficia*.[221] On the other hand, in certain cases, the servants of a monastic family did participate in the criminal endeavor. A sacristan and a cook carried out the poisoning of the Abbot of Saint-Benoît de Quinçay in 1316.[222]

The Involvement of Servants in the Crime of Poisoning

As with links of kinships, links of service are much affected by poisoning. The Justinian Code mainly considers *veneficia* in the context of *domus*.[223] In one-sixth of the cases in our study, the victim of poison succumbed from the action of one of his/her servants. "No threat is to be feared more than that presented by those one knows," wrote Boethius, echoing medieval writers of literature as well as intellectuals.[224] The evangelist Matthew had already said it: *Inimici hominis domestici ejus* (Matthew 10: 36), as John of Winterthur remembers concerning the death of Henry VII.[225] The reason is that the service of a master, whether he be king or artisan, gave ample opportunity to be in contact with his food, his clothing, or his body without arousing suspicion: a familiar person is by definition above suspicion.[226] But if a servant were unfaithful to the law of Christ, every master should be aware of the danger.[227] The servant named Saraceno who poisoned his Venetian master in 1364 with rat poison illustrates this danger.[228] The servant either acted on his own initiative or he carried out a command from the initiator of the homicide. More than 20 percent of those who carried out a poisoning and can be identified were the servants of the man or woman who was poisoned, such as Pierre Flori, who served Master Ricard (1317).[229]

The services carried out in palaces by butlers, chambermaids, kitchen workers, stable hands, palace staff, doctors, and other barbers, confessors, or chaplains made the use of poison very easy. Those with contact to the body of the proposed victim have a particular advantage. Confidence in medical science exposed a princely patient to great danger when he put himself entirely in the hands of his caretaker despite the advice of Aristotle addressed to Alexander: "Oh, Alexander, do not trust a single doctor, for a doctor, be assured without a doubt, has the power to do harm/and could undertake a felony" (*O Alissandre, ne vus afiez/En un sul mire ke vus tiegnez/Kar un mire, satiez sanz doutance,/Ad bien poer de fere nuisance/E une felunie emprendre purreit*).[230] The danger was doubled when the caretaker was a Jew or a Sarrasin. The trust that Charles the Bald (*le Chauve*) had in Sedechias permitted him, according to a vague tradition, to kill his master under the guise of caring for him.[231] In the twelfth century, William of Tyr deplored that the Muslim doctors held the complete confidence of the Latin princes in the Orient, such as King Badouin III (1163), who paid for it with their lives.[232]

The most general service in a residence was affected by the crime of poison.[233] In 1258, the servants of English lords, cupbearers, kitchen workers, and other household staff were particularly under suspicion of having carried out the murderous plots of the members of Henry III's entourage.[234] The most treacherous criminals took advantage of this privileged exposure to suspicion. In 1280, Yolande de Nevers tried to divert attention by claiming that the chefs in the Flemish court had killed the son of the count's heir.[235] Bernard de Montepulciano made the same assertion after the death of the empress at Genoa in 1311.[236] At the time of the death of the Duc de Brabant in 1430, suspicions fell automatically on the duke's servants.[237]

A few cases present the domestic crime in another light: for example, a female servant was killed because she knew about all the previous poison plots against her master Clément la Hure.[238] But the social gradient of *toxicatio* in the vast majority of cases is inverse. It situates the weapon of poison in the universe of master/servant less affected by criminality in general from the time of Charles VI.[239] Poisoning thus emerges first as an inside crime, the opposite of a crime committed in nature or in the street. Commenting on the misadventures he experienced as an abbot persecuted by his monks, Abélard quotes opportunistically the comment of Saint Paul: *Foris pugne, intus timores*.[240] The *domus* and its components engendered, as it were, murders by poisoning committed in familiar surroundings in a narrow setting of familiar relationships which facilitated the identification of women as perpetrators.

Servants were not the only individuals in private homes and courts with the label of familiar figures; there were also individuals in positions of political alliance with the heads of the household who were rewarded with titles of service. About 1160, John of Salisbury already comments on the fact that the service of a prince exacerbates tensions in a court and can lead to the killing of a rival in order to have exclusive rights to the sovereign's ear. One approach was to use potions and enchantments on a prince with the goal of exercising control over him, even to the point of attempting to take the life of his successor from whom was feared exile or disgrace.[241] For example, the enmity between the Sicilian Archchancelor and the Archbishop of Palermo in 1161 inspired such action to settle a dispute between two sets of rival ambitions.[242] The death of Frederick of Austria in 1330 was alleged to have been the result of a bungled attempt by a woman who hoped to preserve the prince's favorable opinion of her husband.[243]

Commercial services in certain categories deemed disreputable exposed clients and users to the peril of poison. We will quickly pass over Christian butchers, whose reputation as poisoners, well anchored in collective folklore, was less related to deliberate homicidal intentions than to the fraudulent habit of selling rotten merchandise.[244] On the other hand, the claimed malice of Jewish butchers, and more generally of the sellers of Israeli products, was considered a threat to Christian consumers. Innocent III in 1208 and Saint Louis at Béziers in 1247 forbad the consumption of their meat.[245] These measures were certainly taken in retaliation—why tolerate the consumption of meat sold by the Jews when they rejected all meat prepared outside their rites.[246] Moreover, in daily life, people did not normally observe the rigorous prohibitions made by the authorities.[247] Nevertheless, mistrust reigned supreme. Another form of commercial relations, medicine practiced by the Jews on Christians was naturally rife with suspicion. The case of a patient supposedly killed by a Jewish doctor exploded in 1161 in Bohemia,[248] followed by numerous other accusations preserved in judicial archives. In 1348, Jewish doctors were reproached for their prescriptions of *potiones venenosae* in the context of an epidemic where the therapeutic failure, however unavoidable, was considered deliberate.[249] In order to avoid this kind of situation, the Council of Trier in 1227 required that Christians abstain from taking potions from Jews.[250]

Poison in Relationships Based on Power

If the circle of relationships is enlarged to include those among the powerful, the use of poison is again found to play a role. This fact is not surprising when the princes of the West were confronted by their heathen neighbors whose enmity was also manifested by the use of poison. From the semilegendary episode concerning the Countess of Castile, the poisonous Ava de Ribagorça in the case of 1321, the Saracens of the West carried out a series of anti-Christian acts with individual or collective attempts at poisoning. Saracens from the Mediterranean area were alleged to have acted against Godefroy de Bouillon,[251] Philippe Auguste (Richard was an ally of the Infidels), Richard of Cornwall, Thomas of Savoie, and Saint Louis, whose supplies failed to be infected.[252] In expectation of the poisonous dangers that Philippe VI was preparing to confront, Guido da Vigevano included in his *texaunus* a discussion of poisons that outlines the way the Infidels set up ambushes.[253] Note that the Arab chroniclers of the tenth to thirteenth centuries that I have consulted lack the least reference to any poisoning of the French, who are, however, always presented in a negative light.

The relationship with the Byzantines, who were in theory less unfriendly, also involved poison used against the Latins whom they had always hated.[254] Allying themselves with the Infidels, the Greeks slowed the advance of the Crusaders through the use of poisonous ambushes. A conspirator, Alexis Comnène poisoned the noble and victorious Robert Guiscard by corrupting his wife. The schismatic Greeks were reputed to have poisoned the water on the path of the Norman warrior.[255] Several anecdotes pertaining to the second and third crusades highlight this *malitia Graecorum* against the Latins, which occurs as a leitmotiv in William of Tyr's chronicle. A vile mixture of lime and chalk disguised as bread was delivered to the Latins wandering in the mountains of Asia Minor (1144 or 1145).[256] At Plovdiv, in 1147, some German knights seated in a tavern, saw a kind of snake charmer, who created panic by pretending to release the snake. The chronicler who reports the incident indicates that this attitude was interpreted by the German soldiers as the desire of all the Greeks to poison the Westerners: *scelus unius omnibus imputant*.[257] This prejudice is all the more interesting because it is not reciprocated: what Anne Comnène remembers about the Latin-Greek relationship is the coarseness, the brutality, and the barbarity of the Greeks, quite the opposite of the subjects of *basileus*.

Poison was also a factor in the relations between powerful Christians. As part of an elected monarchy where murder could redistribute the cards,[258] the members of the Wisigoth aristocracy were quite familiar with the use of poison. Such a situation also existed between the French royalty and the bishops.[259] Those who disputed the plunder from Carolingian power also used poison.[260] D. C. Douglas, proposes that this manner of resolving conflicts belonged completely to the Norman eleventh century.[261] Seeing in this time and place a consequence and a circumvention of the restrictions brought to open warfare by feudal institutions is not very convincing[262]: it was during a traditional siege of Le Mans that Gautier succumbed to the poison of Guillaume le Bâtard.

At the end of the Middle Ages, the conflict between the Valois and their English vassal involved very little *venenatio*. There were only a few accusations in 1348[263] and the English involvement in the case of 1390 is questionable.[264] The anti-English propaganda, which is full of other accusations, does not accuse them of using poison as a weapon of war against the French, even in the case of Robert Wourdreton, or in the case of the French officials alleged to have been poisoned in London in 1400. On the other hand, the King of Navarre, who tried to use the fear of the French expressed by the English valet of an English minstrel, to involve him in one of his conspiracies,[265] used poison in his struggle with the King of France.[266] The quarrels that pitted the house of Orléans and the house of Bourgogne against each other in the course of the fifteenth century involved quite commonly *toxicatio*, from the crimes alleged against Louis d'Orléans to the poisoning attempts that Louis XI and the dukes of Bourgogne accused each other of committing. Internal conflicts among the English aristocracy made use of poison as much under the Plantagenets as under the Lancasters: civil war could have the bitter tastes of poison (1258, 1397–1400, 1419, 1442).

As a continuation of politics in other ways, medieval war in theory permitted the expression of the strength of arms and the skill of laying siege to a town. Nevertheless, in nearly 8 percent of the cases, poison was used to terminate a military conflict. Without considering the use of weapons coated with poison that were found in the feudal era—some attribute the death of Richard the Lion-heart to a poisoned arrow from a crossbow[267] and Pietro d'Abano mentions the use of swords dipped in poison[268]—without taking into account the poisonous reputation of firearms,[269] it appears that the poisoning of a military adversary was a practice frequently alleged from the twelfth to the fifteenth centuries. Certainly, the practice was often attributed to city dwellers, unfamiliar with chivalric values: the citizens of Avignon in 1226, the inhabitants of Kutna in 1304, of Civita Castellena in 1354.[270] But were the soldiers of Charles VI, who were intoxicated in 1412 by mysterious herbs that had been thrown into the river, the only victims of *ignobiles*?[271]

Thus, relationships among the powerful did not exclude the crime of poison. Can it be said then that poison was a weapon used especially in political crimes? Despite the title of G. Minois' book, which associates the knife with political crimes, the response is mostly negative. Poison was not substituted for other combat methods but was added to them, sometimes when the traditional methods failed or proved ineffective. The military context for the use of poison appears to be less important than the domestic sphere, the natural cradle of *toxicatio.*

Our study of the sociology of the crime of poisoning reveals much more about the social imaginary than about criminal statistics. At the confluence of intellectual thought and the opinions in the street, sometimes manipulated by the chroniclers, this imaginary responds to the lack of visibility of this type of homicide and actually frequently creates the crime and organizes it into preestablished categories. Individuals in close quarters from the married couple to state officials were targeted by poison in the hands of persons who were marginal in one way or another. Criminal poisoning implies a hierarchical relationship. It occurred normally in a closed space, very different from the space where brawls occurred among random companions, even from the space where witchcraft was practiced, which was more likely to occur in neighborhood relationships. Murder on the inside, in a household, in the community, or in the palace, the crime was attributed to people defined in one way or another by their exteriority. This exteriority, perhaps conspiratorial, expresses all the horror of *veneficium.*

NOTES

1. See C. Gauvard, "*De grace especial . . .*," pp. 30–31 on the levels of society covered by the jurisdiction of the Parlement of Paris; P. Braun, La valeur documentaire des lettres de rémission, *La faute, la répression et le pardon*, Actes du 107e congrès national des sociétés savantes (Brest, 1982), *Bulletin philologique et historique*, 1984, t. 1, pp. 207–222.

2. C. Gauvard, "*De grace especial . . .*," tableau 15, p. 315.

3. Orderic Vital, t. 2, p. 101.

4. *Histoire des femmes*, p. 78; an idea probably linked to the natural toxicity of the feminine sex that is thereby immunized against poison (C. Thomasset, Le corps féminin ou le regard empêché, *Micrologus*, 1993, nº1, pp. 99–114, p. 112).

5. N. Pancer, *Sans peur . . . , passim.*

6. C. Gauvard, "*De grace especial . . . ,*" p. 306.

7. *Ead.*, p. 308.

8. Froissart, t. 3, p. 243 of the Buchon ed.; *Parlement criminel*, X2a 14, f. 214 v–217 v.

9. Brunetto Latini, *Li livres dou tresor*, ed. F. J. Carmody, Berkeley, 1939–1948, rpr. Geneva, 1998, I, 97, p. 79.

10. Froissart, t. 3, p. 243 of the Buchon ed.

11. *Parlement criminel*, X2a 14, f. 214 v–217 v. Taking up a tradition already present in the writings of Isidore of Seville (*Étymologies*, XI, 2, 32), the *Catholicon* de Balbi, *sv Mors*, distinguishes *mors acerba, mors immatura* et *mors merita*, that of the aged.

12. Guillaume Guiard, *Branche des royaus lignages*, ed. *RHGF*, XXII, Paris, 1865, pp. 211–212.

13. Pierre de Zittau, *Chronique de Königsaale*, ed. J. Loserth, Vienne, 1875, p. 351 and sq. According to biblical tradition, the age of thirty-five is considered to be the exact middle point of a life span. See M. Th. Lorcin, Vieillesse et vieillissement vus par les médecins du Moyen Âge, *Bulletin du centre d'histoire économique et sociale de la région lyonnaise*, 1983, n°4, pp. 5–22, p. 16.

14. *Gesta Trevirorum integra*, ed. J. H. Wyttenbach and M. F. J. Müller, Trèves, 1838, p. 230.

15. Dynter, t. 3, pp. 497–499.

16. Jean de Roye, t. 2, p. 285. See H. Stein, *Charles de France . . .*, chap. 10.

17. *Chronicon Angliae*, p. 333. Numerous examples in the writings of the Religieux de Saint-Denis (t. 2, p. 750), Burchard (t. 2, p. 507, 561 of the Thuasne ed.) or Philippe de Vigneulles (t. 3, pp. 361–363).

18. *Chronique de Sainte-Catherine au Mont Rouen*, ed. *RHGF*, XXIII, Paris, 1875, p. 211.

19. Ferretus Vicentinus, col. 1013: *sic etiam multi orbis principes et probi tirones, quos nulli bellorum tumultus, nulla gladiorum tormentorumque ruina paventes, aut hostibus terga vertentes effecere, latenti morbo subtracti sunt.*

20. Pietro d'Abano, *De venenis . . .*, p. 5; Michele Savonarole, *Libellus de balneis et termis naturalibus omnibus Ytalie sicque totius orbis proprietatibus*, Ferrare's ed., 1485, MS BNF, lat. 7357, f. 83 v.

21. *Cronica de gestis principum*, pp. 45 and 57. Same opinion in the writings of Jean de Winterthur, p. 64: *patet quod a rege Rudolfo omnes reges Alamanie seu imperatores in occisione gladii vel veneni mortui sunt.*

22. *Estoire de Eracles*, p. 179.

23. Y. Hypothèse de Lanhers, Crimes et criminels au xive siècle, *RH*, 1968, n 240, pp. 325–338, p. 335, concerning plots in the time of Philippe de Valois.

24. See M. Senellart, *Les arts de gouverner. Du* regimen *médiéval au concept de gouvernement*, Paris, Le Seuil, 1995, 3e partie.

25. Jean Martin de Ferrara, *De venenis evitandis*, f. 1.

26. Poggio Bracciolini, *De infelicitate principum*, ed. D. Canfora, Rome, 1998, § 32 and pp. 44, 46, 55.

27. Commynes, p. 643.

28. Philippe de Vitry, *Le dict de Franc Gontier*, ed. Tarbé, in *Œuvres*, Reims, 1850, p. 140.

29. Honorat Bovet, *L'apparicion de Jehan de Meun*, ed. E. Nys, Bruxelles, 1883, p. 11.

30. De Vigny's words are well known: "There are two things often questioned about kings: their birth and their death. People don't want one to be legitimate and the other natural" (*Il y a deux choses que l'on conteste bien souvent aux rois: leur naissance et leur mort. On ne veut pas que l'une soit légitime et l'autre naturelle*).

31. Pierre Damien, *Opusculum de brevitate vitae pontificum romanorum et divina providentia*, ed. Migne, *PL* 145, Paris, 1853, col. 471–480.

32. *Vie de saint Samson*, I, 16-19 et 55: see the editor's remarks, p. 93.

33. Grégoire le Grand, Dialogues, III, 5, t. 2, p. 274 and sq., Sabin, Bishop of Canossa.

34. Alvaro Pelayo, *De planctu ecclesiae*, f. 130.

35. Orderic Vital, t. 2, pp. 371–372: Maurille de Rouen; Abélard, pp. 106–107.

36. Guillaume de Tyr, p. 620; Guillaume de Newburgh, t. 1, p. 71 and sq.; Matthieu Paris, t. 3, p. 623.

37. Guillaume de Tyr, p. 686, and *Estoire de Eracles*, p. 61. See H. E. Meyer, Zum Tode Wilhelms von Tyrus, *Archiv für Diplomatik*, 1959–1960, n°5–6, pp. 280–302.

38. Nangis, t. 1, p. 126. See *Chronique anonyme de Saint-Martin de Tours*, ed. RHGF, XVIII, Paris, 1764, p. 297: *statim iniquorum consilio toxicatus ecclesiam beati Martini Turonensis... super juridictione abbatiae Bellimontis aggreditur. Sicque beatus vir qui abiit in consilio impiorum et in via peccatorum stetit, non diu in illa cathedra pestilentie sedit*. Nangis retained only the first four words and the last sentence.

39. *Actes du Parlement de Paris, 1254–1328*, n 2323.

40. Monfrin, p. 231. One could say the same about prelates who were victims of heretics or of witches such as the Archbishop of Embrun (1437), Marx, pp. 131–135.

41. Ambroise Paré, *Traité des venins*, p. 293.

42. *Annales de Fulda*, ed. Pertz, *MGH SS*, I, Hanovre, 1826, p. 398.

43. Guibert de Nogent, *De vita sua*, III, 18, p. 440: *quia ergo palam non poterat* [presbyterum occidere] *hunc veneficio corrumpere parat*.

44. M. McVaugh, p. 158: "Nor was it just the powerful who feared poison: the preoccupation was alive at all levels of society."

45. Albe, p. 164: *Quis locus regiminis poterit esse tutus, quis rector securitate gaudebit, si romanus pontifex et ejus curia talibus subjiciantur casibus?*

46. Leleux, p. 69. J. Nelson, Les reines carolingiennes, *Femmes et pouvoirs des femmes à Byzance et en Occident (vi^e^-xie siècles)*, s.d., S. Lebecq et al., Lille, 1999, pp. 121–132, p. 129.

47. M. Robert, p. 2.

48. Carbonelli, PJ XXXIV, p. 344: *tales agricole, sicut est B., sunt libenter rudes nec possunt vel debent esse ita apti et sutiles ad tales pravas falsitates faciendas*.

49. *Chronique du Religieux de Saint-Denis*, t. 1, pp. 632–635.

50. *Chronique des comtes d'Anjou...*, pp. 124 and 151.

51. *Registres du trésor des Chartes*, JJ 77, f. 90 v.

52. *Parlement criminel*, X2a 6, f. 442–443.

53. *Parlement criminel*, X2a 14, f. 214 v–217 v.

54. See F. Cardini, Le guerrier et le chevalier, *L'homme médiéval*, dir. J. Le Goff, Paris, Le Seuil, 1989, pp. 87–128, on the *ritterliches Tugendsystem* (p. 95).

55. *Parlement criminel*, X2a 6, f. 178–181.

56. Juvénal des Ursins, p. 187 of the ed. of 1614.

57. Cf. Pierre Farget, *Miroir de la vie humaine*, Paris, 1482, f. 113: "If I don't dare to say that all [physicians] are thieves, drunks and poisoners, they kill men" (*Si n'ose dire que tous* [les médecins] *soient larrons, inthoxicaires et empoisonneurs, ilz tuent les hommes*).

58. Dynter, t. 3, pp. 296–297.

59. *Estoire de Eracles*, p. 61.

60. Secousse, p. 374. On this individual, see S. Duvergé, Un empoisonneur aux gages de Charles le Mauvais: Maître Angel, *Bulletin hispanique*, 1936, n 38, pp. 369–373, this reference suggested by P. Jugie to whom we are very grateful.

61. Carbonelli, p. 258, Jean de Grandville's promises to Amédée VII.

62. Richer, II, 59; a miracle of Saint Thomas Becket saves from death "a physician" deliberately given a deadly potion by one of his colleagues who was full of jealousy. (VI, 101, p. 496).

63. Carbonelli, p. 226. The case of Jean de Saint-Nicolas de Bari is similar: his intervention on behalf of a patient offended a Christian doctor: Marx, p. 224.

64. Secousse, p. 499.

65. *Registre criminel du Châtelet*, p. 435.

66. Guibert de Nogent, *De vita sua*, III, 18, pp. 440–442.

67. *Chronique rouennaise* appended to Pierre Cochon's chronicle, p. 325.

68. Cf. J. Michelet, *La sorcière*, p. 131. Lawsuits against charlatans became more numerous in Parlement from the beginning of the fourteenth century (D. Jacquart, *La médecine médiévale*, p. 303 and sq.). Excluded, with some exceptions, from the University, Jewish physicians who were reputed to base their knowledge on the book of Psalms, found themselves also rejected for this reason.

69. Alvaro Pelayo, *De planctu ecclesiae*, Lyon ed., 1517, I, 48, f. 26 v–27.

70. *Chronique parisienne anonyme de 1316 à 1339*, ed. A. Hélot, *Mémoires de la Société de l'histoire de Paris et de l'Île de France*, 1884, n°11, pp. 1–207, p. 158.

71. F. Graus, *Pest-Geissler-Judenmorde*, p. 308.

72. For Cîteaux, see A. Dimier's conclusions, Violences, rixes et homicides . . .

73. *Statuts, chapitres généraux . . .* , t. 5, p. 28, 1410.

74. Abélard, p. 107.

75. M. McVaugh, p. 158.

76. Martin le Franc, *Le champion des dames*, t. 4, v. 18867–18868.

77. Matthieu Paris, t. 4, p. 168.

78. Monstrelet, t. 2, p. 66; Zantfliet, col. 398.

79. Guichardin, II, 3 and VI, 4. See I. Cloulas, *Les Borgia*, p. 156 and sq., 231, 295, 315 and sq.

80. *Statuts . . . de l'ordre de Cluny*, t. 5, p. 28 or *Statuta capitulorum generalium ordinis cisterciensis*, t. 5, pp. 588–589 and t. 6, p. 15.

81. Du Clercq, p. 668 of Buchon's edition.

82. Quintilien, *Institution oratoire*, V, 10, p. 134: *latrocinium facilius in viro, veneficium in femina credas*.

83. Baptista Condrochius, *De morbis veneficis ac veneficiis*, Venise, 1595, p. 102 v.

84. O. Pollak, *The criminality of women*, Philadelphia, 1950, p. 16. F. Obringer, *L'aconit et l'orpiment . . .* , chap. 5, on the association in Chinese written language of women and poison.

85. N. Pancer, *Sans peur...*, p. 237: "There was no form of violence that was specifically feminine such as poison or magic." C. Gauvard, "*De grace especial...*," p. 319: Specifically female crimes do not exist.

86. B. A. Hanawalt, The Female Felon in fourteenth century England, *Viator*, 1974, n 5, pp. 253–268, p. 258: "In later ages, poison gained the reputation of being the woman's weapon, but medieval peasant women seemed to have ignored the possibilities of deadly nightshade and poisonous mushrooms..."

87. G. Duby, *Dames du xiie siècle*, III, pp. 29 and 37 on the woman *inermis* forging her own weapons.

88. Gautier Map, *Contes pour les gens de cour*, tr. and pres. by A. K. Bate, Turnhout, Brepols, 1993, p. 234, on Livia and Lucilia; Boccace, *Des cleres et nobles femmes*, French version (1401) of the *De claris mulieribus*, ed. J. Baroin and J. Haffen, Paris, 1993, XVIII (Médée).

89. Orderic Vital, t. 4, p. 374: *Livor femineus a quo primus Adam est de Paradisi sede projectus.* On the Norman's death, see H. Taviani-Carozzi, *La terreur du monde. Robert Guiscard et la conquête normande en Italie*, Paris, Fayard, 1996, p. 477 et 493.

90. L. Moulinier-Brogi, Plantes toxiques et humeurs peccantes: la pensée du poison chez Hildegarde de Bingen, *Le corps à l'épreuve*, pp. 71–103, p. 79.

91. Orderic Vital, t. 5, pp. 34–35.

92. For a sexual interpretation of this myth, see R. Caillois, *Le mythe et l'homme*, Paris, 1972 (1re ed., 1938), chap. 1: fear would come from the confusion between the blood resulting from the loss of virginity and that of the menstrual flow, considered to be toxic.

93. Burchard de Worms, *Corrector sive medicus*, col. 1004 of Migne's ed.

94. Raban Maur, *Pénitentiels*, ed. Migne, *PL* 110, Paris, 1852, **penitential** of 841, addressed to the Bishop of Auxerre, chap. 30: *De his etiam super quibus interrogasti, id est de illa femina quae menstruum sanguinem suum miscuit cibo vel potui, et dedit viro suo, ut comederet.*

95. Etienne de Fougères, *Le livre des manières*, ed. R. A. Lodge, Genève, 1979, v. 1033 and sq.

96. The character of Rosamund belongs to the standard misogynous rhetoric: see Jean Raulin, *De matrimonio*, following l'*Itinerarium paradisii*, Paris, 1524, sermon III, f. 117 v.

97. Jean de Meun, *Le Roman de la rose*, ed. and tr. A. Strubel, Paris, Livre de Poche, 1992, v. 9151 and sq.: "For their nature commands them / So that each one does her worst / don't they see how step-mothers / Put poison in the food of their stepsons / And make charms and enchantments / and many other works of the devil..." (*Car leur nature leur commande / Que chascune a pis fere entande. / Ne voit-on pas comment les marrastres / Cuisent venins a leur fillastres / Et font charmes et sorceris / Et tant d'autres granz deablies...*).

98. Cited by G. Garcia Teruel, Les opinions sur la femme dans quelques récits du xiie et du xiiie siècles, *MA*, 1995, n 101, pp. 23–40, p. 30.

99. Martin le Franc, *Le champion des dames*, v. 6441–6445 then str. 2467 and 2470.

100. Christine de Pizan, *Le livre de la cité des Dames*, pp. 159–160.

101. B. A. Hanawalt, The Female Felon..., article cited; N. Gonthier, Délinquantes ou victimes, les femmes dans la société lyonnaise du xve siècle, *RH*, 1984, n°271, pp. 25–46.

102. C. Gauvard, "*De grace especial . . .*," p. 307. Women represent 4 percent of the beneficiaries of the **lettres de rémission** (p. 300).

103. *Documents nouveaux*, pp. 29–31.

104. *Actes du Parlement de Paris, 1254–1328*, n 5187.

105. *Registres du trésor des Chartes*, JJ 120, f. 85–85 v.

106. *Registres du trésor des Chartes*, JJ 196, f. 72.

107. *Registres du trésor des Chartes*, JJ 234, f. 107 v–108.

108. C. Gauvard, "*De grace especial . . .*," p. 317; B. A. Hanawalt, The Female Felon . . . , p. 258: in almost 2/3's of homicides committed by women, another person was needed to carry out the crime. See also A. Porteau-Bitker, Criminalité et délinquance féminine dans le droit pénal des xiiie et xive siècles, *RHDFE*, 1980, n°58, pp. 13–56, p. 36.

109. Guillaume de Malmesbury, t. 1, p. 211.

110. Richer de Sénones, p. 300.

111. Nangis, t. 1, p. 340.

112. Vigneulles, t. 3, pp. 301–302.

113. Des Godins de Souhesmes, p. 134.

114. *Documents nouveaux*, pp. 29–31.

115. K. Pratt, The Image of the Queen in Old French Literature, *Queens and Queenship in medieval Europe*, ed. J. A. Duggan, Woodbridge, 1997, pp. 235–259, p. 244.

116. *La vie ancienne de saint Samson*, I, 55; Frédégaire, IV, 50. The editor of the *Vita Samsonis* finds a strong influence from the poisonous Frankish queens on the account (thirteenth century) of the attack on Samson by the wife of King Judwal.

117. Jean de Hocsem, p. 368. Louis de Bavière died in reality from a heart attack (H. Thomas, *Ludwig der Baier*, Graz, Vienne, Cologne, 1993, pp. 378–379).

118. P. Stafford, *Queens, Concubines and Dowagers*, p. 97: "The domestic nature of this world *(le palais)* makes stealth, and especially poison, a normal means. Since Tacitus's Livia if not before, this secret method of encompassing death has regularly been imputed to the queens."

119. *Cronica de gestis principum*, p. 36. J. M. Bak, Queens as Scapegoats in Medieval Hungary, *Queens and Queenship . . .*, pp. 223–233.

120. A factor well demonstrated by M. Aurell, *Les noces du comte, mariage et pouvoir en Catalogne (785–1213)*, Paris, 1994, pp. 103–113 et p. 545.

121. Marguerite de Navarre, *Heptameron*, ed. M. François, Paris, 1960, XXXVI, pp. 261–266.

122. J. Russel, p. 182; see M.-Th. Kaiser-Guyot, *Le berger en France aux xive et xve siècles*, Paris, 1974, pp. 141–147. The author emphasizes, however, the thorough integration of the shepherds into the total community.

123. J. Chiffoleau, *Contra naturam*. For a casuistic and procedural approach to medieval nature, *Il Teatro della natura, Micrologus*, 1996, n IV, pp. 265–312, p. 278.

124. Pietro d'Abano, *De venenis*, p. 33 from the ed. of 1537.

125. Jacques de Vitry, *Lettres de la cinquième croisade*, Lettre II, novembre 1216–février 1217, p. 54. The identity of the women in question is, however, not very clear: Muslim or Christian? Jean de Joinville, *Histoire de saint Louis*, p. 51 from de Wailly's ed.

126. Nangis, t. 1, p. 43. Because of these practices of the people on the Mediterranean coast, there are poisonings that were supposed to have shortened the lives of various prelates of the Holy Land.

127. Carbonelli, p. 278.

128. Orderic Vital, t. 3, p. 175.

129. D. Nirenberg, p. 237: in Majorca, a Muslim slave is accused of having poisoned Christians by spitting seawater on their doors.

130. *Historia peregrinorum*, ed. A. Chroust, Berlin, 1928, p. 146.

131. Liutprand de Crémone, *Relatio de legatione Constantinopolitana*, pp. 185, 196, 200, 205 then 207. He mistook wine with resin in it for a poisonous beverage: see O. B. Rader, Becher oder Tod. Richtig und falsch verstandene Zeichen bei Tisch, *Mahl und Repräsentation. Die Kult ums Essen*, ed. L. Kolmer, Paderborn, 2000, pp. 113–123.

132. See Anne Comnène, *Alexiade*, ed. *RHC; historiens grecs*, t. I, Paris, 1875, part II, pp. 1–204, p. 32; Guillaume de Tyr, II, 14, p. 92 in the ed. of the *RHC*.

133. Brocardus, *Directorium ad passagium faciendum*, pp. 431 then 439. Brocardus speaks of quicklime mixed in bread by the Greeks at the time of the Second Crusade.

134. Eustache Deschamps, *Contre les empoisonneurs*, ballade CCCCLXV, t. 3, pp. 282–283, verse 10 and the next-to-last verse.

135. Thietmar de Mersebourg, p. 401: *Aeris hujus* (de l'Italie) *et habitatorum qualitates nostris partibus non concordant. Multe enim prochdolor ! insidie in Romania et Longobardia sunt... multique toxicato cibo pereunt.*

136. *Estoire de Eracles*, XXVI, 23, p. 210 (a very uncertain allegation, linked to the subsequent hostility of the emperor's wife toward the "Germans": see P. Csendes, *Heinrich VI*, Darmstadt, 1993, pp. 192–193); *Annales de Melk, MGH SS*, IX, Hanovre, 1851, p. 511. Charles IV, *De vita sua*, ed. tr. L. Ölsner, Prague, 1979, p. 37; Thomas Ebendorfer, *Chronica pontificum romanorum*, ed. H. Zimmermann, *MGH, Ss Rer. Ger.*, n. série (16), Munich, 1994, t. 2, p. 521.

137. Orderic Vital, t. 3, pp. 181–182, 187, t. 5, pp. 34–35, t. 2, pp. 57 and 80.

138. Matthieu Paris, t. 5, p. 432.

139. See Olivier de la Marche, *Mémoires*, t. 1, p. 28: Married to the heir of the Lord of Milan, Boniface de Pavia lost a son, who was strangled in his cradle by a snake. Boniface cut the snake into two pieces after a struggle in which he received a large amount of venom.

140. Jean Servion, p. 196.

141. *Chronique du Religieux de Saint-Denis*, t. 2, pp. 86 and 546; t. 3, p. 132.

142. Carbonelli, PJ XXXIV, p. 350.

143. *Chronique du Religieux de Saint-Denis*, t. 2, pp. 86 and 546.

144. Gaguin, f. 167 of the ed. of 1500: poisoning of the heir to the Duchy of Milan by his uncle Ludovic Sforza.

145. Jean Lemaire de Belges, *La légende des Venitiens*, ed. A. Shoysman, Bruxelles, 1999, p. 18, to which can be added allegations of poisoning against the Cardinal d'Amboise (p. 405 of the Stecher ed., t. 4 of *Œuvres*, Genève, Slatkine Reprints, 1969).

146. Pierre Gringore, *Œuvres complètes*, ed. Montaiglon and Rotschild, Paris, 2 vol., 1858–1877, t. 2, p. 247.

147. C.-V. Langlois, Les Anglais du Moyen Âge d'après les sources françaises, *RH*, 1893, n°52, pp. 298–315, p. 314: *Walecome font doucement / Intus sunt pleni fraudibus / scorpionibus similes / Por ce sont dit Anglois coué.*

148. Monstrelet, t. 4, p. 399, Chastellain, t. 1, p. 341.

149. Cited by F. Bériac, *Histoire des lépreux au Moyen Âge*, p. 68.

150. Ibid., p. 189.

151. *Parise la Duchesse*, v. 41 and sq.: "When I was small, I was put into training as a clerk / At Saint Paul of Ravenna, I learned about poison / From an old smelly leper: there is not a worse one in the world" (*Cant je fui petitez, si fui mis a clerçon / A san Pol de Ravane, apris une poison / D'un vies masel puant: il n'a peior el mont . . .*).

152. Ed. *RHGF*, XXIII, p. 354: "The year 1421 was an infamy against the lepers of the kingdom: for healthy people did not want them to take water from their wells or from their fountains . . . " (*L'an M.^{III}.C.XXI fut une infamie contre les ladres du roiaulme de France : car les sains ne voulurent point que ilz puisasent de l'eaue en leurs puits ne en leurs fontaines . . .*).

153. Mentioned by J.-N. Biraben, *Les hommes et la peste en France et dans les pays européens et méditerranéens*, Paris, 2 vol., 1975–1976, p. 59: this act of July 21, 1348 accuses the Jews of meetings and conspiracies with the lepers in order to put deadly poisons in wells and in fountains and other places.

154. Vigneulles, t. 2, p. 107, according to Gaguin: "justice was done against the lepers who wanted to poison the water" (*justice fut faicte des meseaulx qui vouloient empoisonner les eawe*).

155. Cited in *L'imaginaire du sabbat . . .*, p. 325, n. 60.

156. Nangis, t. 2, p. 32.

157. S. Graysel, *The Church and the Jews in the xiiith century*, 2^{e} ed., New York, 1966 and addendum, New York, 1989, t. 1, p. 75, n. 148.

158. *Chronique parisienne anonyme*, p. 58: "works of the devil" undertaken "by the feeding and the introduction of the Jews" (*deablerie* entreprise *par l'ammonicion et introducion des Juifz*).

159. Konrad de Megenberg, *De mortalitate . . .*, p. 868: *non videtur mihi quod ipse gens misera judaïca causa fuerit generalis mortalitatis.* Richard Lescot, *Chronique*, ed. J. Lemoine, Paris, 1896, p. 83: *Corruptio tamen aquarum Judeis fuit tunc imposita . . . quamvis alia causa quam ista assignari potuerit . . .*

160. Trachtenberg, p. 106.

161. This formula is sacred: see Raban Maur, *De universo libri XXII*, ed. Migne, *PL* 111, col. 232; it is used in a chronicle that speaks of a case in which the communion wafer has been defiled (1290), *RHGF*, XXII, p. 32.

162. Burchard de Worms, *Corrector*, col. 1009.

163. See M. Bulard, *Le scorpion symbole du peuple juif*, Paris, 1935 and L. Aurigemma, *Le signe zodiacal du scorpion*, Paris-La Haye, Mouton, 1976, p. 62, who gives a few literary examples.

164. See B. Blumenkranz, *Le juif médiéval au miroir de l'art chrétien*, Paris, 1966, p. 12.

165. According to D. Nirenberg, p. 59.

166. M. Barber, Lepers, jexs, moslems . . . , p. 14; F. Bériac, *Histoire des lépreux*, p. 99.

167. See N. Coulet, Juif intouchable et interdit alimentaire, *Exclus et systèmes d'exclusion au Moyen Âge, Sénéfiance*, 1978, n 5, pp. 207–221.

168. *Décret de Gratien*, 28, 1, 13.

169. M. Kriegel, *Les juifs à la fin du Moyen Âge dans l'Europe méditerranéenne*, Paris, 1979, p. 40.

170. P. Pluchon, *Vaudou, sorciers empoisonneurs...*, p. 147, points out that the Blacks accused of poisoning in the Antilles of the eighteenth century are those who live most separated from the Whites.

171. In 1096, the emperor forbad them to carry arms: R. I. Moore, *La persécution*, p. 101.

172. F. Graus, *Pest-Geissler-Judenmorde*, p. 301.

173. *Sacrorum conciliorum amplissima collectio*, t. 23, col. 1175: *ne forte judaei per hoc christianos... venenent.*

174. Marx, PJ XI, pp. 226–227 and Trachtenberg, p. 82.

175. N. Daniel, *Islam et Occident*, Paris, tr. fr., Cerf, 1993, pp. 144–145. Tabari, *Chronique*, ed.-tr. H. Zotenberg, Paris, 4 vol., reed. 1958, then 1984, t. 3, p. 356.

176. This observation remains true in the seventeenth century: A. Lebigre, *L'affaire des poisons*, Bruxelles, Ed. Complexes, 1989, p. 82.

177. D. Nirenberg, p. 99.

178. Burchard de Worms, *Corrector*, chap. 35.

179. F. Lauwaert, *Le meurtre en famille; parricide et infanticide en Chine (xviii–xix*[e] *siècle)*, Paris, Odile Jacob, 1999.

180. *Registres du trésor des Chartes*, JJ 234, f. 107 v–108.

181. C. Gauvard, "*De grace especial...*," p. 318 et 573. Crime between spouses represents only 2 percent of total criminality observed in the ***lettres de rémission*** granted by Charles VI and 1 percent of the total number of homicides (p. 609 et tableau 34, p. 619).

182. See the brief overview by N. Gonthier, Les rapports du couple d'après les documents judiciaires à la fin du Moyen Âge, *Le mariage au Moyen Âge (xi*[e]*–xv*[e] *siècles)*, Actes du colloque de Montferrand (mai 1997), textes réunis par J. Teyssot, Montferrand, 1997, pp. 155–164. Poisoning is mentioned *in extremis*.

183. B. A. Hanawalt, The Female Felon..., p. 259.

184. *Registres du trésor des Chartes*, JJ 68, f. 485 v. Another alibi could be the plague.

185. Geoffroi de Vendôme, *Œuvres*, ed. Migne, *PL* 157, Paris, 1854, letter 24 to his monks (1095), col. 168: *Sexus iste nostrum primum venenavit parentem...*

186. The *Policraticus* of John of Salisbury, IV, 11, takes up again a story of familial and conjugal poison taken from Book IX of the *Facta memorabilia*.

187. Boccace, *De casibus illustrium virorum*, ed. P. G. Ricci and E. V. Zaccaria, Milan, 1983, VIII, 22.

188. *Lex Thuringorum*, ed. K. F. von Richthoffen, *MGH, Leges*, t. 5, Hanover, 1872, art. 55; Alain de Lille, *Liber poenitentialis*, II, 36, t. 2, p. 66. Reginon de Prüm, *Libri duo de synodalibus causis*, II, 84, pp. 246–247: *Si mulier maritum suum causa fornicationis veneno interficit...*

189. On the subject of wives as viewed by Orderic Vital, see D. Lett, Les épouses dans l'aristocratie anglo-normande des xie–xiie siècles, *Le mariage au Moyen Âge...*, pp. 15–27.

190. *Registres du trésor des Chartes*, JJ 234, f. 107 v–108.

191. *Registres du trésor des Chartes*, JJ 84, f. 145.
192. Christine de Pizan, *Le livre de la cité des Dames*, pp. 157 then 159–160.
193. Eustache Deschamps, *Mirouer de mariage, Œuvres complètes*, t. 9, p. 64, v. 1859–1860. From the same inexhaustible vein, see Chaucer, *Wife of Bath's Prologue, Canterbury Tales*, pp. 565–576.
194. C. Gauvard, *"De grace especial . . . ,"* tableau 13 *b*, p. 308: 83.5 percent of the victims of conjugal crimes are women.
195. *Leges Burgundionum, lex romana*, titre XXI, *De divortiis*, pp. 143–144.
196. *Annales de Fulda*, p. 392.
197. C. Gauvard, *"De grace especial . . . ,"* tableau 34, p. 619: the victim is a relative of the guilty party in 6 percent of the cases.
198. Etienne de Bourbon, *Tractatus de diversis materiis praedicabilibus*, III, n°174, pp. 153–154.
199. C. Gauvard, *"De grace especial . . . ,"* tableau 34, p. 619.
200. *Digeste*, 48, 9, 1 and 7. Placentin, *In codicis libris IX summa*, p. 435, au titre *De his qui parentes vel liberos occiderunt*. Case of a son buying poison to give to his father.
201. Alvaro Pelayo, *De planctu ecclesiae*, f. 27 v.
202. Y. Brissaud, L'infanticide à la fin du Moyen Âge: ses motivations psychologiques et sa répression, *RHDFE*, 1972, n 50, pp. 229–256.
203. Matteo and Filippo Villani, *Istorie*, Florence ed., 2 vol., 1581, t. 2 p. 150. Boccacio refers to his poisonous acts against Theseus in the *Généalogie des dieux* (livre IV).
204. Jacques Fournier, t. 2, p. 56.
205. Alvaro Pelayo, *De planctu ecclesiae*, f. 149, vice 78. Jean de Meun, *Le Roman de la rose*, p. 547. Ser Giovanni Fiorentino, *Il pecorone*, 23e journée, pp. 212–218.
206. Grégoire de Tours, t. 1, p. 226 of the Büchner ed.
207. Orderic Vital, t. 3, pp. 181–182, and t. 4, pp. 196–197.
208. J. de Gaulle, Pièces sur Pierre de la Brosse, *Bulletin de la Société de l'Histoire de France*, 1844, pp. 87–100, deposition from the legate Simon.
209. *Le livre de Baudoyn conte de Flandres et de Ferrant filz du roy de Portugal*, BNF, ms. fr. 1611, f. 180 and sq.
210. Guillaume de Malmesbury, t. 1, p. 183.
211. Orderic Vital, t. 5, pp. 34–35.
212. *Registres du trésor des Chartes*, JJ 196, f. 72.
213. Grégoire de Tours, III, 31, p. 102 of Poupardin's edition.
214. *Actes du Parlement de Paris, 1254–1328*, n°5224.
215. *Chronique du Religieux de Saint-Denis*, t. 3, p. 210.
216. Bernardino Corio, *Storia di Milano*, ed. Morisi Guerra, Turin, 1978, p. 1376. Concerning this case see M. Nicoud, Expérience de la maladie et échange épistolaire. Les derniers moments de Bianca Maria Visconti (mai–octobre 1468), *MEFRMA*, 2000, n°112-1, pp. 311–458.
217. Froissart, t. 12, pp. 81–88 from the ed. *SHF*.
218. *Li bastard de Bouillon* presents in effect, as in the Foix case, two half-brothers who are enemies, one of whom wishes to poison their common father. The hero of the novel kills the poisoner then goes to inform his incredulous father while the second son of Phoebus denounces his brother who is then killed by his father.
219. *Parlement criminel*, X2a 18, f. 11 v–14, 1423.

220. Bartole, *Commentaria in Digesti partes*, t. 2, p. 177 v–178.

221. Observation of L. Moulinier-Brogi, Plantes toxiques et humeurs peccantes..., p. 98.

222. *Actes du Parlement de Paris, 1254–1328*, n°5048. See also the baker of the monastery where Saint Samson lived, *Vie ancienne*, I, 16.

223. *Codex justinianus*, IX, 16, 8 and IX, 41, 3.

224. *Chronique des comtes d'Anjou...*, p. 124: *Nulla pestis efficacior est ad nocendum quam familiaris inimicus (Chronique des sires d'Amboise); Li roumans de Dolopathos*, v. 1535–1538; Nicolas Falcucci, *De dispositionibus venenorum*, f. 83.

225. Jean de Winterthur, p. 65.

226. Zantfliet, col. 417: *familiarissimus et ob hanc causam nequaquam suspectus.*

227. Sante Ardoini de Pesaro, *Opus de venenis*, p. 8.

228. S. Chojnacki, Crime, Punishment and the Trecento Venetian State, *Violence and Civil Disorder in Italian Cities...*, p. 213.

229. *Actes du Parlement de Paris, 1254–1328*, n 4826.

230. *Le secré de secrez*, éd. O. A. Beckerlegge, Oxford, 1944, p. 33. The text is perhaps inspired by the *Politique*, III, 7, where Aristotle speaks of physicians who fall into crime because of corruption.

231. *Annales de Saint-Bertin*, ed. Clémencet, Grat, Vieillard, Paris, 1964, p. 216.

232. Guillaume de Tyr, XVIII, 34, p. 879: *Nostri enim Orientales principes, maxime id efficientibus mulieribus, spreta nostrorum Latinorum physica et medendi modo, solis Judaeis, Samaritanis, Syris et Sarracenis fidem habentes, eorum curae se subjiciunt imprudenter, et eis se commendant...*

233. Albe, PJ XI; Isarn d'Escodata and Pons de Vassal, butlers in the pontifical palace, were supposed to administer the poison to John XXII.

234. Matthieu Paris, t. 5, p. 702 and sq.

235. *Chronique de France et de Flandre*, f. 11 v–12.

236. Jean d'Outremeuse, t. 6, pp. 140–146.

237. Monstrelet, t. 4, p. 399.

238. *Parlement criminel*, X2a 4, f. 143, 1341.

239. C. Gauvard, "*De grace especial...*," tableau 34, p. 619: total of 5 percent.

240. II *Cor.* VII:5, in *Historia calamitatum*, p. 106.

241. Jean de Salisbury, *Policraticus*, I, 10 and II, 28. See E. Peters, *The Magician, the Witch and the Law*, pp. 47, 54, 113.

242. Hugo Falcandus, *Historia sicula*, ed. Muratori, *RIS*, VII, Milan, 1725, col. 279.

243. Jean de Viktring, pp. 135–136: *fertur etiam quod a quadam nobili muliere confectum quoddam cibarium sumpserit, quo ipse rex in favorem sui mariti moveretur, in morbum impetiginosum corporis est mutatum, mortis materiam secum ducens.*

244. Cf. Étienne de Bourbon, *Tractatus de diversis materiis praedicabilibus*, n 434, p. 377.

245. See W. C. Jordan, Problems of the Meat Market of Béziers, 1240–1247, *REJ*, 1976, n°135, pp. 31–49; the papal text is p. 32, n 5; p. 43 for Béziers.

246. N. Coulet, Juif intouchable et interdit alimentaire, p. 215; Grayzel, t. 1, pp. 72–73 and p. 336, Council of Albi, 1254; let us recognize that the texts that Grayzel publishes rarely inspire prohibitions due to the risk of poisoning.

247. W. C. Jordan, Problems of the Meat Market..., p. 43: the meat sold by the Jews constitutes a supplement that is sometimes quite useful to the Christian market.

248. Grayzel, p. 74.

249. *Registres du trésor des Chartes*, JJ 81, f. 258 v.

250. S. Grayzel, p. 72, n 139 then p. 318.

251. Orderic Vital, t. 4, p. 130. Literary tradition gives in any case a Christian identity to the murderer (imaginary) of the confessor of the Holy Sepulcher. P. Aubé, *Godefroy de Bouillon*, Paris, Fayard, 1985, p. 336, completely invalidates the version of the poisoning of which Foucher de Chartres and Guillaume de Tyr are unaware.

252. Rigord, *Gesta Philippi Augusti*, ed. H.-F. Delaborde, Paris, 2 vol., 1882–1885, t. 1, pp. 116–117. Matthieu Paris, t. 5, p. 432 and p. 740; *Grandes chroniques de France*, t. 7, p. 140.

253. Guido da Vigevano, *Texaurus*..., f. 39: *Sarraceni omnibus modis conantur christianos interficere, specialiter veneno.*

254. *Grandes chroniques de France*, t. 6, p. 19: "they have always hated our people" (*de toz jors heent nostre gent*).

255. Aubry de Trois-Fontaines, *Chronique, MGH SS*, XXIII, Hanover, 1874, p. 805; Salimbene, p. 358.

256. Brocardus, *Directorium*..., p. 439.

257. Eudes de Deuil, *La croisade de Louis VII roi de France*, ed. H. Waquet, Paris, 1949, p. 36.

258. Rodrigo Jimenez de Rada, II, 17 (according to the *Historia Gothorum* d'Isidore de Séville), and III, 12.

259. See J. Heuclin, Violence et meurtres dans le clergé gaulois pendant le haut Moyen Âge, *Violence et religion*, s.d. J.-M. Delmaire et P. Cazier, Lille, PUL, 1998, pp. 131–150.

260. *Annales de Saint-Bertin*, p. 216; *Annales de Fulda*, p. 414; Flodoard, *Annales*, année 950 claimed poisonings of Louis le Bègue (879), Arnulf (899), and Lothaire d'Italie (950).

261. Douglas D. C., *William the Conqueror*, Londres, 1964, p. 408: "Poisoning as a method of political action in eleventh century Normandy."

262. J. Gillingham, 1066 and the introduction of chivalry into England, *Law and Government in Medieval England and Normandy*, Festschrift für J.-C. Holt (ed.), G. Garnett, J. Hudson, Londres, 1994, pp. 31–55. My thanks to the author of this study who kindly shared it with me.

263. S. Krüger, Krise der Zeit als Ursache der Pest? Der Traktat *De Mortalitate in Alamania* des Konrad de Megenberg, *Festschrift H. Heimpel*, Göttingen, 1972, t. 2, pp. 839–883, p. 841: Anglais accusés à Narbonne. See also J.-N. Biraben, *Les hommes et la peste*, t. 1, p. 58.

264. *Registre criminel du Châtelet*, t. 1, p. 474: Pierre de Thoulouse said that he received his poisonous mission from a certain hermit surrounded by Jacobins working for the English and the Flemish.

265. Secousse, p. 499: " 'I have in France few friends and many enemies who are also yours' said the King of Navarre to the Englishman" (*J'ay en France peu d'amis et beaucoup d'ennemis qui aussi sont les vostres* dit le roi de Navarre à l'Anglais).

266. Id., p. 410, confession of Pierre du Tertre: questioned about the coded language in the orders received from *le Mauvais,* he said that he did not know if the word "merchandise" involved treason, poison, or another evil deed (*a ce mot "marchandises" se tapisse traïson, venin ne autre malefaçon*). Further on, the accused party answered that he doubted that the word referred only to poison (p. 425).

267. Matthieu Paris, t. 2, p. 300 of the translation.

268. Pietro d'Abano, *De venenis,* chap. 4.

269. N. G. Siraisi, *Medieval and Early Renaissance Medicine,* Chicago-Londres, 1990, p. 176.

270. Matthieu Paris, t. 5, p. 23; Pierre de Zittau, p. 176; J. Glénisson, G. Mollat, *L'administration des États de l'Église au xive siècle. Correspondance des vicaires généraux Gil d'Albornoz et Androin de la Roche (1353–1367),* Paris, 1964, n 90, p. 39.

271. Monstrelet, t. 2, p. 273.

4

Horrendum scelus. An Abominable Crime

In the instructions given for the pretrial investigation for the trial of Hugues Géraud, April 22, 1317, at Galhard de Riez, Pope John XXII qualified the act that the Bishop of Cahors was preparing to commit against him as *horrendum scelus.*[1] This expression can be applied to crimes other than the crime of poisoning, in particular bewitchment, and is used especially with reference to a victim of high rank. It conveys the feeling of horror associated with poison unlike the more honorable crime of murder committed against an adversary able to defend himself and with cognizance of the accepted rules.[2] Somewhat different from contemporary society, which evaluates the atrocity of a murder by the number of wounds and the quantity of blood that has been spilled, such a sentiment of horror did not reflect only the emotion of the moment. The expression used by the pope is rooted in a judicial tradition coupled with a sensitivity based in medieval civilization. It is appropriate to see how horror was expressed before trying to understand what in the Middle Ages of the West made *toxicatio* a *horrendum scelus.*

A CRIME DESCRIBED IN SUPERLATIVES

In 895, the participants in the Council of Tribur considered the act of killing with poison, herbs, or evil spells of various sorts a *pessimus homicida*.[3] If the association of the crimes of poisoning and witchcraft suffices to prove that poisoning is not considered separately, it does not indicate that poisoning was not considered the most serious of all crimes, as early as the Carolingian era. Jurists of later centuries would classify poisoning precisely at the top of the list of all crimes of treason. This negative identity was expressed in different ways.

A *terribilis casus*[4] between the Extreme and the Unspeakable

Homicide by poisoning calls for an extreme vocabulary. Certainly, since the Late Empire, the rhetoric of horror is omnipresent and the vocabulary of high treason, in full revival after 1200, includes a generous amount of hyperbole.[5] The clerk who wrote the chronicle of Saint-Pierre d'Erfurt calls the alleged poisoning of Henry VII *scelus inmanissimum*.[6] But the comparative preceded the superlative in the qualification of *veneficium*.

The response by Antonin mentioned above stipulates that killing with poison is more serious than killing with a sword: *Plus est hominem veneno extinguere quam occidere gladio*.[7] Used again in 1317 by the distinguished scholar of civil law Jacques Duèze, the formula is not confined to the highest circles of the clergy. Present in certain prescriptive texts or in judicial commentaries from the end of the Middle Ages,[8] the expression can be found in acts coming from sometimes humble jurisdictions.[9] But the adverb "more" is only relative in its use with *veneficium*, this term often being used without a precise qualifier. Perhaps inspired by the *Theodosian Code*, Balde understands that this crime is "more appalling."[10] Aimini, Bishop of Avignon, believes that it is "more terrible" (1305) than a murder *cum gladio*.[11] About 1360, the statues of Forli state, like the majority of contemporary texts, that poisoning is "more" serious (*gravius*).[12] The expressions *scelus gravissimum* or *malum enormissimum* appear often.[13] The comparative is replaced by the superlative. Certainly, this vocabulary is shared among a vast group of crimes and has an objective connotation that is hard to define.[14] This fact does not prevent *venenatio* from belonging to the highest category of crime. As Jouvenel said during a trial in Parlement in 1423, it is a question of a *cas maxime*.[15]

Attached almost automatically to the very notion of crime,[16] the horror expressed by *horrendum scelus* is a moral obligation: *toxicatio* is to be abhorred and despised. Bertrand Aimini considers his canons' intrigues as *orrenda et detestabilia*.[17] A letter written by Charles V similarly qualifies the poison plot of 1378 as "*horrible et detestable*."[18] The Parlementary decree against Jehan Hardy, in 1474, multiplies the epithets to condemn the accused's "very horrible, execrable, damned, unjust, and detestable deed"(*tres horrible, execrable, damnee, inicque et detestable entreprise*).[19] Thomas Basin is of the opinion that the death of Charles of France is a *detestandum* crime.[20]

The idea that *veneficium* is a crime of extreme cruelty comes from the *Theodosian Code*.[21] *Saevitia* and *crudelitas* (a term that is etymologically inappropriate since it is linked to spilled blood) are used to characterize murder by poison. Grégoire de Tours called the death of the Bishop of Angoulême "cruel."[22] A Parisian chronicler spoke of the cruel conspiracy of the lepers,[23] the enemies of Louis XI grieved the "the cruel and inhumain death" (*mort cruelle et inhumaine*) of Charles de Guyenne.[24] John XXII expressed indignation at the *feralis sevitia* of Hugues Géraud and his accomplices.[25] Linked to this notion of savage bestiality, the idea of the lack of human qualities also emerged.[26] In the eyes of Ferretus de Vicenza, *toxicatio* was contrary to the sense of humanness,[27] not only by its high degree of cruelty but also because it reduced the poisoner to the rank of an insect or a reptile. The Creator provided certain animals with *venenositas*, but not men. Individuals who poison others thus committed a crime "against nature" in the broad sense that this expression took on at the end of the Middle Ages.[28] In 1305, the act of inquiry against the canons of Avignon ranked their crime among the *crimina quasi contra naturam*[29] as much in regard to the status of their victim as in their *modus operandi*. This hyperbolic language was also used in more obscure cases. It is with a "cruel and inhumane" poison that a monk of Ourscamp planned to kill his abbot in 1411.[30] In itself, poisoning took on a frightening dimension that words could scarcely describe.

Ferretus de Vicenza commented shortly after 1300 that poisoning constituted an unspeakable kind of death.[31] The category of *nefandum* incorporated the crime of poisoning serious beyond words.[32] This term was not reserved strictly for acts committed against the *majestas* but can be found with reference to the modest level of a Cistercian monastery where certain members were thought to have committed *plura nefanda* against an abbot, certainly the representative of divine authority.[33] However, it is necessary to admit that the term *nefanda* or *nefandissima* linked to this or that *venenatio* was used to label, in the vast majority of cases, poisonings committed against royal victims. For the inhabitants of Vaud [a Swiss canton], Amédée VII's physician perpetrated a crime that was *nefandissimum*.[34] The fact that the Religieux of Saint-Denis used this adjective concerning the poisoners of 1390 results from the fact that the attack on the common good, such as the poisoning of the waters of the kingdom, was equivalent to a crime of high treason, as the edict of June 1321 had already indicated, according to the Roman tradition (*Digeste*, XLVII, 11).[35]

Far from judicial science and from political speculation, the obscure Pierre du Tertre, the henchman of Charles the Bad (*le Mauvais*), gave the common perception of the hideousness of the crime: "the most evil in the world and the most heinous that there could be, no one would consent to kill him with poison" (*le plus mauvais du monde ou le plus hayneux qu'il pourroit avoir, il ne voudroit consentir a mourir de poisons*). Everyone agreed on the horror of "such a villainous and evil act" (*tel fait si vilain* [and] *si mauvais*).[36]

The Worst Kind of Treason

Speaking of poisonous plots brewing at the court of Bourgogne in the 1460s, the monk Adrien de But, a witness of these events, delivered this observation: poisoning is considered as treason of the worst kind.[37] Applied to many crimes in the Middle Ages, the qualification of *proditio* appears to be particularly linked to the crime of poisoning.[38] Specialists in law were the first to point it out: he who poisons mixes betrayal with homicide. With Balde, Italian jurists in the years 1300–1500 emphasized this relationship.[39] It is even essentially in its link with *proditio* that the extreme seriousness of murder by poison resided.[40] Legal texts agree with this opinion. The reproaches addressed to the poisoners of the Bishop of Avignon in 1305 were related to the *crimen proditionis*.[41] Poisoning was considered so nearly the equal of *proditio* that, in a letter addressed to the nobility of Florence, Alexander VI used the double expression *proditionem et veneficium* to designate the crime that nearly ended his life.[42]

In England, the *Act for Poysoning* of 1531 put poisoning temporarily at the rank of high treason after it had been catalogued earlier as a felony or *petty treason*.[43] This kind of betrayal with a floating definition was not at all limited to feudal law;[44] *venenatio* was also considered a felony. This was the word that came to Pierre du Tertre to designate the projects attributed to his master Navarre.[45] The poisonous plots of the king of England against Philippe Auguste were named in the same way.[46] This terminology was also favored in literary texts: the *Roman d'Alexandre* used it to describe Antipater's act.[47] Its use in the *Chronique parisienne anonyme* concerning the case of 1321 placed it in a clearly broader context.[48]

Whatever the words, the attachment of *toxicatio* to betrayal, the term that described the relationship of the victim and the guilty party, recurred constantly in stories and testimonies, and not only in the upper levels of society. The individual who poured the *virus mortiferum* for Alexander was called significantly *Proditio* in the *Alexandréide* of Gautier de Châtillon.[49] The expression "*occire en traïson*" (to kill in betrayal) in *Gaydon* means "to poison."[50] The case in 1313 puts in the forefront and brings to a climax the betrayal that was inherent in the murder of the emperor. The Jacobin accused of regicide was overwhelmed with abusive terms many of which emphasized the treachery of his deed: *pejor Juda traditore . . . traditor et insidiator pessimus, malignissimus traditor* or *infidelissimus*, all this to describe the "false" Preacher.[51] A chronicler from Languedoc considered the lepers to be unfaithful subjects acting against the common good and also against the royal majesty and called their plot *summa et inenarrabilis et nephanda proditio*.[52] Guillaume de Machaut called the act attributed in 1348 to Jews treason (*traison*) because, through the sovereign's goodwill, they were considered guests of the kingdom who turned against their benefactor.[53] Instinctively, a servant of Amédée VII cried out to the physician of Jean de

Grandville: "False traitor, you have killed our master."[54] Far from the political universe, the term came naturally from the pen of the tutor from Mantua, Italy, of 1379 plagued by the schemes of a wily student. The traitor in question, a simple agent of murder, was a kitchen worker but nevertheless *proditor*.[55]

Poisoning was in other respects often considered the manifestation of a general proclivity for treason. Treacherous by nature, the Lombards, like the Greeks were also recognized by most as poisoners.[56] The use of poison against Louis VIII by Thibaud de Champagne represented a more general felony manifested by giving up the *ost* before the end of the prescribed forty days. That was also the consequence.[57] Traitor to his king whose son he may also have poisoned, Pierre de la Broce was also in collusion with the King of Castille.[58]

Poisoning "signified... treason, trickery, total disloyalty" (*senefie..../ Trahison, tricherie, toute desleaute*) stated a poem about 1300[59] : treason not only of a "public" kind, by which one or several murderers attack the prince or his status, but also a private treason, committed in the heart of the *familia*.[60] Situated at the extreme end of abomination, close to the unspeakable, *veneficium* was nevertheless described as the *summum* of treason. One chronicle described Hugues Géraud as a "very bad traitor who had formulated a plot to kill Pope John with poison" (*tres pesme traistre qui avoit procuré à occhire pappe Jehan par venin*).[61] The use of the superlative owed as much to the kind of crime as to the rank of the victim.

Once again, the crime of poisoning was considered to be an absolute abomination. Its use was prohibited even among the worst of men. This treachery was so despicable that its use was forbidden even against a person who has returned illicitly from banishment.[62] The question of its use against tyrants received a mostly negative response. As for the murder of Tiberius, the opinion of John of Salisbury was ambivalent: even if detestable, *veneficium* can prove to be beneficial.[63] This idea is found in the writings of those individuals who talked about the poisoning of the "fiscal tyrant" that Philippe le Long was on the way to being,[64] and one can guess the same perspective behind the later account that Ranulf Higden gave concerning the murder by poison of John Lackland (*sans Terre*), killed by a lay person who was alarmed about the extravagant taxes planned by the Plantagenet.[65] It was shared at the beginning of the fourteenth century by Ferretus de Vicenza, based on theories from antiquity in a region where the "tyrants of usurpation" like the "practicing tyrants" were legion.[66] But, leaving pagan history and individual cases in order to discuss generalities, John of Salisbury adopted a clearly more negative position when he commented that poison is not lawful even against the most tyrannical prince: "I never read that permission was given to kill with poison" (*je ne leu onques que conge fust donné de occire par venin prendre*) says his text faithfully translated by Foulechat under Charles V.[67] As to be expected, the reasons he gives pertain to the treachery and disloyalty that were inherent in the crime of poisoning, which was totally contrary to Christian ethics. The expulsion of tyrants from power was permissible, provided that the operation did not occur to the detriment of the faith. But, poison was reserved for those who had nothing to do with divine law, the Infidels.[68] In the context of the assassination of Louis d'Orléans and connected to the dangerous theories developed by Jean Petit, Gerson cites the *Policraticus* in his **decretal** *Pro humani* in order to condemn, with *De assassinis* as support, all recourse to means contrary to morality even against someone immoral.[69] Consequently, poisoning was prohibited. Faithful to the opinion of John of Salisbury, the Gerson's statement expresses magnificently the absolute abomination of the crime of poisoning.[70]

THE REASONS FOR AN ABOMINATION: HOW TO KILL

No text explicitly develops the reasons for the appearance of *veneficium* in the category of horrible crimes. Its mention was sufficient in itself. Medieval thinkers obviously did not possess an anthropology of criminal poisoning, which would miraculously facilitate the task of assembling all the elements in a coherent mass. But it is likely that they had in their minds a certain number of these elements. Without a doubt, the particular modalities of the crime constituted a fundamental motif of its ranking among the *horrenda scelera*.

An Insidious and Secret Crime

The first operational characteristic of *veneficium* was its insidious nature. But, as Balde said, its clandestine nature increased the offense[71] and contributed to the perception of poisoning as an extremely serious act, *insidia*, par excellence.

In the Scriptures as in Canon Law and its commentaries, the formula *per insidias* was associated with *veneficium*.[72] Using a somewhat paradoxal vocabulary, Thomas Aquinas classified *veneni exhibitio* among hidden (*occulte*) aggressions.[73] Lay legislation repeated the idea if not the vocabulary. In an article on law enacted at the beginning of the eleventh century as a complement to the Lombard code of Rothari, the emperor Henry II included *veneficium* as a secret, hidden way of killing, the opposite of open combat.[74] Balde ranked the crime of poisoning in the category of *crimen occultum*, the opposite of acknowledged criminal acts committed openly.[75] Conforming to this perception, and probably also inspired by civil law,[76] legal texts used the term *insidias venenosas*.[77] The poisoner was a false *incidiateur*, an *insidiator pessimus*.[78] The superlative can be explained by the very process involved in poisoning. Armed with a sword or a dagger, the hidden aggressor was obliged to come out in the open upon the arrival of the person he wanted to eliminate. Aggression with poison, however, went beyond the stage of ambush, for it hid the murderer and his weapon and never revealed them.

The opposite of the sword, the dagger, the arrow, or the club, poison was hidden from sight and, if possible, from taste. Prepared according to hidden recipes, in out-of-the-way places and shrouded in the night,[79] it acted by means of a "hidden ingredient." Hard to distinguish in its effects from various illnesses, it left neither a wound nor a cut and ate away secretly at the victim from the inside. Ferretus de Vicenza condemned without appeal such a *modus necandi*: detestable and pernicious, poison meanders secretly through the body, consuming noiselessly intestines and entrails.[80] In this regard, as G. Duby has suggested, it is similar to enchantments and bewitchment.[81]

Poisoning also finessed violence and challenges, which were so closely linked to medieval homicide. Significantly, the assassins of Gilles de Bretagne contrasted poisoning and methods of "killing" (*fait meurtrier*).[82] Contrary to Roman law that curiously perceived *veneficium per vim infusum*, medieval texts observed the absence of *violentia extrinseca* in poisonous schemes.[83] Let us repeat the wording of *L'Estoire de Eracles empereur* concerning Richard of England: he wanted to attack Philippe Auguste "without laying a hand on him" (*sanz metre en lui main*)[84] : deprived of the ritual of challenge that normally preceded an aggression, poisoning goes against the norms of homicide. The *Etablissements* of Saint Louis contrasted "murder" (*murtre*) to homicide committed "in a scuffle" (*en mêlée*) and defined the first by the absence of a challenge or a quarrel.[85] This absence was the essence of the crime of poisoning. By disposing of a preliminary altercation, poisoning left the world of admitted homicide. By avoiding the challenge, it left the ritual of enmity practiced on the battlefield and also in a tavern or on the street.

Without having met obvious hostility, the victim was trapped, receiving innocently (*simpliciter*) and without realizing it (*incaute*) the fatal drink or food.[86] A passage from the *Miracles de Notre-Dame* presented in Paris during the fourteenth century contrasted bloodshed with herbs and poisons that were considered as the worst ways to make an attempt on someone's life.[87] That is because the struggle against the secret action of herbs and poisons was more difficult than dressing a wound. Hidden poison put the victim into a state of extreme vulnerability and made him incapable of defending himself. For Hippolite de Marsilis, the formula *Plus est* is partially explained by this.[88] In addition to the ignorance of the victim, the ambush with poison made use of his involuntary complicity. Of course, even in the early Middle Ages when the crime was treated most objectively, no text accused the person poisoned of inadvertently killing himself by taking the fatal poison. One finds only pity for the person who was rushed into death by emptying in one gulp the *poculum mortis* or by biting with enthusiasm the apple that has been poisoned.[89] A ***lettre de remission*** depicted a poor carder who drank a "full cup" (*pleine tasse*) of poisoned wine because of a fierce thirst from soup that was too salty.[90] One of the great cruelties of *venentio* lay in this involuntary collaboration of the victim with his own death. Moreover, the quick action of certain poisons mortified a second time the man or woman who absorbed it by depriving them of the rituals of a good death. "Often the good mouthful [poison] /...causes death to come suddenly" (*Souvent le bon bouquon /...la mort fait souldainement descendre*) observes Eustache Deschamps.[91] Composed at a time when the model of a good death was being disseminated, the *Chroniques de France* remarked concerning the poisoning of Thierry d'Austrasie: "the king drank the poison...he died immediately without confession and without repenting his great sins" (*le roy beut le venin...tantost fut mort sans confession et sans repentance des grans peches qu'il avoit fait*)[92] : a disastrous death that put the salvation of a soul at risk after having destroyed the health of the body.

Thus, the clandestine and insidious character of poisoning had multiple consequences. The least was not that it put everyone at risk of a sudden death, and in particular the most powerful: "No one can protect himself from a deadly traitor (*Nul ne se poeut garder de traître mortel*).[93] This situation spread terror. *Eramus omnes territi*, wrote Charles de Luxembourg concerning the episode of 1331.[94] The horror of *venenatio* came from its invisibility that made it a universal threat and equalized all social status.

Premeditated Homicide

In the fifteenth century, following an already long tradition, the jurist Felino Sandeo classified poisoning among the crimes committed *per industriam*, that is a crime committed deliberately and with planning, the opposite of "murder by chance" or an impulsive crime committed in a "free-for-all."[95] The canon had probably read the formula in the **decretals** or in the Bible that associates it with *per insidiam*, the turn of phrase examined above. Let us consider on what grounds poisoning constituted a homicide *per industriam* and what characteristics contributed to the horror it elicited.

Very early, **penitentials** and canon law were able to distinguish an act resulting from sudden anger (*iracundia subita*) from an action committed after premeditation, *ex odii meditatione*.[96] The ethic of intention, which was recognized first in the twelfth century, made the second kind of crime infinitely more serious than the first because it assumed a conception and a perseverance of the murderous will (*animus occidendi*) foreign to any examination of conscience.[97] Under the influence of the canonists and thanks to the rediscovery of Roman law that did not ignore the aspect of intention, medieval judicial thought slowly but surely began to consider this factor. Poisoning came out not only as a *homicidium voluntarium* but especially as a crime that is necessarily premeditated. Even if, in terms of penal classification, the notion remained uncertain and unclear for a long time,[98] it was inherent to *toxicatio*.

The story of the cobbler of Freiburg who decided to give poison to his wife in a sudden fit of temper was exceptional.[99] All other criminal poisonings appeared, even in the texts that tried to soften this aspect, as acts conceived over a long period of time and accomplished by *perseveracions et continuacious* as was stated about the accused of 1390.[100] In the twelfth century, Hugo Falcandus wrote that Amiral Majo thought about poisoning the Archbishop of Palermo, waiting for the right moment and the ideal place to commit his act.[101] "For a long time they had prepared deadly poisons" (*De long temps avoient appareillez poisons mortieux*) stated a chronicle about the criminals of 1321.[102] According to Michel Pintouin, the act that the King of Navarre had financed against the Ducs de Valois in 1385 was *precogitatum*.[103] The female protagonist of a case that occurred in 1493 "thought day and night how she could kill him [her husband] with poison" (*jour et nuyt pansoit comment elle le* [son mari] *pouroit faire morir par poison*).[104] Premeditation cannot be better illustrated; here it was almost an obsession. The delay between the decision to commit murder and the deed itself was evidence of a long preparation. The canons of Avignon who were planning a poisoning aborted their plan in March 1305 and committed the crime in August.[105] The chamberlain of Philippe le Bon, Jehan Coustain, who had planned his murder a long time in advance, gives evidence of a similar foresight.[106]

This slow maturation cannot be conceived without the presence of an inextinguishable and deeply rooted feeling of hate. Along with revenge that was linked to it, one encounters hate as an explicit motive in one out of nine cases. The Normandie of Orderic Vital is the setting of a veritable toxic feud.[107] As a judicial idea considered basic in the history of medieval criminality,[108] hate was certainly expressed in ways other than the use of poison, but at this time it reached its most extreme point, a fact already underscored by Quintilian.[109] Many poisoners shared the sentiment of Charles the Bad (*le Mauvais*) who declared to the agent he hired that he wished to poison "the one whom he hates the most" (*celui qu'il hait le plus*), that is, Charles V.[110]

The word *industria* also included the idea of the elaboration of a crime according to a murderous process that included its preparation, its organization, and its execution. The making or the acquisition of the poison, its transport, access to the victim, the concealment of the substance, the eventual recruitment of other agents—all the factors had to be taken into account, along with tests of the toxic material or of the victim's vigilance.

In his treatise written soon after the Black Plague, Konrad of Megenberg reported that the Jews had tried on pigs, dogs, and chickens the very violent poison (*toxicum mordacissimum*) that they planned to put into streams and wells.[111] Jehan Coustain took care to have the Comte de Charolais drink first a harmless *poculum* in order to confirm the possibility of a later poisoning.[112] The illustration of an Anglo-Norman manuscript of the *Roman d'Alexandre* from the beginning of the fourteenth century highlights this series of steps, for it presents, along with the scene of the fatal banquet, the moment of the preparation of the poison.[113]

It is not surprising that among the words frequently used to denote criminal poisoning one finds *machinatio* and its derivatives. Once again, this does not indicate that the vocabulary of "machination" studied closely[114] is exclusively linked to *veneficium*. Elsewhere, this vocabulary is associated above all with the higher levels of society. Nevertheless, it can be used for many different kinds of situations, but it is particularly well adapted to *venenatio*. Abélard used the term many times in his account of his ordeals at Saint-Gildas-de-Rhuys.[115] Orderic Vital spoke of the *machinamenta inimicorum* concerning the poisoning of the Comte du Mans and his wife.[116] Bernard Gui wrote concerning Hugues Géraud that he had "conspired" (*machiner*) with the goal of killing the sovereign pontiff.[117] Christine de Pizan said that a "certain prince" wanted "to plot with poison or other methods" (*machiner par poison ou autrement*) against Charles V.[118] In his defense of the killing of tyrants, Jean Petit used the word *machinatio* to designate the ensemble of the criminal activity of Louis d'Orléans. The account of Edmond de Dynter on the attempt of Jehan Coustain featured the terminology that had become almost consecrated to the crime of poison in condemning his *detestanda et abhominanda intoxicationis machinatio*.[119]

A poisoning implied debates and multiple contacts to organize the ruse (*fraus, nequitia*),[120] as well as *dolus*, a Roman judicial category that appeared often in writing,[121] and it is not without significance that the officially recognized poisoner Charles de Navarre had himself called *callidus* in his coded language.[122] The enemies of Benoît de Nursie met together in consultation. "Abominable negotiations" united various individuals around Hugues Géraud.[123] The members of the cathedral chapter of Avignon, led by the dean, the treasurer for the affair, discussed in the Episcopal palace itself the amount of money to give to the person who carried out the poisoning.[124] Jean de Hocsem, who was well acquainted with the law passed by Orléans, qualified with the words *nefancum commercium* (with the judicial meaning of connivance or collusion) the criminal process that ended up with the presumed poisoning of Henry VII, where money also played an important role.[125] The inquest held for Jean de Grandville condemned his dealings and deliberations that were quite well thought out.[126] The plotting, like the conspiring—another word often used by the chroniclers or legal judicial texts[127] —was not done alone. It presumed another common dimension of *intoxicatio*: criminal association.

Poisoning and Villainous Associations

Studies devoted to medieval criminality have shown that poisoning involves groups more often than individuals working alone.[128] At the end of the thirteenth century, *Britton* ranked the crime of poisoning among murders that required numerous accomplices,[129] the opposite of homicide *cum gladio*, which was more discrete and more direct.[130] In a ***lettre de rémission*** obtained in 1481 by a laborer in Agen, the supplicant admitted to having brutalized "a little" the witch-poisoner considered responsible for his suffering in order that she reveal why and with whom she had committed the poisoning of which he thought himself to be the victim.[131] The crime of poison was instinctively perceived as involving multiple actors. In a rather important proportion (about 20 percent of the cases), although less than for other forms of homicide, the crime of poisoning implicates several individuals in a long chain of complicity. This association with the goal of poisoning contributed to the evocation of horror, especially at the end of the Middle Ages. Behind the person who actually handled the poison was perceived the shadowy presence of the originator of the plot. In the earliest periods, the act of a Sédéchias against Charles the Bald (*le Chauve*) or that of the Sarrasin baker who murdered a Norman abbot of Calabria involved only them. Starting in the thirteenth century, however, with the cases that occurred in the entourage of the Staufens, the worrisome idea of a poisonous plot became clear. Few sources were satisfied with the identification of Bernadin de Montepulciano, but many saw acting in the shadows the Guelphic powers that were hostile to Henry VII. In the same way, the action alleged to have been committed by Jean de Grandville, "the main player on the job" (*le principal de la besongne*), reflected the behavior of powerful individuals who ranked above him in society.[132]

The villainous groupings had variable dimensions. They united poisoners who were lovers, personified at the top by the magnate Zawisch and Cunégonde, the queen mother of Bohemia (1278) or Jacqueline de Brabant and the Duke of Gloucester (1415).[133] At a lower rank in society, remarried couples formed similar criminal associations. Jehan de Bourgeauville and his new wife (criminal Parlement, 1402), Jeanne Beaupoux and Jehan Droillaut (1492), or the lovers from Lorraine Jehan Jacquot and Françoise le Noir in 1493 belong to this category.[134] Friendly or family ties united poisoners of all ranks. Several knights attacked the brother of the Lord of Amboise in 1152, two Visconti brothers against the third (1355).[135] Joining together with the purpose of poisoning went so far as uniting all, or at least part, of a monastic community: against Benoît de Nursie, Maurille, the future prelate of Rouen (about 1060) or a priest from Metz in 1399.[136]

Without taking proportions similar to those that Titus-Livy[137] mentioned, with one or two exceptions, and without uniting as many people as in the criminal gangs pursued by the authorities at the end of the fourteenth century, the association of poisoners on a large scale gave the crime worrisome proportions. A good example of this phenomenon was the tens or even hundreds of persons who were alleged to have wanted to poison the wells in the West in 1321. Seventy-five persons here, fifty persons there received instructions that were then transmitted to several patients back in the leper-houses.[138] As for the Jews in 1348, their involvement in poisonings was supposed to have operated in proportion to their presence in Western countries. The number of Jews created the same number of poisoners. Fourteenth-century minds were not far from convincing themselves of the existence of groups of "poisoners" (*gens venimeux*) who specialized in *veneficium* just as brigands and thieves were organized in another kind of criminality.[139]

In more than 40 percent of the cases, toxic homicide was not carried out by the instigator. This phenomenon was present from the beginning to the end of the Middle Ages but was accentuated from the thirteenth to the fifteenth centuries. This phenomenon did not reach this scope for other forms of homicide. It was at the origin of "contracts" that in general associated a powerful director and a humble executor. Hildebrand was provided with an executor of low poisonous works in the person of Brazutus.[140] Charles the Bad (*le Mauvais*) of Navarre almost always delegated the execution of his numerous poisonings, including one committed "at a supper in his own room" (*a un souper en la propre sale*) in 1365.[141] Recourse to others to execute the crimes, that is, to professional assassins, did not discourage the most determined. Certainly, the *modus operandi* of these hired killers that terrorized the Western princes depended on the use of daggers, sometimes dipped in poison.[142] But the Christian princes did not hesitate to turn toward the followers of the Old Man of the Mountain (*Vieux de la Montagne*) in order to skillfully give a poisonous substance to their enemies. King Richard was involved in intrigues in the Orient to eliminate Philippe Auguste in this way[143]; if one believes a pontifical letter, Manfred sent assassins armed with poisons to his enemy Charles d'Anjou (1264).[144] Those who sold poison in Venice were truly merchants of poison: ten million ducats were promised to a poisoner sent to kill François Sforza (1453); remuneration varied in proportion to the rank of the person to be killed.[145]

Complicity in a plot involving *veneficium* had as a more or less formal setting a clandestine *societas* with the goal of murder of which Aristotle speaks in *Nicomachean Ethics*.[146] The criminal pact associated the protagonists in a reflected and organized way, sometimes including an oath.[147] In 1321, one reads, an agreement (*accordement*) was passed with the goal of poisoning all of Christendom.[148] Certain sources mention the meetings of four "councils" or "chapters" during which lepers passed an accord with the Jews.[149] This ecclesiastic vocabulary, used also for heresy, illustrates the institutionalization of the crime. In 1348, the Jews were alleged to have constituted a sort of assassination "company" whose mission was set at a meeting held in Toledo.[150] On a regional scale, the authorities of Breisach claimed to have discovered a sort of league that united the Jews of the town to those of Strasbourg, Bâle, and Freiburg.[151] The same idea of the organization of a poisonous enterprise is seen again in 1390 with the declarations of the well poisoners who spoke of a large meeting held in Cherbourg. An accused man confessed: "there are several masters and governors who direct the job" (*ils sont plusieurs maistres et gouverneurs a gouverner la besongne*).[152] Linked like heresy and later witchcraft to the idea of a plot, which was at its height in the fourteenth century, poisoning proved to be a ramified *maleficium*. Even on a much more modest scale than the large cases of 1321, 1348, and 1390, it assumed a criminal dialogue with despicable terms. Without speaking of the Venetian methods mentioned above, the criminal association involved a concrete agreement. Sordid financial transactions added the scandal of a murderous negotiation to the horror of homicide. Transactions between equals: the canons of Avignon passed an agreement to organize and finance the elimination of their unfortunate bishop[153]; there was agreement on salary: "We will make you a rich man," said men in religious habits to a poor wretch in 1390, who was seduced by this promise heard through the ages.[154]

Poisoning and Criminal Practices

Contemporary criminality has pointed out the frequent tendency of subsequent offenses of users of poison, who were encouraged to confine themselves to this method of killing because of the inherent discretion of this *modus necandi*.[155] A certain Clément la Hure appeared before Parlement in 1341, accused of killing or having killed with poison Guillaume Ythier, his wife, a female servant, the parents of the plaintiff, and finally hired men who had become irritating.[156] This example of a *serial poisoner*, who had other ways to murder at his disposal, poses the question in an immediate way concerning the singularity of the poisonous act: does it occur only once or repeatedly?

In more than 75 percent of the cases, the accused claimed to have committed, attempted, or planned only one single poisoning in his whole "career as a murderer," which is certainly often difficult to know in its entirety. A toxic *habitus* linked to the horrible result of the crime is difficult to present as evidence, not only in regards to "objective" criminal behavior but also as a category of firmly held judicial opinion on the existence of a *habitus* offender deduced from Aristotlean and Thomist philosophy.[157] In the case of Etienne *de Vallibus*, accused of a triple poisoning spaced out over time,[158] as in the case of the poisoner of 1341, the proclivity to use poison did not elicit comment. In truth, the crime of poisoning was rarely the act of important criminals or individuals who were specialists in the use of poison. When individuals have committed several murders by poisoning, no discourse points out a special profile.

The question of singularity is posed in another way. To what degree was the *toxicator* adept at other methods of killing? Were these methods in harmony with the evilness of this deed? Only about one-seventh of those accused of multiple homicides used other weapons besides poison. As the weapon of a first murder, poison could be the last recourse because of the inadequacy of other methods. In the early Middle Ages, Brunehaut combined poisoning with several other forms of homicide.[159] Fredegonda diversified methods of killing to the point of mixing them up. While attesting the daggers plunged into poison used against Childebert or Sigebert,[160] Abélard claimed that his monks set various sorts of ambushes for him, as violent as they were clever.[161] In more modest milieux, poisoners also combined other ways of killing with their poisonous activity. The canon accused of having poisoned the Cistercian monks of Bellevaux-en-Bauges (1410) expressed the malice he felt toward other members of the community by numerous and diverse violent methods.[162] In the same way, Guillaume Gerfa of Freiburg brutally killed a little girl of four years before using poison on his wife (1483).[163] These forms of homicide appear to have only one thing in common with *venenatio*: the criminal, because of his evil nature, was ready to commit all sorts of murders, and he did not choose poison because he wished to avoid spilling blood. An example of this situation is the poisoner of 1404 who decided to have hired men kill his wife before coming up with the more practical idea of having her poisoned.[164] Other murderous methods did not necessarily have an intrinsic link with *toxicatio*, they sometimes were used simply as a result of its failure or its impracticality. The enemies of Pope John VIII went from poison to a hammer in order to achieve their goals and those of the heir of the throne of Jerusalem. Believing that they would not succeed with a potion, they decided to attack their victim during a chess game.[165] The assassins of Gilles de Bretagne "seeing that they were not likely to kill him with poison" (*voyans qu'ilz ne l'avoient peu faire mourir par poisons*), moved on to strangulation committed in the prince's private quarters.[166] The enemies of Guillaume de Flavy used in turn toxic substances and hand weapons to achieve their goal while their victim slept.[167] After observing that "no poisons could kill him" (*nulles poisons ne lui povoient nuyr*), René Colinet's mother-in-law massacred him literally in his bed (1469).[168] Like the Breton prince, like Charles VII's captain, the unfortunate man was killed in private. The criminal similarity is obvious here. This approach to murder preserved its insidious nature.

Philo d'Alexandria believed poisoners to be more reprehensible than those who murder with violence because of the connection of their deed with magic.[169] As stated above, witchcraft maintained a close lexical, judicial, and material relationship with poisoning. In the sixteenth century, Jacques Grevin still maintained that witchcraft seemed "to have some connection with poison" (*avoir quelque convenance avecque venins*).[170] The combination of the two crimes appeared effectively, as much against the same victim as against different victims. The lack of success of evil spells was supposed to have resulted in a recourse to poison with Bertrade de Montfort[171] and Louis d'Orléans who, "seeing that he had not obtained his damnable goal by evil spells, decided to have him (Charles VI) poisoned" (*voyant que par les diz malefices n'avoit point obtenu sa damnable intention, se converti a le* [Charles VI] *faire empoisonner*),[172] before resorting to violence.[173] Guichard de Troyes, Hugues Géraud (in case the poison didn't work),[174] Pierre de Latilly also associated *maleficium* and *veneficium* at the beginning of the fourteenth century. Individuals from lower ranks in society just as often committed both types of crime, such as Emeline la Hanriotte (1319) or Jeannette Nova, who was reputed to be adept with both poison and enchantments (1390).[175] A woman, who thoroughly disliked her husband, first used enchantment, then a potion, and finally mixed **realgar** with crushed glass, in a sort of *crescendo*, having gone from words to poison, passing by the intermediate mixture of a potion (1382).[176] In 1464, Perrissone Gapit, from the diocese of Lausanne, attacked her son-in-law with *verba sinistra et injuriosa* whose failure led to the use of poisoned pears.[177]

The witchcraft trials in the fifteenth century demonstrated the connection of the two crimes. In 1437, a woman appeared before the ***juge-mage*** of the Briançonnais region accused of being all at the same time *maleffica, veneffica, appostata, invocatrix demonum, filicida, fachureria, ydolatra*, etc.[178] Incantations gave a diabolic dimension to poisoning. Powder made concrete one of the possible forms of aggression by witchcraft.[179] However, an immense majority of the "acts" of witchcraft that appeared in court prove to lack any connection to poison, and the opposite is also true. In narrative sources, only about 7 percent of all cases of poisoning include witchcraft as well. In the archives of Parlement from 1281 to 1423, that I consulted, poison and witchcraft are associated in only one case out of ten. Out of all the poison cases collected, with all the sources mixed together, fewer than 15 percent of the cases pertain to poisoners who have also been accused of the crime of witchcraft. Hansen's collection contains no more than about ten cases (2.9 percent) that relate witchcraft to crimes of poisoning. Finally, out of nineteen trials of male and female witches from the shores of Lake Geneva between 1448 and 1498, only five present both crimes together. The association of the two crimes probably reinforced the contempt showered on the *veneficus*, who was contaminated by the hideous connotation of *maleficus*. It is doubtful that witchcraft was the origin of the accusation, even during the times of energetic prosecution of witches. If *veneficium* appears to be a crime associated with witchcraft (one of fifteen, as Bodin asserts[180]), witchcraft is far from appearing to be systematically a practice associated with poisoning.

The crime of poison had a reputation of singular horror for many reasons. First of all, the crime required both premeditation and perseverance for its accomplishment.[181] Secondly, from its point of conception, motivation for the crime inspired fear that was increased by the large number of cases that involved an organized plot carried out by several individuals. And finally, a whole range of occult activities could play a role in the act. The connection of *venenatio* with other dreadful deeds appears, however, far from being the first reason for the horrific perception of this crime. It was, first of all, the method of killing that put poisoning among the worst of crimes. But the horror that *veneficium* inspired was also linked to the goals that it served.

THE REASONS FOR THE ABOMINATION: OBJECTIVES AND EFFECTS OF POISONING

Since the time of John of Salisbury, medieval theoreticians of the terrestrial Cité often used organic metaphors. Gerson resorted to one when he stated that tyranny attacks the social body like a poison that circulates in an organism and finally destroys it.[182] In addition to illustrating the problem that retained the attention of the Parisian academic, the image offers a good example of the profound apprehension of *veneficium*, particularly during the last centuries of the Middle Ages. A common point united all the presumed poisoners: they used poison to destroy the link of trust that unites people.

The Destruction of Basic Social Units

We have seen how the crime of poisoning was a weapon of proximity that was often used among family members. Still, it is important to understand the criminals' motives and the social range of their acts. The crime of poisoning constituted an attack on the basic nucleus of medieval society that included the married couple, parents, and the *familia*.

In slightly more than 10 percent of the cases, the crime of poisoning occurred for family reasons with the vast majority involving spouses. Poisoning became a factor in a marriage disrupted either by infidelity or by dissension. Far from being an ordinary method to deal with adultery, poison was even so completely consistent with marital disputes.[183] A kinship existed between sexual deception, sometimes by the use of make-up or seduction potions very close to poison,[184] and dietary or pharmaceutical deception, which the criminal used when he abused the confidence created by intimacy. Emma, a fickle woman who was supposedly the poisoner of Lothaire in 986,[185] illustrates the coalescence of the two crimes that one also sees associated in judicial archives from the end of the Middle Ages[186] or in the brief news items dear to the chroniclers.[187] The link between intimacy and poisoning is also illustrated by men such as the Sire d'Ormoy in 1308, who became a murderer because of his misguided love (*ob amorem inordinatum*)[188] or the knight Robert Gui on trial before Parlement 1358–1360 for having sacrificed his legitimate spouse to his passion for a nun.[189] Several very young wives, such as Jehanne Gaigne (18 years) tried in 1382 or Willemine la Barbière (16 years), beneficiary of a ***lettre de rémission*** in 1459, wanted to escape from a situation that had become unbearable because of the brutality of their aged husbands whom they had married against their will.[190] Against nature and divine law, the poisoning of a spouse was a way to destroy a legal marriage, which was increasingly difficult to dissolve. The death of a spouse permitted a subsequent marriage, which had all the appearances of legitimacy. At the end of the ninth century, Boson, Marquis of Provence, dissolved in this way his marital ties in poisonous acid in order to be able to marry the daughter of Louis of Italy, whom he abducted[191]: a radical way to get around the prohibitions and avoid the problems of divorce experienced by Lothaire II.

In omni fratre tuo non habeto fiduciam (Jeremiah 9:4): with these words from Scripture John of Winterthur justified, in a somewhat forced manner, the presumed murder of Henry VII, who was certainly killed by a brother, but not his own, which the chronicler knew very well[192] but who wanted in this way to condemn the infidelity of a close associate. Hostiensis confirmed that parricide and fratricide surpass in horror all other murders.[193] In his discourse on the killing of tyrants, Jean Petit commented on the crimes of Louis d'Orléans made worse by his link with the victim[194] whereas the accusers of Louis XI were not mistaken to condemn the horrible fratricide represented by the poisoning of Charles de Guyenne "by someone who was naturally assumed to love him" (*par celluy qui naturellement estoit tenu de l'aymer*).[195] There also, poisoning represents a crime, which, the opposite of violent homicide, tries to appear as a work of nature in order to mask a murder that is against nature. And the same idea would apply to cases of parricide or infanticide by poison. *Toxicatio* then served lust that is no longer sexual but material. The stepmother "who causes the death" (*fait mourir faulcement*) of the child of a previous marriage was often motivated by a desire to deprive him of his father's inheritance[196]; similarly, the inheriting nephew advanced the date of the death of his aged aunt.[197]

By affecting the ties of *familia*, poisoning attacked another fundamental relationship in a society founded on the confidence placed in servants and their loyalty. Poisoning was based on a perversion of *fides*, an act of treachery, a word that was used sometimes to denote *toxicatio*.[198] Confidence and loyalty were not only diverted, but craftily exploited in order to commit a homicide. The alleged poisoner of the Bishop of Châlons in 1405 was his barber Guillaume de Béthune, in whom the prelate had complete confidence, to the point of making him the executor of his will.[199] Those who made an attempt on the life of Charles de Guyenne were those closest to him whom he trusted completely.[200] By corroding this link of service from the inside, the poisoner called into question not only one of the bonds between individuals but, at the same time, the psychology of social relationships, for he sowed a ravaging suspicion that led all masters to exclaim as did Frederick II when faced with the treason of Pierre de la Vigne: "Whom can one trust and with whom can one feel safe?"[201] If it is true that, different from the Antilles of the eighteenth century,[202] no conspiracy with the goal of overturning masters by poisoning them is known at the end of the Middle Ages, that did not prevent masters from being appalled by cases of trusted servants whose loyalty was undermined by promises and who subsequently poisoned them.

The bond that united the monastic family cracked in the same way under the action of *venenum*. The crime of poisoning often targeted an abbot bent on reforming his abbey: Benoît de Nursie was exposed to the refusal of his brothers to comply to his program of additional discipline (*illicita non lecere*)[203]; Maurille de Rouen was considered hateful by his rigor against those who transgressed the Rule Book,[204] and Abélard, who was concerned with improving the lifestyle of his Breton monks.[205] The crime of poisoning often targeted the reforming abbot. He was considered an intruder in the community that sought to expulse him as a foreign and disturbing body, because he brought a powerful spiritual medicine to a sick body, which in this case was the monastic group. The use of poison was the ultimate expression of disobedience. Brought into the heart of the Church, it threatened to dissolve the very fundamentals of communal life and it was not by chance if the correspondent of Pierre de Celle used, in the twelfth century, the image of *toxicum mortis* planted in the center of the cloister garden to speak of the peril that threatens life within a monastery.[206]

The Corrosion of the Political Body

Amidst the superior social organization found in the political community, the use of poison put immutable and providential order at risk. Poison worked to corrode the links forged by institutionalized loyalty and also the links put in place by hierarchy, which was disturbed by the unjustified rise of unworthy people. Poisoning was distinguished from other forms of political crimes, for, from the very fact of its dissimulation, it delivered no message, quite the opposite of the murder of the Duc d'Orléans by the men of John the Fearless (*sans Peur*). Neither claimed nor justified, poison served unmentionable and illegitimate ambitions, which reflected an imbalance in the institutions of power in the grip of tyrants and usurpers.

Whatever their particular goal, the immense majority of political poison cases were naturally motivated by a thirst for power, which motivated, for example, Charles de Navarre.[207] The desire for power was at the source of more than 18 percent of the crimes (30 percent of the indicated motives) and it played a role throughout the whole era. Sabin was killed by a man burning with the ambition of becoming bishop.[208] The murderous monks of Raffred de Farfa operated *ob ambitum honoris* against an abbot who was an energetic reformer of the worldly side of his abbey, which through worldly connections had become a more profitable entity.[209] The Countess of Castille betrayed her father and her son with poison because of her ambition to possess a "royal" title, in this case that of the wife of an emir[210]; Robert Guiscard's wife was supposed to have poisoned her husband in the hope of becoming *basilissa* by favoring the victory of Alexis Comnène over the Normans in Sicily.[211] The foolish and blind ambition and greed for domination for which Basin reproached Louis XI, at the time of his brother's death,[212] motivated a large number of poisoners. Poisoning manifested and demonstrated an imbalance in the exercise of power.

At the top of the hierarchy of the Church, the unlimited ambition of Hildebrand, who was known later for his authoritarianism through the proimperial sources, led him to have a half-dozen pontiffs poisoned. The very rigorous Episcopal government of Bernard de Castanet was manifested, in the words of his enemies, by the poisoning of numerous persons who resisted him.[213] Among the poisonous princesses, recourse to poison reflected a *cupiditas dominandi* that followed the natural bent of all authority.[214] It exemplified the figure of the domestic tyrant denounced by preachers at the end of the Middle Ages.[215] Inspired by the "malice" of Eadburh, the people of Wessex refused to accept an appointed queen, who sat at the side of her husband, before the feeble Ethelwulf, who was totally subservient to the daughter of Charles the Bald (*le Chauve*), could restore the title and dignity of the queen.[216] Louis d'Orléans' appetite for power was blamed for his crime of *toxicatio*. Certainly, poison was included among enchantments and other methods claimed to have been used against Charles VI, but its repeated use particularly indicated the nature of a man who was accused of wanting with all his being to "wear the hat of fine gold" (*porter le chapeau d'or fin*), as the *Pastoralet* says.[217] An imminent figure among Italian despots during the Renaissance, Sigismond Malatesta made poison an integral part of his tyrannical reign.[218]

The link between tyranny and poison is illustrated by a famous fresco executed at the end of the 1330s by Ambrogio Lorenzetti in the public palace in Siena. On the wall that represents Bad Government, the tyrant is shown with a devil's features carrying a cup of poison and surrounded by allegories that include *Proditio*.[219] The painting reflects without doubt the thought of political poisoning as a manifestation of tyranny. John of Salisbury's *Policraticus* linked poison to tyranny by a simple metaphor.[220] The representations are more precise. Whereas Aristotle spoke of the physical elimination of his enemies without granting real importance to the methods when writing about the misdeeds of a tyrant, Gilles de Rome wrote at the end of the thirteenth century, in his *De regimine principum*, faithfully translated by Henri de Gauchy, that tyrants "destroy and poison their own brothers as well as those who are close to their lineage in order to have their possessions and their heritage" (*detruient et enveniment lor propres freres et ceux qui lor sont pres du lignage por avoir lor possession et lor heritage*).[221] This comment shows a particular sensitivity to the poison used by tyrants, echoing perhaps the problems of the Staufen with the papacy of whom Gilles was to be an ardent defender. Note, however, that the translation of the *Politique* made by Nicole Oresme nearly a century later gives a disappointing gloss of the word "tyran."[222] A passage in Gerson's famous *Vivat Rex* also uses the poison metaphor to describe tyranny and its devastating effects on the body of the kingdom that it literally empties of its vigor by drawing everything to itself.[223] And in the Italian coups d'état, Pogge considered *toxicatio* a vice linked by nature to the abusive and excessive power of tyrants.[224]

Poison contributed to the insidious establishment of a new order that obeyed in appearance the laws of nature and divine power while in reality human will was being substituted for them. In the highest ranks of the Church, the usurpation of the tiara was in play: the only motive for the poisonings alleged to have been done by Hildebrand was his desire to become pope, realized only after six murders because the pontifical elections did not satisfy his desires and ambitions. On lower levels of the ecclesiastic world, the poison of usurpation appeared just as often. According to Grégoire le Grand, the Archdeacon Frontin acted surreptitiously to take the place of the aging Bishop of Canossa.[225] The same motivation pushed Fonton to have the Bishop of Angoulême poisoned.[226] Among the regular clergy, the ardent desire to seize abbatial or priorial functions motivated the *toxicatores*: at Farfa, the poisoners of Abbot Raffred, even though he was quite aged, did not have the patience to wait for him to follow the path of all flesh, so great was their appetite for power,[227] an extremely serious way to force the hand of God, if it can be said that way. From the twelfth century on, the tensions caused by the growing stakes of ecclesiastical power were settled notably by the means of *poculum mortis*.[228] Even prioral dignity inspired secret homicide: for example, Guichard de Troyes in Provins.[229]

In lay political society, controlled in numerous places by the laws of nature (such as primogeniture succession), poison was a way to violate them while leaving the impression that they have acted. During the late Middle Ages especially, there were numerous examples. In 1317, Mahaut d'Artois was suspected of having used poison against Louis X in order to open the way to the royal throne for his son-in-law Philippe le Long.[230] The prince on the throne of Armenia set a poisonous trap for the widow and children of Jean de Lusignan (1344) in an attempt to maintain his illegitimate position of power by killing the legitimate heirs of the previous king.[231] During the Valois regime, a similar attempt was attributed to the members of the royal family who were inconsolable that their birth put them in a secondary position. According to the late account of the canon Zantfliet of Liège, a person very close to the crown (Louis d'Anjou?) poisoned Charles V, who was then without an heir.[232] The poisonous attempts against Charles VI and also against the Dauphin attributed to Louis d'Orléans had the purpose of changing the succession to a throne also desired by his wife. Nasty tongues said that the Duchesse Valentine Visconti "was jealous and envious... and wanted her husband to have the crown of France, by whatever means was necessary" (*estoit envieuse et convoiteuse... et volontiers eust vu que son mari fust parvenu à la couronne de France, ne lui chailloit comment*).[233] This scenario is so ordinary that, from the distant town of Lucerne where he was writing his chronicle, Diebold Schelling attributed, almost by instinct, the death of Charles VIII to the second Louis d'Orléans who became Louis XII.[234]

Queens and princesses who instigated poisonings entered into these usurpation plots for themselves or for their progeny. They abandoned an auxiliary and/or occasional role of legitimate substitute for a weak or immature masculine authority in order to exercise an unwarranted authority or influence. Because they were more often implicated in power struggles, the Frankish queens appeared to have been involved in more poisoning schemes than the princesses of the fourteenth or fifteenth centuries. The texts that tell the story of Eadburh explain that she used poison to get rid of her husband's advisor who had become too influential.[235] Centuries later, it is said that the wife of Philippe de Valois "acted like a king and caused to be destroyed those who displeased her" (*estoit comme roy et faisoit destruire ceulx qui contre son plaisir aloient*),[236] notably by poison.[237] These princesses are the reincarnation of the *venefica* Jezebel,[238] the queen of Israel who remained pagan and having achieved through enchantments (this is the meaning of *venefica*) a complete hold on her husband Ahab—the inversion of the natural order of a couple—whose seal she hid in order to be able to command at her will,[239] like Bertrade de Monfort and Jeanne de Bourgogne.[240] The other plan of usurpation pursued by the poisoning princesses is to promote their progeny at the expense of the natural heirs. Marcatrude eliminated a son that her husband Gontran, King of Bourgogne, had with a first wife, with the goal of assuring her own son a royal future.[241] Bertrade de Montfort, the stepmother of the future Louis VI, was thought to have attempted to poison the legitimate heir of Philippe I, who succumbed to her charms, in order to put one of her own children on the throne.[242] Nearly two centuries later, Marie de Brabant, the second wife of Philippe III, was thought to have caused the death of the heir Louis de France "with the intention that the children that the king has and will have with this queen be the heirs of the kingdom of France" (*en cele intencion que li enfant que li roi a et aura de cestre roine soient hoir dou reaume de France*).[243] With this same goal, Yolande de Nevers disposed of the only son of Robert de Béthune, who cried out at the news of the death of his heir: "his stepmother caused his death wrongfully so that her children could have my heritage" (*sa marastre l'a fait mourir faulcement affin que ses enfans ayent mon heritaige*).[244] Furthermore, the murder of the stepson brings up hypothetically the question of an uncertain future for the stepmother: a question of physical safety, of course, but also an issue of political position that was strengthened by the ascension to the throne of a young son who would need his mother as regent.

Political society was composed of those who served the prince to whom the crime of poisoning permitted not the accession to the supreme power but a reinforcement of their influence on him or at least a maintaining of this influence. In this way, they managed to escape unlawfully their subordinate social position acquired at birth. From the end of the twelfth century, the *Roman d'Alexandre* asked its reader to extract the lesson from the misfortune of the Conqueror: "never must a man glorify a serf nor raise him above his station" (*ja nus hom ne doit serf essaucier ne lever*).[245] Under Philippe III, the story of Pierre de la Broce is interesting. Those (Guillaume Guiart and Primat) who presented him as the poisoner of Prince Louis implied that the fear of a succession that might take away his eminent position, *secundus post regem*, was not strange as a motivation for his action.[246] Born into a lowly social state, Guichard de Troyes incarnated another example of a poisoner who wished to maintain his position near the height of power. He held a seat in Parlement, in the Council, and was a party to the secrets of the queen Jeanne.[247] Vexed by a first disgrace that occurred following a murky financial affair[248] and anxious about the accession of Prince Louis to the position of Comte de Champagne,[249] he was alleged to have had killed with poison or enchantments the two princesses of Navarre, and to have attempted to attack the sons and the brother of King Philippe le Bel in order to regain his positions. Jehan Coustain, an influential person in the duchy of Bourgogne and "totally unworthy of his high position" (*tout indigne de son eslevement extreme*), was reputed to have used poison in order to prevent the ascension of the heir of Philippe le Bon. The hostility of the Comte Charles de Charolais, who wanted "order in his house," toward the wife of Coustain, Isabeau Machefoin, a member of the countess's household, gave a foretaste of what awaited the *valet de chambre* after the disappearance of a protector for whom he served as first valet.

His ascension blinded him to the horror of a crime that served unlimited ambition.[250]

In Roman Antiquity, recourse to poison did not occur, in theory, to influence the result of a battle. As Thomas Basin remembered, the enemy of Pyrrhus, Fabrice, had proudly refused this detestable method of scoundrels, commenting on the duty to win by the single virtue of regular combat, for *toxicatio* was the crime of cowards and the depraved.[251] In the Middle Ages, the use of poison reflected the crisis in chivalry when it intervened in military conflicts among Christians. It was not by chance that a work that was supposed to illustrate this crisis, *La mort le roi Artu* (*The Death of King Arthur*), presented a knight who wanted to poison his enemy Gauvain.[252] The opposite of a fair combat on an enclosed field, the poisoning of warriors conveyed scorn of the ideals underlined by the ideology of the sword that promoted the challenge in a prescribed form, respect for the enemy and loyal confrontation in order to win a cause. For poison to disturb this order of things falsified not only the scale of military values but muddled the judgment of God. Its use sanctioned the powerlessness of weapons (the original meaning of *nequitia*) to the benefit of deceit.[253]

Late Breton historiography explains that in 981, the Comte de Bretagne Conan had poisoned the Bishop and Comte de Nantes Guérech because he was unable to defeat him "on the battlefield" (*par bataille*).[254] The *Roman de Brut* by Wace presented the poisonous scheme of the Saxons who fought against Uther at the end of the fifth century: "They want to kill Uther by poison, / By poison or by treason / For they do not trust their weapons / To kill him" (*Murdir le[Uther] vulent par puison, / Par venim u par traïson / Kar en lur armes ne se fient / Tant que par lur armes l'ocient*).[255] The Comtesse de la Marche sent agents to poison the food of Saint Louis because her husband was incapable of conquering him on the field of battle.[256] According to the continuator of Géraud de Frachet, the allied enemies of the emperor Henri de Luxembourg employed Bernardin de Montepulciano because they were unable to oppose the sovereign's victorious campaign.[257] The confession of Jacques de Rue in 1378 shows that, having decided against making open war against Charles V after the battle of Cocherel, his rival from Navarre planned to act by a more discreet and perhaps more efficacious method. In 1382, Louis d'Anjou's rival, Charles de Tarente, preferred to send a poisoner to the Valois prince rather than to confront him in a combat whose outcome was in question. But, in order to hide his cowardice, he ordered the criminal to simulate a battle challenge to his victim in order that he might be able to approach him[258]: one cannot be further from the rules and rites of noble warfare while pretending to follow them. It was the Anglo-Flemish military weakness that, according to an accused in 1390, was at the origin of the plot to poison the wells: "The people of Flanders do not see how they can harm and get revenge on the king of France and his allies if not by poison" (*Les gens de Flandre ne regardent pas et ne pevent veoir que autrement ils puissant grever ne avoir vengeance du roy de France ne de ses alliez se ce n'est par empoisonnement*).[259] Jean de Roye finally explained that the Duc de Bourgogne came to the point of wanting to poison Louis XII when he "understood that he did not have the strength to succeed in destroying the kingdom of France" (*voyant qu'il n'avoit pas puissance de parvenir a destruire le royaulme de France*).[260] These multiple examples, which concern significantly more the end of the Middle Ages, certainly do not support the arguments of those who are nostalgic about chivalric war and who blame the decline of values. They illustrate nevertheless the threat against the rules of ethical combat that the princes of the West tended to forget when they lowered themselves to behave like pagan potentates.[261]

As Eustache Deschamps said in a striking oxymoron, the poisoner is only a "bold coward who lacks courage" (*hardi couard failli de cueur*), bold because of the impudence of his deceit, coward by the cowardly method that he used because he lacked virtuous courage.[262] *Couart* (Coward) was the name of the senechal who was the accomplice of the vague poisonous desires of the evil empress in *Florent et Octavien*.[263] And significantly, cowardice was used to characterize certain of the groups that were reputed to be adept at poison, among which the Lombards held an important position. On the contrary, the chivalric heroes of literature never used poison, even for coating the surface of their weapons. By becoming involved in war, poison, like mercenaries, put chivalry seriously at risk. It is possible that those who condemn "poisonous Italy" as the country of the *condottiere*, preoccupied with saving their strength by any way possible, are unconsciously linking the use of mercenaries to replace citizens who no longer used arms with the use of poison as another way to avoid the battlefield. The chroniclers of Savoie related the strategy of the Visconti against Comte Amédée VI at war in his States (about 1375).[264] As for the Aragonese inhabitants of Naples, they would not have found any other means than poison put in the water supply by the Jews and the Moors to resist the French invaders in 1495.[265]

Especially in France where the prince owed his crown solely to the divine will that caused his birth, reign, and death, recourse to poison was seen as originating in conceptions of power totally against nature. Practiced in the entourage of the Prince, the crime served the evil ambitions of upstarts who, as one chronicler wrote about Coustain, poisoned the air, a superb image of the almost pathological corruption of political society.[266] Practiced by the Prince, it lowered him to the rank of the ignoble, the varlet,[267] and the Infidels, far from the true path of virtue (Thomas Basin),[268] and thus seriously disturbed the order of the Christian world. In this way, poison invaded the organism. Gerson's image is decidedly well chosen.

The Poisoning of Christianity

The modalities and the motives of *venenatio* explain for the most part the horrified perception that most people held for the crime. But at the end of the medieval era, the crime was all the more abhorred because it referred to a double enterprise, external and internal, of the destruction of Christianity in the grip of the enemies of the Cross and of the Devil, the enemy of all good things.

Beyond the quarrels among the Christian princes, the relations of the Christians with those disloyal to the law of Christ were marked, as we have seen, by the use of poison by this last group. The weapon appeared as an element of massive destruction—upon reflection, the only one of the Middle Ages—that attacked from the exterior as from the interior "those of the West" (Eustache Deschamps), as an insidious and disarming virus. The Infidels, strangers to the norms of combat and incapable of conquering the Christians militarily, used poison in their attempt to destroy Christianity. The emir of Cordoba (al-Mansour, a powerful supporter of the califat of the Omeyyade dynasty from the second half of the tenth century) intended to destroy Christian power in the North by doing away with the Count and his son, with the help of the poisonous Countess of Castille Ava de Ribagorça. This treacherous princess began by giving her husband's horse bran to eat, so that in the heat of battle, the animal would weaken under its master putting him at the mercy of the enemy. As for the son, he was to eat a *poculum mortis*.[269] The desire to poison Christians with powders becomes evident at the time of the alert of contaminated pepper in 1245 and then again during the absence of Saint Louis who had left on Crusade: in 1250, poison was found on the cadaver of one of the leaders of the the Shepherds' Crusade (*les Pastoureaux*) as well as on letters from the Sultan of Babylon with whom the "Master of Hungary" had made an agreement with the goal of giving up the kingdom to the Muslims by poisoning the inhabitants.[270] This phase in the middle of the thirteenth century announced the crises of the first half of the following century. In 1321, the "Sultans" of Grenada and Babylon (or Tunis) believed that poison was the ideal way to annihilate the combativeness of the Christians, who were in the process of chasing the Infidels out of Spain.[271] A letter indicated that as soon as the Christians were weakened by the powders thrown into the wells, Muslim forces were to besiege the West that would then be delivered into the hands of the Islamic Empire.[272] The fruit of fantasy and manipulation, the document nevertheless reflected the association of poison with the destruction of Christianity.

The Muslims of the Orient used the same methods. In the Holy Land, the Infidels put poison in the Christian camps: the death of Godefroy de Bouillon, the difficulties of Richard of Cornwall or of Saint Louis whose food was the object of poisoning attempts[273] are examples of the enemy's use of poison against Christians. When the Turkish threat succeeded that of the sultans of Egypt or of Spain, the master of Constantinople was thought capable of attacking Christianity by poisoning it in its heart, in the fountains of Rome (1490).[274]

Inside the West, the Infidels had relays and accomplices whose goal was to put the populations out of condition to defend themselves. After the affair of the Shepherds' Crusade (*les Pastoureaux*), several linked episodes conveyed, in the course of the fourteenth century, the fear of the destruction of Christianity by the work of a poisonous enemy nestled in its bosom and increasing in size. In 1321, the lepers' plan was to infect the healthy population in order to seize the kingdoms and domains of the West in order to eventually turn them over to the Infidels. Although skeptical, Bernard Gui indicates that the lepers were dividing up villages and castles in advance.[275] Also solicited by the King of Grenada to help conquer Christian kingdoms,[276] the Jews had had for a long time the reputation of maintaining a close alliance with Islam for whom they appeared to be the advanced column in the West.[277] The specter of a fearful, poisonous coalition of Jews and Muslims was operating at full tilt. The reunion of two incarnations of corporal and spiritual poison with a third armed with literal poison nearly destroyed the world.

In 1348, this destruction became concrete in the plague. In an extension of the affaire of 1321, the accusations grew to a universal scale against *Judée la honnie* (Guillaume de Machaut), a peril barely avoided twenty-seven years earlier. The accused gave astounding confessions revealing that the basic reason for the crime ascribed to them went beyond the simple hate invoked for the particular poisonings.[278] This time the goal was to take back the scepter of monotheism from the Christians. Gilles Li Muisit tells that a Jew from the entourage of the Duc de Brabant, who had falsely converted to Christianity, confessed to having sought the triumph of his sect by poisoning water, which Jean le Bel affirms that he did "in order to have the authority and wealth of the entire world" (*pour avoir la seignourie et l'avoir de tout le monde*).[279] The episode of 1348 inspired a discourse certainly contested by a number of physicians or political leaders, but significant in that it demonstrated an obsessive fear of poison, a weapon that made concrete the great anti-Christian conspiracy that appeared as early as 1321. This perception of the world with apocalyptic ramifications[280] can also be seen in the fear of a plot by witches in which poison also played a role.

For Chaucer, recourse to poison demonstrated the presence of the Devil in the world.[281] Linked indeed in many ways to the devil, the crime of poisoning constituted in several respects a manifestation of the hold that he (the devil) attempted to extend over all Christians. The Sarrasin baker of Orderic Vital acting *instinctu diabolico*[282] could lead one to believe that the devil is behind every poisoner. But it is a question of a stereotype that can be seen also in the ***lettres de rémission***. Other evidence exists of the relationship of poisoning with satanic conspiracy with the goal of wiping out Christianity. Even if it was not furnished by Lucifer, all poison was somewhat *venenum diaboli*, a figurative expression that frequently appears in the Scriptures, the **penitentials** or the religious works that designate sin sometimes represented by poison: thus the enemies of Saint Samson, full of satanic poison, attempted to use literally a poisoned substance.[283] The figure of the snake, the poisonous and diabolic animal par excellence,[284] as well as the figures of the toad, a demonic and toxic creature[285] found in various potions, refers back to both the devil and poison. The iconography of Saint John reflects perfectly this equivalence since small dragons, representing the spirit of Evil, are escaping from the cup from which the apostle is removing the poison with a sign of the cross.[286]

The hand of the Devil was behind the gigantic poisoning attempted in 1321. Interrogated by the inquisitor Jacques Fournier, Guillaume Agasse, the commander of the leprosarium of Lestang, spoke of the poisons, charms, and potions destined to kill those who drank from the infected water.[287] When the composition of the powders included communion wafers, witchcraft immediately came to mind. As part of the plot, the Jews had been considered for a long time as the followers of Satan.[288] In 1390, the interrogators at the Châtelet suspected strongly that the poisoners of the water had drawn magic signs on the wells and fountains that were to be infected, thus showing that they were serving the Devil.[289] The trials of witches in the fifteenth century demonstrated that the judges were convinced that the Devil acted invisibly and secretly. C. Ginzburg has established a clear parallel between the accusations of 1321 and 1348 and the collective accusations of witchcraft that became more frequent during the following century,[290] for example against the the Vaudois (or Waldenses) accused of using enchantments and poisons against the Dean of Notre-Dame d'Arras, Jacques Dubois, (1461) or the wells and fountains.[291] While many other means were available to the *malefici*, poison belonged to the weapons of conspiracy whose goal was to help the Prince of Darkness triumph.

The demonic threat did not come only from the servants of the Devil who were acting en masse. The characters in Chaucer's tale have nothing to do with demon worshippers. They reflect simply the alarming extension of the sin with which the Devil *venenator* has infected man since the Fall. According to Alexander Nequam, sin inspired by the devil has the status of a spiritual poison much more virulent than a material poison.[292] The crime of poison was a way to satisfy the most serious yearnings to sins, which were, in fact, poisons of the soul. Envy was sometimes invoked as the motive for murder.[293] Grégoire le Grand went so far as to depict the crime of poisoning as the highest expression of envy.[294] For Laurent d'Orléans, envy poisoned everything, from the heart to words, and from words to acts,[295] a concept that is not surprising after consideration of several cases. In the *Speculum exemplorum*, the first *exemplum* of the section dedicated to *invidia* is the poisoning of Saint Benedict.[296] There are many factual examples. Benoît de Sainte-More wrote that the enemies of the Norman Richard III "poisoned him because of envy" (*l'empoisonnerent par envie*).[297] The Bishop of Valence succumbed in 1239 to *insidiae invidorum*.[298] The murderers of Gilles de Bretagne attempted to poison him "because of greed, envy, ambition, and unbridled desire" (*pour cupidité, envye, ambicion et desir desordonné*).[299] Of course, another important sin, greed (or covetousness) could motivate generously rewarded poisoners as well as vile persons like Coustain or Chaucer's valets. But this sin infected also Charles the Bad (*le Mauvais*) or Louis d'Orléans[300] and, linked to the betrayal of the worst kind,[301] it motivated equally those who in principal were committed to poverty. It was the greed for gold that led Roman monks to poison a religious of Saint-Evroult, despite all monastic values.[302]

A poem of uncertain date (about 1280?) entitled *De triacle et de venin* (*Concerning* treacle *and poison*) indicates that the word "*poison*" ("*venin*") means pride, envy, covetousness, gluttony, lust, a way of saying that "venin" refers to sin as such.[303] In a certain sense, crimes of poisoning committed by all levels of society symbolized a spiritual poisoning. "The world is sown with the poison of sin" (*Par venin de pechié est enherbez li mons*) says the same poem.[304] It could be added that heresy was another poison that had crept into the Christian community. In the rhetoric of the clerks, the heretic had had the reputation for a long time of sowing the poison of his evil doctrine by coating the most noxious words with honey.[305] Accused of having poisoned Benedict XI, the heretic Bernard Délicieux was among those who, with the appearance of lambs, acted like wolves.[306] The ability of people like him to mask their true nature led them eventually (but, in fact, rather rarely[307]) to participate in hidden crimes. However it may be, Satan and his servants introduce Evil into the universe just as a poisoner introduces surreptitiously poison into the organism of his victim. *Malitia* has good reason to be a common term used by theologians and authors of treatises on poison.[308] The poisoning of Christianity is implied in all the meanings of the expression.

The horror of *toxicatio* was linked, in a more or less explicit way, to the goals that its enthusiasts pursued. C. Boujot observes correctly that poison decomposed the social body as it did the human body.[309] The users of poison appeared to launch an assault against the medieval social body, in all its parts. The perils that obsessed people's minds no longer appeared to be the residues of paganism, as they were seen to be in Carolingian times: in 829, in a message addressed to Louis the Pious, the bishops of the empire blamed the persistence of enchantments, divinations, and other *veneficia* on the incomplete eradication of pagan practices and beliefs.[310] *Veneficium* had become a faceless threat in the process of annihilating Christianity without a warning shout.[311]

In a fictional defense speech in the *Declamationes* by the pseudo Quintilian, the defender of a man accused of poisoning points out that after all, this crime is the gentlest of all: no blood, no violence, no wounds or mutilation, no fear felt by the victim who is killed by surprise.[312] One would have difficulty finding similar comments written by a medieval pen in the Western world. Without any doubt, *veneficium* was a "horrible and wrongful deed" (*horrible méfait*).[313] To explain this perception, it is necessary to reconstruct a cultural substratum, of which the sociology of the imaginary is only one of the components. There is a judicial tradition that goes back farther than the Middle Ages. There are industrious, insidious, and treacherous dimensions of a *modus necandi* that contradict all the values of Christian and chivalric civilization. Hospitality and personal relationships were turned upside down by hidden hostility. *Potatio* that was supposed to solidify links or restore peace ends up in death.[314] The goal of poisoners was the destruction of the order established by God, from the conjugal nucleus to the whole universe. Competing with the Almighty, they infringe on nature. The process was all the more frightening because it was clandestine. It can be said that it was part of the mythology of the occult that flourished at the end of the Middle Ages.[315]

Does poisoning then reach the top of the scale of crimes? The answer is complex. On the one hand, the social level of the victim and the kind of relationship that linked him to the aggressor appear to be more important criteria than the *modus necandi* in the evaluation of the seriousness of crimes. On the other hand, an evolution seems to have occurred in the course of the fourteenth and fifteenth centuries. Starting with the enchantments that were fatal to Jeanne de Navarre and continuing on with the planned poisoning of the son and brothers of Philippe IV, the Bishop Guichard de Troyes went "from bad to worse" as a mandate for an inquiry states.[316] The hierarchy seems to reverse in proportion to the intensification of the fight against witchcraft. Bewitchments were placed at a higher level than poisonings because the former, involving the Devil, took on a universally sacrilegious character, independent of the targeted victim. When witchhunts were at their height, it was evident that Satanism ranked well above the crime of poisoning on the scale of horror: the mortal powders of Jaquet Durier took second place behind his devil worship (1448).[317] In the sixteenth century, Bodin described the situation very clearly in his *Scourge of Demons* (*Fléau des démons*): "it is still more serious to kill by witchcraft than with poison" (*il est encore plus grief de faire mourir par sortilege que par poison*).[318] When the antisatanic fever cooled down, criminal poisoning logically took its place at the top of the list. According to the the Edict of Versailles of 1682, poisoners committed "the most detestable crimes of all."[319]

NOTES

1. Albe, p. 163.
2. C. Gauvard, Les sources judiciaires de la fin du Moyen Âge..., p. 475.
3. *Concilium triburiense*, 895, chap. 50, t. 2, p. 241.
4. Balde, *Consilia*, cons. 221, p. 44.
5. See the words of Frederick II's letter (March 1249) denouncing an attempted poisoning: *per secula ingentem nequiciam a seculis inauditam... inde procedit fraus et nephas, inde iniquitas detestanda, inde perniciosum exemplum... ; fuit inhumaniter et nepharie machinatus...* (*Constitutiones regni Siciliae*, t. 6-2, p. 705).
6. *Chronique de Saint-Pierre d'Erfurt* (1072–1335), ed. O. Holder-Egger, *MGH SS*, XXX-1, Hanover, 1896, p. 145.
7. *Corpus juris civilis...*, IX, 18, t. 2, p. 379.
8. Examples *Coutumes et institutions de l'Anjou et du Maine*, t. 1, respectively pp. 491–492 and p. 435. However, it must be noted that the *Liber augustalis* does not use this formula and neither does the *Siete partidas*. Pietro d'Ancharano, *Commentaria in decretalium libros*, t. 5, p. 73. Balde, *Commentaria*, p. 219.
9. Shatzmiller, pp. 88–89, acte de la cour de Manosque, 1300; *Spicilegium brivatense. Recueil de documents historiques relatifs au Brivadois et à l'Auvergne*, ed. A. Chassaing, Paris, 1886, p. 443, a judicial document from the monastery of Saint-Chaffre, 1390.
10. *Code théodosien*, IX, 38, 7 and XI, 36, 1. La *Rhétorique à Herennius*, ed.-tr. G. Achard, Paris, 1989, II, 30, defined *crimen atrocissimum* as a crime that touches all men. Balde, *Commentaria*, p. 219. *Atrocius* also appears in the act of John XXII.
11. Labande, p. 140: *cum longe sit abominabilius interficere...*
12. *Statuto di Forli*, II, 46.
13. Balde, *Consilia*, cons. 221, p. 44. Concerning the word *scelus*, C. Gauvard, "*De grace especial...*," t. 1, p. 117.
14. *Ead.*, t. 2, p. 790. The author points out how much the list of these "horrendous crimes" varies from one text to another. The jurists themselves use the terms rather imprecisely, for example, Angelus Gambiglione.
15. *Parlement criminel*, X2a 18, f. 12.
16. C. Gauvard, "*De grace especial...*," p. 802.
17. Labande, pp. 137–144.
18. *Chronique des règnes...*, t. 2, p. 285, n 4.
19. A. Vitu, *La chronique de Louis XI dite* Chronique scandaleuse *faussement attribuée à Jean de Troyes et restituée à son véritable auteur*, Paris, 1873, Ruling made against Jehan Hardy , p. 59.
20. Basin, p. 132.
21. *Code théodosien*, IX, 38, 7 and XI, 36, 1: *scelera saeviora*.
22. Grégoire de Tours, V, 36, t. 1, p. 300 from R. Latouche's tr.: Marachaire *crudeliter enecatu: nephanda crudelitas* than the death of Bishop Frédéric de Liège (*Vita Frederici episcopi Leodiensis*, ed. W. Wattenbach, *MGH SS*, XII, Hanovre, 1856, p. 502 and sq.).
23. *Chronique parisienne anonyme*, p. 58.
24. *Preuves des mémoires de Philippe de Comines*, ed. N. Lenglet du Fresnoy, Paris, 1747, pp. 199–200.
25. Albe, p. 163.

26. For example, the pope plots to poison *inhumaniter* Frederick II: *Constitutiones regni Siciliae*, t. 6–2, pp. 708–709.

27. Ferretus Vicentinus, col. 1013: *omni prorsus humanitati contraria.*

28. Jean de Saint-Victor, p. 651. See J. Chiffoleau, *Contra naturam...*

29. Labande, pp. 137–144.

30. *Statuta capitulorum generalium ordinis cisterciensis*, t. 4, p. 152: *inhumano crudelique toxico.*

31. Ferretus Vicentinus, col. 1013: *nefandum mortis genus.*

32. Cf. J. Chiffoleau, Dire l'indicible...

33. *Statuta capitulorum generalium ordinis cisterciensis*, t. 6, p. 15.

34. Carbonelli, p. 268; *Chronique du Religieux de Saint-Denis*, t. 1, p. 632: *rem nephandissimam* that the plot to poison the Comte de Foix conceived by the King of Navarre and carried out by the parricidal son of Gaston Phoebus.

35. H. Duplès-Agier, Ordonnance de Philippe le Long contre les lépreux (21 juin 1321), *BEC*, 1857, pp. 270–272: *leprosi ipsi crimen lese majestatis nostre ac contra rem publicam commiserint.*

36. Secousse, pp. 408–409.

37. Adrien de But, *Cronica dunensis*, ed. Kervyn de Lettenhove, Bruxelles, 1870 (coll. de chroniques belges inédites, t. XIII-1), p. 245: *[Intoxicatio] pessimae traditionis genus habetur.*

38. Pointed out by M. Sbriccoli, *Crimen laesae maiestatis...*, p. 171 and p. 150 and sq.

39. Balde, *Commentaria*, f. 10: *Ille qui venenat aliquem dicitur eum proditorie occidere. Consilia*, p. 44: *In veneno est proditio cum homicidiis juncta.* Felineo Sandeo, *Commentaria super toto quinto decretalium*, f. 194 v. Andrea Barbazza, *Consilia, consilium* n 70, f. 154 v.

40. Hippolite de Marsiliis, *Commentaria...*, f. 2 v: *ratio [gravitatis] est quare occidens*[sic] *veneno proditorie et clam delinquunt*; Jacoppo Butrigario, *Lectura*, f. 6.

41. Labande, pp. 137–144.

42. Pasolini, n 1096.

43. W. Stacy, Richard Roose and the Use of Parliamentary Attainder in the Reign of Henry VIII, *Historical Journal*, 1986, n 19, pp. 1–15, p. 3. J. G. Bellamy, *The Law of Treason in England in the Later Middle Ages*, Cambridge, 1970, does not imply that the statute of 1352 included comments concerning *modus necandi*, which interests us here.

44. Philippe de Beaumanoir, *Coutumes de Beauvaisis*, t. 1, pp. 429–430: felony is defined as secret hate.

45. Secousse, pp. 408–409: questioned about "a terrible and detestable act associated with poison that the King of Navarre...was supposed to have caused to be given to the king, he answered that in this case..., he is not nor wants to be in the company of anyone considering such a felony" (*un gros fait et detestable touchant poisons que le roy de Navarre... devoit faire administrer au roy, il respont que en ce cas..., il n'est ne ne veult estre avecques lui ne avecques autre pensant telle felonnie*).

46. See *Estoire de Eracles*, XXVI, 4, p. 179: *King Richard planned a serious felony...*

47. *Le Romand d'Alexandre*, v. 4403–4404: "Hear what felony and what evil they will do / With the poison with which they will kill him" (*Oés quel felonie et quel mal li feront / Le venim appareillé a qoi il l'occirront*). Same usage in *Godefroid de Bouillon*, p. 316.

48. *Chronique parisienne anonyme*, pp. 57–59.

49. J.-Y. Tilliette, l'*Alexandréide* de Gautier de Châtillon: *Énéide* médiévale ou "Virgile travesty," *Alexandre le Grand dans les littératures occidentales et proche-orientales*, s.d. L. Harf et al., *Littérales*, numéro spécial, 1999, pp. 275–287.

50. *Ciperis de Vignevaux*, v. 4346; *Gaydon*, v. 265.

51. *Imperator Heinricus. Ein spätmittelalterlicher Texte über Kaiser Heinrich VII. in kritischer Beleuchtung*, ed. K. U. Jäschke, Beiheft zu Hémecht, Luxembourg, 1988, pp. 128–129; Jean de Winterthur, p. 65.

52. Amalric Auger, *Chronique*, in *Vitae paparum avinionensium*, ed. Baluze, t. 1, Paris, 1914, p. 193.

53. Guillaume de Machaut, *Jugement du roi de Navarre*, in *Œuvres*, ed. P. Tarbé, Reims-Paris, 1849, repr. Genève, 1977, v. 231, p. 70.

54. Carbonelli, p. 240: *False proditor, tu interfecisti dominum nostrum*; the surgeon in charge of preparing the corpse of the prince exclaimed "*O de prodictore !*" in reaction to the frightful condition of the cadaver (p. 262).

55. Monfrin, lettre V.

56. *Livre des Trahisons de France envers la maison de Bourgogne*, ed. Kervyn de Lettenhove, Bruxelles, 1873, p. 148: "Treason in this country is much more common than it ever was in Lombardie" (*Trayson est en ce païs plus commune que jamais ne fust en Lombardie*).

57. Matthieu Paris, t. 3, p. 116. The count allegedly poisoned the monarch in order to avenge the ban that the monarch had imposed on him to prevent him from leaving the royal army.

58. Primat, *Chronique*, translated by Jean de Vignay, ed. *RHGF*, XXIII, Paris, 1876, pp. 99–100.

59. *De triacle et de venin*, ed. A. Jubinal, in *Nouveau recueil de contes, dits, fabliaux et autres pièces inédites des xiiie, xive et xve siècles*, Paris, 1839, p. 362.

60. On the two meanings of treason, one "private," the other political, H. Wolff, Traîtres et trahisons d'après quelques œuvres historiques de la fin du Moyen Âge, *Exclus et systèmes d'exclusion au Moyen Âge, Sénéfiance*, 1978, n 5, pp. 41–55. She speaks of Jehan Coustain without detailing the form of his crime.

61. *Chronique parisienne anonyme*, p. 32. Originally the superlative form, "pesme" (de *pessimus*) took on the meaning of "cruel," "fierce." Therefore, there is no redundancy in the superlative here.

62. Hippolite de Marsiliis, *Commentaria super titulis . . .*, f. 4 v.

63. Jean de Salisbury, *Policraticus*, VIII, 19, t. 2, p. 366 of the Webb ed.: *licet veneficium detestabile semper fuerit, venenum quo ille extinctus est orbis censuit esse vitale.*

64. I. Guyot-Bachy, *Expediat ut unus homo moreretur pro populo*. Jean de Saint-Victor et la mort du roi Philippe V, *Saint-Denis et la royauté. Études offertes à Bernard Guenée*, Paris, Publications de la Sorbonne, 1999, pp. 493–504.

65. Ranulf Higden, t. 8, p. 196: *tradit autem vulgata fama quod apud monasterium de Swynesheved, alborum monachorum intoxicatus obierit. Juraverat enim, ut asseritur, ibidem prandens, quod panem tunc unum obolum valentem faceret infra annum si viveret duodecim denarios valere. Quod audiens unus de conversis fratribus loci illius venenum confecit, regi porrexit.*

66. Ferretus Vicentinus, col. 1013: *nec iniquum sed honestum esse viros perfidos et humanum cruorem sitientes vi dolisve necare.*

67. Jean de Salisbury, *Policraticus*, VIII, 20, traduction de D. Foulechat, p. 105.

68. Id., ed. Webb, t. 2, p. 377: *...nec veneni, licet videam ab infidelibus aliquando usurpatam, ullo umquam jure indultam lego licentiam. Non quod tirannos de medio tollendos esse non credam sed sine religionis honestatisque dispendio.*

69. Jean Gerson, *Œuvres complètes*, t. 10, p. 185 and sq., in particular p. 200. Some members of the Council of Constance believe, on the other hand, that any method is suitable for killing a tyrant (G. Minois, p. 97).

70. Jean Gerson, *Œuvres complètes*, t. 10, p. 213, among the propositions to be rejects is the following: *cum contingat ab omni coetu et politia tyrannidem exerceri, sicut papa potest esse tyrannus super ecclesiasticos et abbas super monachos et capellanos, et maritus contra uxorem et servos, ecce quanta datur licentia quod quilibet possit ut tyrannus interficitur... subito sine diffidatione et per veneficia et per mendacia, etc.*

71. Cited by Hippolite de Marsiliis, *Commentaria...*, f. 2 v.

72. *Exode*, 21, 14: *si quis per industriam occiderit proximum suum et per insidias, ab altari meo evelles eum; Corpus juris canonici, Décrétales* de Grégoire IX, V, 12, *De homicidio voluntario vel casuali*, t. 2, col. 793. Pietro d'Ancharano, *Commentaria in Decretalium libris*, t. 5, p. 73.

73. Thomas d'Aquin, *Summa totius theologiae, Secunda secundae*, q. 61, art. 3, vol. 1, p. 179 in t. 3; the word *exhibitio*, with the double meaning of presenting and nourishing is in no way incompatible with the idea of being hidden.

74. *Leges Langobardorum*, p. 584: *si quicumque veneficio seu quolibet modo furtivae mortis aliquem peremerit*... This idea appears also in the *Liber augustalis*, II, 33: *veneficio vel quolibet genere furtive mortis.*

75. Balde, *Commentaria in libro VI codicis*, f. 124: *Nota quod venenatio est crimen occultum.*

76. *Code théodosien*, IX, 38, 4: *insidiae venenorum.*

77. Rigault, n°XVII, p. 289.

78. Jean de Roye, t. 2, p. 285; *Imperator Heinricus*, p. 127 and sq.

79. A. Provost, p. 438, deposition of Jean Margot for the trial of Guichard de Troyes.

80. Ferretus Vicentinus, col. 1013: *Detestabilis quidem est et res perniciosa venenum... quae solutis animi sensibus invisibiliter corpus extinguit, viscera nostra morsu rodit, et velut ignis medullas exurit et dum venis serpit, vix est qui potenti medela subveniat.*

81. G. Duby, *Dames du XII*[e] *siècle*, III, p. 29.

82. *Mémoires pour servir de preuves à l'histoire de la Bretagne*, col. 1550 et sq.: "it is appropriate that we kill him" (*il convient que nous le facions mourir de fait*) they said in the hypothetical case that poison would fail to be fatal.

83. Godefroy Ménilglaise, acte du 9 octobre 1317 finding Mahaut d'Artois innocent of poisoning Louis X , p. 208: *Rex morte naturali et non violenta aliqua violentia extrinseca nec aliquo veneno nature debitum solverat.*

84. *Estoire de Eracles*, p. 179.

85. *Etablissements de saint Louis*, ed. P. Viollet, Paris, 4 vol., 1881–1886, I, 26, t. 2, p. 38: "murder is the killing of a man or a woman without quarrel or challenge" (*murtres si est d'ome ou de fame quant l'en la tu... sanz tencier à lui et sanz lui deffier*).

86. Case of the Bishop of Angoulême described by Grégoire de Tours p. 300 of Krusch's edition; the poisoning of the Bishop of Amiens, Richer, II, 59.

87. *Miracles de Notre-Dame par personnages*, t. 5, p. 178, miracle de Berthe, v. 650 and sq.: to a woman who was terror-stricken at seeing her blood flow, King Pépin answered that it was not very serious because her aggressor could have killed her "either by herbs or by poison" (*ou par herbe ou par venin*) (v. 654), that is to say, without her being aware of it.

88. Hippolite de Marsiliis, *Commentaria super titulis . . .*, f. 2 v: *non potest fieri aliqua defensio ab ipso recipiente venenum . . . Ideo magis dicitur delinquere veneficus quam sicarius.*

89. Numerous examples of this scenario exist; see for example the case of Francillon Bishop de Tours: *venenum haustum* (Grégoire de Tours, III, 17); Orderic Vital, t. 2, p. 28 then 73.

90. *Registres du trésor des Chartes*, JJ 196, f. 105.

91. Eustache Deschamps, *Contre les empoisonneurs*, verses 10 and sq.

92. *Grandes Chroniques de France*, t. 2, p. 78. It is noteworthy that the sources that precede this passage (Aimoin ou le *Liber historiae Francorum*) neglect this dimension that reflects the realities of the thirteenth century.

93. Cf. *Ciperis de Vignevaux*, v. 3053.

94. *Charles IV*, p. 37. The same terror is expressed in the text by John XXII that has already been cited when he wonders, faced with the plot of Hugues Géraud, whom poisoning can spare if even the pontiff is threatened by it.

95. Felineo Sandeo, *Commentaria super toto quinto decretalium*, f. 194 v.

96. *Die Bussordnungen . . .*, p. 104; *Décrétales* de Grégoire IX, V, 12, 5, t. 2, col. 794 of the *Corpus juris canonici.*

97. Pierre de Blois, *Speculum juris canonici*, ed. Th. A. Reimarus, Berlin, 1837, p. 85.

98. See the reflections of C. Gauvard, "*De grace especial . . .*," especially in Chapter 18.

99. Gyger, PJ 27: angry with his wife, the guilty party hurried to the shop of a Jewish apothecary to buy poison. Here the impulsiveness cannot be considered as an argument that would lessen the seriousness of the crime. The guilty party asked nothing from the authorities since he killed himself with poison.

100. *Registre criminel du Châtelet*, t. 1, p. 469; t. 2, p. 6.

101. Hugo Falcandus, col. 279: *Admiratus enim pestifera veneni potione meditabatur illum extinguere . . . ad idque tempus ac locum praestolabatur idoneum.*

102. *Chronique parisienne anonyme*, pp. 57–59.

103. *Chronique du Religieux de Saint-Denis*, t. 1, pp. 355–357.

104. Vigneulles, t. 3, pp. 301–302.

105. Labande, pp. 137–144.

106. Du Clercq, p. 637. Executed in July 1462, the chamberlain allegedly killed his victim in mid-August. He had planned his crime for a long time since he had been absent from court for many months in order to obtain the poison.

107. Orderic Vital, t. 2, p. 107 and t. 3, p. 419.

108. See D. L. Smail, Hatred as a social institution in late medieval society, *Speculum*, 2001, n 76-1, pp. 90–126. The author shows that hate becomes internalized when the procedures for accusations no longer exist, rendering accusations based on hate more difficult to make. It is doubtful that this situation encourages hidden vengeance with poison because the publicity of the act, that *toxicatio* excludes by its nature, is an essential element of the vindictive system.

109. Quintilien, *Institution oratoire*, V, 13, t. 3, p. 192: *venenum...paratum, quod summi odii argumentum est.*

110. Secousse, p. 374 and sq.

111. Konrad de Megenberg, p. 866.

112. Chastellain, t. 4, p. 242.

113. Ch. Raynaud, Une criminalité d'exception: les meurtres royaux dans le *Roman de toute chevalerie. Histoire et criminalité de l'Antiquité au xx*[e] *siècle, nouvelles approches*, Actes du colloque de Dijon-Chenove (1991), s.d., B. Garnot, Dijon, 1992, pp. 47–55.

114. M. Sbriccoli, *Crimen laesae maiestatis*, p. 339.

115. Abélard, pp. 106–107: *dolosa machinamenta.*

116. Orderic Vital, t. 2, p. 101.

117. Bernard Gui, *Flores chronicarum*, éd. *RHGF*, XXI, Paris, 1855, p. 727: *in mortem summi pontificis fuerat machinatus.*

118. Christine de Pizan, *Livre des fais et bonnes mœurs*, t. 1, pp. 137–139; same language in the letter from the wise king to his brother in Bourgogne, *Chronique des règnes...*, t. 3, p. 210: "the King of Navarre had plotted against the welfare of our person..., and among other things wanted to kill us with poison" (le *roy de Navarre avoit machiné contre l'estat de nostre personne..., et entre les autres choses nous vouloit faire morir par poisons*).

119. Adrien de But, p. 245.

120. Exemples Matthieu Paris, t. 5, p. 702 and sq.: Gautier de Scotenny poisoned the Count of de Gloucester *nequiter et proditiose*; Mathias von Neuenburg, p. 354: Bernardin *nequiter intoxicavit* the emperor Henri VII.

121. *L'Épit. Aegidii* that summarized the breviary of Alaric associates *venenum, ingenium* et *dolus* (p. 435). In a letter to the Comte de la Marche, John XXII calls the crime of Hugues Géraud *dolus*. (*Lettres secrètes et curiales du pape Jean XXII*, ed. A. Coulon, S. Clémencet, Paris, 1900, n°329, t. 1, col. 248); Nangis, t. 1, p. 43: Alphonse de Saint-Gilles is *dolo male potionatus.*

122. *Chronographia regum Francorum*, t. 2, p. 348.

123. Grégoire le Grand, *Dialogues*, II, *Vita Benedicti*, 3, t. 2, p. 140 and sq.; Albe, note placed at the top of the manuscript that includes the legal account of the trial of Géraud, cited p. 7: *nephandis tractatibus prehabitis.*

124. Labande, pp. 137–144.

125. Jean de Hocsem, p. 129.

126. Carbonelli, p. 220: *longevo tractatu prehabito et deliberacione matura cum nonnullis ipsius domini nostri comitis malivolis et inimicis de ipso domino comite veneno finaliter extinguendo.*

127. Examples *Chronique du Religieux de Saint-Denis*, t. 1, p. 467: *in interitum regis Karoli per veneficia conspirando...* ou Chastellain, VI, 79: "Coustain is the one who conspires against you" (*Coustain est celuy qui en vous conspire*) two knights said to Charolais, to whom Coustain's complicity would reveal everything. *Parlement criminel*, X2a 14, f. 173–177 v: "conspired and agreed to kill Cordeilly with poison" (*conspirerent et furent d'accord de faire mourir de poisons*) Cordeilly.

128. For the period 1380–1422 studied by C. Gauvard, the murderer or murderess have accomplices in their action in about 70 percent of the cases (tableau 24, p. 469).

129. *Britton*, I, 6, t. 1, p. 34.

130. Cf. Ps Quintilien, *Declamationes XIX majores*, n°2, p. 29: *Venenum, inquit, paravit. Cur, per fidem, si sufficit ferro, facinus adgreditur cui adhibere conscium, cui praestare debeat ministrum, cum maius habere possit in gladio parricida secretum.*

131. *Registres du trésor des Chartes*, JJ 207, f. 148.

132. Carbonelli, p. 218: letter of 1392 from Jean de Berry to the Prince of Morée: "We have in our prisons the poisoner-physician who is probably the instigator of the deed" (*Nous tenons en noz prisons le phisicien empoisonneur qui doit estre le principal de la besongne*).

133. *Cronica de gestis principum*, p. 36; Dynter, t. 3, p. 441, and Zantfliet, col. 417.

134. *Parlement criminel*, X2a 14, f. 173–177 v; *Registres du trésor des Chartes*, JJ 226 *b*, f. 2; Des Godins de Souhesmes, p. 135.

135. *Chronique des comtes d'Anjou...*, p. 124. Froissart, t. 3, p. 241 of Buchon's edition.

136. Grégoire le Grand, *Dialogues*, II, *Vita Benedicti*, 3, t. 2, p. 140 and sq.; Orderic Vital, t. 2, pp. 371–372; Vigneulles, t. 2, p. 122.

137. Tite-Live, *Histoire romaine*, 39, 41, 5 and 40, 24, 5: cases that implicate thousands of people.

138. Vidal, p. 513; Jacques Fournier, p. 143: in Toulouse in this case.

139. C. Gauvard, "*De grace especial...*," p. 470 and sq.

140. Benno, p. 51.

141. *Chronique des règnes...*, t. 2, p. 301; Secousse, p. 381: poisoning of Séguin de Badefol.

142. See the story of Prince Edward in 1272, *Chronographia regum Francorum*, t. 1, p. 4. Cf. B. Lewis, *Les Assassins*, tr. fr. Paris, Berger-Levrault, 1982.

143. Guillaume le Breton, *Chronique*, t. 1, p. 193 and *Philippide*, t. 2, p. 107 or Philippe Mousket, *Chronique rimée*, ed. F. de Reiffenberg, Bruxelles, 3 vol., 1836–1845, t. 2, p. 280.

144. *Novus thesaurus anecdotorum*, ed. U. Martène, t. 2, Paris, 1717, p. 86. Does the Capetien use *assassini* in the exact sense of the word or in the wider meaning of "paid killers?"

145. Neri di Gino Capponi, col. 1211; see also C. de Cherrier, *Histoire de Charles VIII*, Paris, 1870, PJ III, pp. 492–493.

146. Aristote, *Éthique à Nicomaque*, V, 3, in *Opera omnia*, Paris, 5 vol., 1862–1874, t. 2, p. 55. Other crimes support the conclusion of a clandestine pact.

147. Jacques Fournier, p. 138.

148. Vidal, p. 513: letter to the "King of Tunis" attributed to a Jew.

149. Nangis, t. 2, p. 34.

150. Mathias von Neuenburg, p. 268: *scilicet in Hyspania habito per eos dudum consilio de veneficiis convenisse...*

151. Trachtenberg..., p. 104.

152. *Registre criminel du Châtelet*, t. 1, p. 474 and p. 438.

153. Labande, p. 142.

154. *Registre criminel du Châtelet*, t. 1, p. 420.

155. O. Pollak, *The criminality of women*, p. 19.

156. *Parlement criminel*, X2a 4, f. 143.

157. On the notion of "professional criminal" at the end of the fourteenth and the beginning of the fifteenth centuries, see C. Gauvard, "*De grace especial...*," p. 457 and sq.

158. *Parlement criminel,* X2a 6, f. 368 v–369 et X2a 7, f. 33–34, 1357–1361.

159. Nicole Gilles, t. 1, f. 29: speech by Clotaire addressed to Brunehaut, "woman cursed among all women, subtle plotter able to find skill and deceit to deceive the world" (*femme mauldicte entre toutes les femmes, subtile engineresse a trouver art et engin pour le monde decevoir*), who is not afraid "to kill, to poison, and to murder even the kings of France…, as many as ten kings: among whom some were killed by your advice with knives; and other by your hands and others by poison…" (*d'occir, d'empoisonner ne de meurtrir si noble generacion qu'est celle des roys de France…, jusques a dix roys: dont les uns sont mors par ton conseil, par glaiv; et les autres par tes mains et les autres par poisons…*).

160. Grégoire de Tours, ed. Büchner, t. 1, p. 270 and t. 2, pp. 196–198.

161. Abélard, p. 106: *tam violenta quam dolosa machinamenta.*

162. *Statuts de l'ordre de Cluny,* t. 5, p. 28.

163. Gyger, PJ 27.

164. *Parlement criminel,* X2a 14, f. 153–155 v.

165. Salimbene de Adam, *Cronica,* ed. O. Holder-Egger in *MGH SS,* XXXII, Hanover, 1913, p. 43.

166. *Procédures politiques du règne de Louis XII,* ed. R. de Maulde, Paris, 1885, p. 411.

167. Escouchy, t. 3, p. 346 and sq.

168. *Registres du trésor des Chartes,* JJ 196, f. 72.

169. *Lexicon für Antike und Christentum,* art. Gift, X, Stuttgart, 1978, col. 1231.

170. Jacques Grevin, *Deux livres des venins,* p. 31.

171. Orderic Vital, t. 4, pp. 106–107: *machinatio imperfecta deseruit… Deinde procax noverca veneficos adhibuit…*

172. Jehan Petit, *Apologie du tyrannicide,* in Monstrelet, t. 1, p. 231.

173. *Chronique du Religieux de Saint-Denis,* t. 4, p. 123. Jean Petit proclaims *ducem ipsum in mortem regis primo per sortilegia, supersticiones et maleficia, inde per pociones venenosas, iterum ac tertio per ignem et alias violentas injectiones machinatum fuisse.*

174. *Lettres secrètes et curiales,* col. 102: *propinationis habilitate negata.*

175. *Confessions et jugements,* p. 30. *Spicilegium brivatense,* n°160: skilled in *sortilega* and *fachineria,* the accused woman makes potions that can become poisons.

176. *Registres du trésor des Chartes,* JJ 120, f. 85–85 v.

177. Modestin, p. 276 and sq.

178. Marx, pp. 131–135.

179. F. Graus, *Pest-Geissler-Judenmorde,* p. 332, wonders why poison is associated with witchcraft when it is totally superfluous for inflicting harm *sine ullo veneni haustu.*

180. Jean Bodin, *Fléaux…,* p. 199 v: "the twelfth [crime] is exceptional, killing with poison or enchantment" (*le douziesme* [crime] *est particulier, de faire mourir par poisons ou sortileges…*).

181. However, it should be noted that in contrast to cases in the twentieth century, those in the Middle Ages do not present the slow and progressive poisoning of a victim who has swallowed small toxic doses.

182. Gerson, *Œuvres complètes,* t. 7, p. 1158.

183. See for the early Middle Ages, the excellent clarification by G. Bührer-Thierry, La reine adultère, *CCM,* 1992, n 35-4, pp. 299–312.

184. A link had been established since Antiquity between the fabrication of make-up and poison (*Digeste*, 48, 8, 3), since both were meant to deceive by imitating nature. Cf. Alvaro Pelayo, *De planctu ecclesiae*, f. 149 v: *mulier si se depinxerit, et oculos hominum ad se traxerit, vindictam dabit extremam. Venenum enim obtulit etsi non fuit quod biberet*. See the remarks of G. Duby, *Dames du XII*[e] *siècle*, III, p. 14.

185. Adémar de Chabannes, *Chronique*, ed. J. Chavanon, Paris, 1897 and ed. P. Bourgain et al., Turnhout, 1999, p. 150 of Chavanon's edition.

186. *Parlement criminel*, X2a 15, f. 224 v et X2a 16, f. 35 v–36 ou *Registres du trésor des Chartes*, JJ 226 *b*, f. 2.

187. *Filippo Villani*, t. 2, p. 150 and 308.

188. Jean de Saint-Victor, p. 651.

189. Geoffroy de Salagny, t. 1, f. 113 and t. 3, f. 107 v.

190. *Registres du trésor des Chartes*, JJ 120, f. 85–85 v and *Documents nouveaux*, pp. 29–31. See also Des Godins de Souhesmes, p. 134: Hawis Brunet, young poisoner of an old, unwanted husband (1491).

191. *Annales de Fulda*, p. 392.

192. Jean de Winterthur, p. 65.

193. Hostiensis, *Summa aurea*, Bâle, 1573, col. 1229: *omnia homicidia excedit parricidium vel fratricidium, et gravius reputatur*.

194. Coville, p. 222; cf. *Le Pastoralet*, ed. Kervyn de Lettenhove, Bruxelles, 1873, p. 634: "His brother was not at all his brother / But his enemy..." (*Son frere frere n'estoit mie / Mais anemis...*).

195. Jean de Roye, t. 1, pp. 303–309 of Mandrot's edition.

196. Example of Yolande de Flandre in *Le livre de Baudoyn*, f. 180 and sq.

197. *Parlement criminel*, X2a 18, f. 11 v–14, affaire Anne, 1423.

198. The one who attempted to kill the canon Guarneri was called by him *perfidus proditor*. See Monfrin, letter V. Jean de Grandville was called the *perfidus medicus* of the Comte de Savoie (Carbonelli, p. 255).

199. *Parlement criminel*, X2a 14, f. 257 v.

200. Basin, t. 2, p. 118: *familiares de quibus plurimum confidebat*.

201. *Constitutiones regni Siciliae*, t. 6-2, mars 1249, pp. 708–709.

202. P. Pluchon, *Vaudou, sorciers empoisonneurs*, p. 251.

203. Grégoire le Grand, *Dialogues*, II: *Vita Benedicti*, 3, t. 2, p. 140 and sq.

204. Orderic Vital, t. 2, pp. 371–372: *exosus trangressoribus pro rigore disciplinae*.

205. Abélard, p. 106.

206. Letter from Nicolas de Clairvaux to Pierre de Celle, who was a victim of the hostility of his monks, ed. Migne, *PL* 202, col. 477: *ab antiquo plantatum est toxicum mortis in horto illo... ex quo ibidem regularis rigor elanguit...*

207. *Chronique du Religieux de Saint-Denis*, t. 1, p. 467: *Ad regni fastigium aspiravit*.

208. Grégoire le Grand, *Dialogues*, III, 5, t. 2, p. 274 and sq.: *ambitione adipiscendi accensus episcopatus*.

209. Hugues de Farfa, *De destructione monasterii Farfensis*, ed. *MGH SS*, XI, Hanover, 1854, p. 535.

210. Rodrigo Jimenez de Rada, V, 3, p. 151.

211. Roger de Hoveden, *Chronique*, ed. W. Stubb, 1868–1871, t. 3, p. 162.

212. Basin, t. 2, p. 130 and sq.: *ceca et stulta ambicio et cupiditas dominandi*.

213. Théry, p. 42 and sq.

214. Concerning the theologians' fear of power, see P. Buc, *L'ambiguïté du Livre. Princes, pouvoir et peuple dans les commentaires de la Bible au Moyen Âge*, Paris, 1994.

215. Antonin de Florence, *Summa moralis*, Strasbourg edition, 1490, lettre T, *Truculenta tyrannis*.

216. Guillaume de Malmesbury, t. 1, p. 43: *non enim West-Saxones reginam vel juxta regem sedere, vel reginae appellatione insigniri patiuntur, propter malitiam Edburgae filiae Offae regis Merciorum;* in Castille, the story of the poisonous princess served to introduce the custom of having the women drink first (M. C. Guerreri, L. Chalon, *L'histoire et l'épopée castillane au Moyen Âge*, Paris, 1976, p. 531).

217. *Pastoralet*, p. 639.

218. Pie II, *Commentarii*, ed. A. van Heck, Rome, Cité du Vatican, 2 vol., 1984, II, 32, p. 154.

219. See R. Starn, *Ambrogio Lorenzetti. Le Palais communal, Sienne*, Paris, Hazan, 1995, p. 48.

220. Jean de Salisbury, *Policraticus*, VIII, 17 to 20.

221. Gilles de Rome, *De regimine principum*, ed. of the French translation of Henri de Gauchy, III, 10, p. 319. The Latin text states, in the edition of Rome of 1607, *immo etiam proprios fratres et nimia sibi consanguinitate conjunctos venenant et perimunt*.

222. Aristotle, *Politique*, tr. de N. Oresme, ed. A. D. Menut, Philadelphie, 1970 (*Transactions of the American Philosophical Society*, vol. 60, part. 6), V, 26 et 27, et V, 29: he observes simply that "tyrant" comes from *tyro* that means "strong." No link is made to the word taken to mean "snake."

223. Gerson, *Œuvres complètes*, t. 7, p. 1158: "as venom or poison kills the human body, similarly tyranny is the venom and the poison and the sickness that puts to death all political and royal life. Why? Because tyranny wants to do everything for its own benefit." (*comme venin ou poison occit le corps humain, pareillement tyrannie est le venin et le poison et la maladie qui met à mort toute vie politique et royale. Pour quoy ? Pour ce que tirannie veult tout tirer a son propre prouffit*). The image is based on the wordplay of the words tirer/tyran. Christine de Pizan mentions in the *Livre de Paix* the tyrant "full of venom and cruelty" (cited by C. Gauvard, *"De grace especial . . . ,"* p. 225).

224. Poggio Bracciolini, *De infelicitate principum*, p. 20.

225. Grégoire le Grand, *Dialogues*, III, 5, t. 2, p. 274 and sq.

226. Voir J. Heuclin, Violence et meurtres dans le clergé gaulois . . . , p. 138: "The Episcopal function gives rise to jealousy . . . Bishoprics and monasteries were in this sense stakes for considerable power."

227. Hugues de Farfa, p. 535: *ipsi miserrimi ob ambitum honoris . . . mortifero eum viru interfecerunt*.

228. Cf. A. Boureau, La preuve par le cadavre qui saigne au xiiie siècle. Entre expérience commune et savoir scolastique, *Il cadavere, Micrologus*, 1999, n°7, pp. 247–283, p. 255. One illustration is the case of William of York whose intended elimination by poison confirmed lesser divergences between two visions of Episcopal power in the England of the twelfth century: see D. Knowles, The case of saint William of York . . .

229. Provost, p. 246 (deposition by the Prior of Saint-Ayoul).

230. Godefroy Méniglaise, pp. 181–230.

231. Jean Dardel, *Chronique d'Arménie*, ed. Ch. Kohler, in *RHC; Documents arméniens*, II, Paris, 1906, pp. 1–109, p. 32: "Because the said King Constant was not of the royal line of Armenia and never had been part of this ligneage, it annoyed him that the said lady and her said children lived as such; so he considered how he could cause their deaths secretly without the people noticing, and he desired especially the death of the said children, in order that the the royal line and the noble blood of Armenia be totally cleansed and that his own children would reign after him. So he had a pot of honey prepared and had them poisoned" (*Pour ce que le dit roy Constant n'estoit mie de la lignie royal de Armenye ne oncques pret de son lignaige n'en avoit esté, il luy ennuya que la dicte dame et ses diz enfans vivoient tant; si se pourpensa comment il les pouroit faire mourir secretement sans ce que le peuple s'en apperçust, et desiroit par especial la mort des diz deux enfans, affin que la lignie royal et le noble sanc d'Armenye fut du tout extirpée et que ses enfans regnaissent apres lui. Si fist emplir un pot de miel et le fist empoisonner*).

232. Zantfliet, col. 288–289.

233. Froissart, t. 3, p. 243 in the Buchon ed..

234. Diebold Schilling, *Luzerner Bilderchronik*, ed. of 1513 reprinted in facsimile, Genève, 1932, f. 169 v.

235. Roger de Hoveden, p. 18; Bishop Asser emphasizes that after her marriage, she did away with royal personages (Asser, *De rebus gestis Aelfredi*, ed. W. H. Stevenson, Oxford, 1904, pp. 12–13). On this queen, see P. Stafford, *Queens, Concubines and Dowagers . . .*, pp. 17–18.

236. *Chronique des quatre premiers Valois*, p. 17.

237. Pierre Cochon, pp. 62–63.

238. J. Nelson, Queens as Jezebels: the careers of Brunhild and Balthild in Merovingian history, *Medieval Women*, ed. D. Baker, Subsidia, I, Oxford, 1978, pp. 31–77, p. 58.

239. I *Rois*, 21–25.

240. Bertrade sent to England, without the knowledge of her husband, an order sealed with the royal seal to have Prince Louis detained at the English court (A. Luchaire, *Louis VI le Gros*, Paris, 1890, p. xxvi); Pierre Cochon, p. 59.

241. Grégoire de Tours, t. 1, p. 226 of the Büchner edition.

242. Orderic Vital, t. 4, pp. 106–107. Suger writes, p. 123: *Hoc etiam unum et matrem et filios efferebat et totam progeniem ut si de regis ruina quacumque occasione contingeret, alter fratrum succederet et sic tota consanguinitatis linea ad solium regni, honoris et dominae participatione cervicem erigeret.*

243. De Gaulle, p. 88.

244. *Le livre de Baudoyn*, f. 180 and sq.

245. *Roman d'Alexandre*, v. 139, p. 752.

246. Guillaume Guiard, pp. 211–212; Primat, pp. 99–100; Bernard Gui, *Flores chronicarum*, p. 724.

247. Geoffroi de Paris, *Chronique rimée*, ed. *RHGF*, XXII, Paris, 1865, p. 117. *De ses secrets il savoit et estoit son compere.*

248. A. Rigault, *Le procès de Guichard de Troyes . . .*, chap. 3 et 7: the bishop expressed his bitterness at having been sent away from the king's council and his desire to see revenge.

249. Id., chap. 4.

250. Du Clercq, pp. 636–637: Coustain began by claiming that the beverage given to the heir of Bourgogne was a simple potion of conciliation. Chastellain, VI, 82: "for he was powerful and so blinded by fortune that nothing could shock him" (*car estoit puissant et si aveuglé en sa fortune que nulle rien ne pouvoit l'espouvanter*).

251. Basin, t. 2, p. 117 *(ignavorum et pravorum esse solet)* et 134. Probably taken from Titus-Livy, *Histoire romaine*, 39, 52, 8.

252. *La mort le roi Artu*, p. 75 and sq.

253. Nicolas de Florence, *De dispositionibus venenorum*, f. 83; Jean Martin de Ferrare, *De venenis evitandis*, f. 1.

254. Pierre le Baud, t. 3, p. 167; Bouchart, t. 1, p. 381.

255. Wace, *Roman de Brut*, v. 8957–8961.

256. Nangis, *Gesta Ludovici*, p. 334.

257. Géraud de Frachet, *Chronique et continuations*, ed. *RHGF*, XXI, Paris, 1855, p. 39, and *Continuatio zwetlensis tertia*, *MGH SS*, IX, Hanover, 1851, p. 664: the inhabitants of Brescia wanted to poison the emperor, *videntes . . . viribus non posse resistere*.

258. *Chronique du Religieux de Saint-Denis*, t. 1, p. 166 and Juvénal des Ursins, p. 27 from the edition of 1614.

259. *Registre criminel du Châtelet*, deposition of Pierre de Toulouse, p. 470.

260. Jean de Roye, t. 1, pp. 303–309.

261. See *Le livre des ruses*, tr. R. R. Kawam, Paris, Phœbus, 1976, pp. 286–287. Le *Secretum secretorum*, written about 1150 for a Sultan, advises in book VIII to poison the water of those under siege in order to take a location with minimum losses.

262. Eustache Deschamps, *Contre les empoisonneurs*, v. 7.

263. *Florent et Octavien*, v. 8865 and sq., t. 1, p. 286.

264. Jean Servion, p. 196.

265. Lewin, p. 545.

266. Chastellain, t. 4, p. 248.

267. Jehan Petit, *Apologie du tyrannicide*, in Monstrelet, t. 1, p. 232: words put by Petit into the mouth of Queen Blanche addressing Louis d'Orléans: "Are you there, good varlet? Are you a hypocrite?" (*Estes vous la, bon varlet? Faites vous bien le marmiteux?*).

268. Basin, t. 2, p. 117: *vera et virtutis via quod eorum proprium est in quibus laudis et gloriae prevalet appetitus*.

269. Rodrigo Jimenez de Rada, V, 3, p. 151.

270. Matthieu Paris, t. 4, p. 490 and t. 5, p. 252.

271. Nangis, t. 2, p. 32: *dolens se per christianos saepius superatum nec potens ad libitum vindicare quod vi armorum non potuit, excogitata nequitia perficere machinavit*.

272. Jacques Fournier, p. 143.

273. Matthieu Paris, t. 5, p. 432; *Grandes chroniques*, t. 7, p. 140.

274. Infessura, col. 1231.

275. Bernard Gui, t. 1, p. 163 in the Baluze ed.: *Et quod dictu incredibile videbatur, in villarum et castrorum dominium aspirabant*. The interrogation of Guillaume Agasse indicates that he already saw himself as the Comte de Foix but also that

the initiative of the plot resided with the lepers, who were solicited by the sultans (Jacques Fournier, pp. 142–143).

276. Pierre de Zittau, p. 414, said that he saw at the monastery of Morimond a copy of the letter from John XXII to all of Christianity. It contained this letter of Philippe de Valois to the pope whom he warned of the discovery at the home of a Jew named Bananias of a document that confirmed the alliance between the Jews and the Muslims (Freher, p. 36).

277. B. Blumenkranz, *Histoire des juifs de France*, Toulouse, Privat, 1972, p. 28.

278. Gaguin, p. 66, concerning Sédéchias, the poisoner of Charles the Bald (*le Chauve*): *motus religionis christianae odio, cui maxime Judaei infensi sunt.*

279. Gilles li Muisit, p. 225, and Jean le Bel, *Chronique*, ed. J. Viard and E. Deprez, Paris, 1904–1905, t. 2, p. 225. See also Konrad de Megenberg, p. 866: *propter hoc precipue ut christiane religionis defuncto populo sceptrum et unctio in judaicam gentem referantur.*

280. *Apocalypse*, 8, 10–11: poisoning of the waters provoked by the fall of the star Absinthe.

281. R. W. Ireland, Chaucer's toxicology, p. 88.

282. Orderic Vital, t. 3, p. 175.

283. *La vie ancienne de saint Samson*, p. 172: *diabolicis repleti venenis.*

284. On this pertinent association, numerous examples taken from patristic writings can be found in *Materials toward a History of Witchcraft*, ed. Ch. Lea, repr. New York, 3 vol., 1957, for example t. 1, p. 50 where a sentence taken from *De Paradiso* of Saint Augustin is cited: *in serpentis autem figura diabolus est.*

285. See J. Berlioz, Le crapaud, animal diabolique: une exemplaire construction médiévale, *L'animal exemplaire*, s.d. M.-A. Polo de Beaulieu et J. Berlioz, Rennes, pur, 1999, pp. 267–289.

286. R. Kieckhefer, *Magie et sorcellerie*, p. 22. Jacques de Voragine, *Légende dorée*, IX. It is a question of a widespread iconographic theme (L. Réau, *Iconographie de l'art chrétien*, III, t. 2, p. 709).

287. Jacques Fournier, p. 138.

288. See Trachtenberg, p. 26 puis 102 and sq. A Jew serves as the intermediary between Théophile and the devil in certain versions of the *Miracle de Théophile.*

289. *Registre criminel du Châtelet*, t. 1, p. 467: one of the accused men revealed that he made a circular sign on the places that had been poisoned.

290. C. Ginzburg, *Le sabbat . . .*, chap. 1 and 2.

291. Du Clercq, p. 632 from the Michaud et Poujoulat edition; *Traité anonyme sur la Vauderie*, partial edition in *Quellen und Untersuchungen . . .*, p. 167.

292. Alexandre Nequam, *De naturis rerum*, II, 121, p. 199, concerning Envy: *Habet enim invidia suum venenum veneno materiali longe detestabilius . . .* Robert Grosseteste wrote a *Tractatus de veneno peccati.*

293. See M. Vincent-Cassy, L'envie au Moyen Âge, *AESC*, 1980, pp. 253–271: in the *Pèlerinage de vie humaine*, Guillaume de Digulleville depicts Envy as an old woman carrying on her back Treason with her box of salves and her hidden knife. On capital sins, see lastly C. Casagrande and S. Vecchio, *Histoire des péchés capitaux au Moyen Âge*, Paris, Aubier, 2003.

294. Grégoire le Grand, *Dialogues, Vita Benedicti*, 27, 3: it is said about the enemy of the poisoned man who was cured by Benedict: *aemulatione gravissima... odium ad hoc prorupit ut ei venenum daret.*

295. Laurent d'Orléans, *La somme le Roi* ou *Livre des vices et des vertus*, ed. of the English tr. W. Nelson Francis, London, 1942, p. 22.

296. *Speculum exemplorum*, p. 474.

297. Benoît de Sainte-More, *Chronique des ducs de Normandie*, ed. F. Michel, Paris, 3 vol., 1836–1844, v. 29993.

298. Matthieu Paris, t. 3, p. 623.

299. Maulde, p. 413.

300. *Chronique du Religieux de Saint-Denis*, t. 1, pp. 355–357, et Coville, p. 207 and sq. Jehan Petit refers to a sentence of Saint Paul that makes lust the mother of all evil.

301. *Chronique du Religieux de Saint-Denis*, t. 1, p. 682: *nulla est turpior proditio cui avaricia causam dat.*

302. Orderic Vital, t. 2, p. 57.

303. *De triacle et de venin*, strophe 5. This poem is found in ms. fr. 837 de la BNF, which also contains poems of Pierre de la Broce composed in 1278–1279.

304. Id., strophe 11.

305. E. Mitre Fernandez, Muerte, veneno y enfermedad...

306. *Processus Bernardi Delitiosi*, p. 55, apostolic letters of John XXII concerning the alleged poisoning of Benedict XI: *voto regularis professionis astricti sub agni species gestant lupum.*

307. Matthieu Paris, t. 5, p. 23, indicates that the inhabitants of Avignon were dealt with in 1248 by knights of the royal army, by Albigenians and by *potionatores* in memory of the illness contracted by Louis VIII during a siege of the town, a sickness attributed to poisoning.

308. See for example M. Salvat, La présentation du diable par un encyclopédiste du xiiie siècle: Barthélémy l'Anglais, *Le diable au Moyen Âge, Sénéfiance*, 1978, n°6, pp. 473–492.

309. C. Boujot, p. 113.

310. *Capitularia regum Francorum*, t. 2, p. 44: *Extant et alia pernitiosissima mala, quae ex ritu gentilium remansisse non dubium est, ut sunt magi, arioli, sortilegi, venefici...*

311. In this way, poisoning perfectly represents the *crimen pestiferum* evoked by Nicolas de Clamanges (C. Gauvard, "*De grace especial...*," p. 217 and sq.).

312. Ps Quintilien, *Declamationes XIX majores*, n 17, p. 346: *cur non veneno? sed nihil est delicatius exitu quem non supplicia, non metus, sed collecta de calamitatibus commendat infirmitas... non spargit cruorem, nec trucem cadaveris relinquit aspectum; placida est, quieta est...*

313. Eustache Deschamps, *Contre les empoisonneurs*, pp. 282–283: speaking of the murderers who commit treason, he wrote: "When they kill valliant hearts, by their outrageous acts, / it is a horrible misdeed" (*Quant ainsi font mourir par leur oultrage / Les vaillans cuers, c'est horribles meffais*).

314. In 1498, Nycod Magan was poisoned during a drinking bout whose purpose was to reconcile him with his murderer (Pfister, p. 190).

315. See on the subject of heresy the words that can be transferred to poisoning by D. Barthélémy and J. Chiffoleau, Les sources cléricales et la notion de clandestinité au Moyen Âge (France, xie–xive), *Histoire et clandestinité du Moyen Âge à la première guerre mondiale*, Actes du colloque de Privas (mai 1977), numéro spécial de la *Revue du Vivarais*, 1979, pp. 19–39.

316. Rigault, p. 58 and PJ, n XII: *de malo labens in pejus*. The formula appears again on p. 68. However, it is possible to explain it by the increasingly higher social rank of the victims as does A. Provost (p. 445).

317. Ostorero, p. 204. The suspicious death of a man against whom he allegedly used powders disappears from the series of accusations against Jaquet, replaced by charges of witchcraft and interacting with the devil.

318. Jean Bodin, *Fléaux des démons et sorciers*, p. 199v.

319. *Recueil général des anciennes lois françaises*, ed. Isambert, Paris, 29 vol., 1822–1833, t. 19, p. 398.

5

Pursuit and Punishment

Veneficium is a crime that inspires such horror that authorities felt a deep obligation to fight hard against it[1]; however, this struggle is not easy to study. Only prescriptive and narrative information is available for the periods preceding the thirteenth century. More information is available for the later centuries of the Middle Ages, but most of the time, legal texts refer to such cases only briefly. The methods of the pursuit of *toxicatores* are equally unclear. Did the crime inspire an organized repression of information such as the one against witchcraft? Who decided how the pursuit and prosecution of the poisoners would be handled? Did poisoning inspire procedures and sanctions in proportion to the feelings it elicited?

THEORETICAL BASES AND EFFECTIVE PRACTICE

Specialists in medieval witchcraft have discovered the process of "criminalization" through which behaviors and beliefs formerly considered reprehensible, but later tolerated, turned into crimes that had to be prosecuted within the framework of the value system of the populace. This phenomenon led to witchhunts during the fifteenth century with jurisdiction in many places disputed between the prince and the Church. On what grounds and what structures is the repression of the crime of poisoning founded, a crime that targets another uncovering? Is it valid to speak of an outbreak of trials?

Permanence of Principles and the Extension of the Field of Repression

Veneficium never left the theoretical horizon of repression. It has always been considered a crime to prosecute in the name of the universal repression of homicide. The *Lex Cornelia de sicariis et veneficis* provides for vigorous pursuit of a murderer and his accomplices and Byzantine law did the same.[2] In the kingdoms built on the rubble of Rome, the principle of punishing *crimen veneficii* was maintained. The texts that pertain to the barbarian populace mention this crime essentially to set the sanctions incurred by those who are convicted of it.[3] In Book VI of the Law of the Visigoths, entitled *De sceleribus et tormentis*, the punishment deserved by the *venefici* is recorded.[4] Carolingian times did not lose sight of the necessity to pursue and to punish these criminals. In 829, the bishops of the Frankish Church proclaimed that these criminals must be pursued and punished by imperial authority.[5] In 873, a capitular of Charles the Bald (*le Chauve*) proclaimed that it was the responsibility of the royal minister to crack down on the *maleficos et veneficos*.[6] Parallel to this public mission, the ecclesiastic authorities were obliged to inflict on practitioners of *veneficia* appropriate penances.[7] The **penitentials** recommended that the users of poison be identified by means of skillful interrogations. The *Ordo ad dandam poenitentian* of Reginon de Prüm includes therefore stipulations on the spiritual penalties to be given to those who are guilty of using poison to kill.[8]

In feudal times, poisoning remained on the list of crimes that had to be suppressed. Advanced monarchies in the twelfth century such as those in Sicily or England affirmed the necessity to prosecute these criminals.[9] The diffusion of texts of Roman law enabled judicial authorities to take up again, in one way or another, the idea according to which the crime of poisoning required punishment. The *Siete partidas*[10] or certain French common law texts steeped in civil law[11] recalls this principle that no expert in civil law could ignore. Many of the rare commentaries on *toxicatio* concern its repression.[12] Like their antique model, the *Liber augustalis* and the legislation of Alphonse X target the user, the preparer, and the seller of the poisonous substances. Therefore, it is certain that the necessity to pursue and to punish the poisoners was maintained more or less consistently all during the Middle Ages. At the end of this period, the need to punish this crime was even more solidly grounded.

Princely ideology presumed the implementation, by means of a powerful justice system and new procedures, of a program of eradication of the crime that damaged the grandeur of the sovereign, affected the common good, and therefore diminished his power.[13] Without the goal of linking judicial practice and juridical doctrine, it is possible that the elevation of poisoning to a level of a crime of great seriousness by Roman law motivated the sovereigns, who were then quite aware of imperial legislation, to pursue poisoning more actively, in the same way that witchcraft was pursued. In addition, the blemish on the kingdom by the *scelus*, literally in the case of the poisoning of the water, required the Christian monarch to undertake purification by eradication. Such a program presumed an extension of the sphere of the struggle to activities formerly left unpunished. In the Paris of 1408, the authorities decreed it illegal to be present near the gallows with the pretext of protecting the "poisoners," who were supposedly there to buy supplies.[14] This interdiction demonstrates the extension of the repression to acts, previously ignored by law, and still tolerated elsewhere.[15] The composition of potions with suspicious ingredients, the purchase and possession of more or less mysterious powders also came to the attention of the justice system. In 1348[16] and 1390,[17] individuals were arrested and prosecuted for possessing herbs. Bernard de la Roche, who was at first arrested for being a foreigner, was carrying powders that resulted in torture and a prison sentence in the 1390s.[18] The failure of remedies provided by practitioners became subject to prosecution in cases where formerly misfortune or bad luck were simply lamented. One only needs to compare the fate of the physician of Henri I of France with that of Amédée de Savoie to be convinced: the unfortunate swallowing of a potion made by the first resulted only in moaning; the second was prosecuted for the deliberate murder of his patient.[19] Denounced by Honorat Bovet at the end of the fourteenth century, the "criminalization of inexplicable death," played a role in the increase of prosecutions of poisonings,[20] murders that were previously prosecuted but within narrower boundaries. We can note that the step of the intensified uncovering of the crime coincides with the development of material and intellectual means that joined together to detect poison.

Which Courts? Which Procedures?

As with other crimes, criminal poisoning could be dealt with in a totally legal way, outside courts of justice, unofficially or under the distant control of judicial authorities. This type of resolution existed in the Republic of Rome: Valère Maxime cites the case of wives who were poisoners and who were legally strangled, so to speak, in their homes to avoid a long investigation (154 B.C.).[21] As a good reader of the *Memorable Acts and Words* (*Faits et dits mémorables*), John of Salisbury quotes another example that questions judicial intervention in the case of a murder by poisoning that was often left to the private sphere. A woman had poisoned her husband and her stepson. Should the governor of Smyrna have called upon public power, or should he have left the affair to be resolved in the domestic realm where it all started?[22] Such a question was still discussed in twelfth-century England. The laws called those of Henry I stipulate that the person who is accused of poisoning (or bewitchment) must be subject to the mercy of the victim's relatives, who will decide his fate in a context considered vindictive but nevertheless a private act.[23] About 1380, in the case between the relatives of the Lord of Grammont and Pierre Gerbais, his presumed poisoner, the prince's justice intervened only after an undertaking of vengeance—a veritable private war—apparently unimpeded, even if more difficult in the States of the late Middle Ages.[24]

The absence of an *ad hoc* structure characterized the prosecution of *toxicatio* during the Middle Ages. It had not always been like that. In order to better repress this crime, Sylla had created a permanent and special investigative bureau that also served as a jury: the *questio de veneficiis*.[25] Cicero pleaded in front of such a *questio* for Cluentius.[26] But the *questiones* system collapsed under the Antonins.[27] There was no reason for the medieval judicial systems to use the Syllanian system with which the most eminent specialists in civil law seem not to have been familiar. However, the principle of a law court in charge of a certain kind of wrongdoing had reappeared during the struggle against heresy with the Inquisition, which was also charged with the repression of witchcraft (1326).[28] Because of the lack of a strong juridical consistency, poisoning was not given its own judicial agency. Therefore, like homicide in general, the knowledge of this crime is based on diverse examples, from the most ordinary to the most exceptional.

An order to prosecute addressed by the Parlement to the bailiff of Bourges in 1317 demands that cases of escaped poisoners be subject to the king's justice, instead of leaving them, as we are made to understand, in the hands of a noble victim, who perhaps possessed legal rights, or was assuming the right to retaliation.[29] If this act demonstrates a refusal to permit bypassing royal jurisdiction, does it also reflect royal desire to be aware of all cases of this kind? The answer is very likely negative. If the crime of *toxicatio* was committed or planned by ordinary people against ordinary victims, it was delegated to local jurisdictions, who possessed the judicial power. In 1281, a decision in Parlement sent back the poisoner Férinet to the lay court of the Bishop of Amiens.[30] The justice system of Manosque in the 1300s, the lay court of the monastery of Saint-Chaffre in 1390, and the justice system of Aire-sur-la-Lys in 1459 were all authorized to take jurisdiction of crimes of poisoning and to judge them.[31]

These cases also came first before ***bailliages*** and ***sénéchaussées***, or even before a lower level of military police or their equivalent outside France. In 1477, local judges considered the case of a servant girl who was accused of poisoning her mistress, the Duchess of Clarence. If the grandson of the victim brought the case before the English Parliament, he did so because of the pressure that the victim's husband, the Duke of Gloucester, had put on the local justice system after having the suspect kidnapped.[32] Let us go back to France. The case of Etienne *de Vallibus* was first referred to the seneschals' court of Toulouse (1357).[33] It was the bailiff of Mâcon who conducted the investigation and decided the punishment for the poisoner of Geoffroi de Salagny.[34] Despite the fact that the Châtelet followed a particular system that in certain periods extended its responsibility beyond simply the *prévoté* and *vicomté* of Paris, it also acted as a local jurisdiction: in 1308, as well as in 1355, the provost considered the case of poisoners in his jurisdiction.[35] In 1402, his action against the supposed poisoners of a prosecutor in Parlement was the subject of an appeal whose result validated the decision of the provost whom the people of the Parlement required the lay-councilors of the court to appoint before giving the sentence.[36] Indeed, on occasion, the superior court did intervene.

In England, it is the social rank of the victims of the poison, the kings Henry IV and Henry V, that explains Thomas Stanford and Roger Oliver being sent before the King's Bench in 1402 and 1419.[37] In France, more than half of the cases that concerned individuals of privilege were submitted to the court of the sovereign, because the act was considered as being his business or because it followed an appeal. The rank of the suspect Mahaut d'Artois, who was accused of poisoning Louis X, required the supreme court to deal with the case after the accused asked to be judged before a court of his Peers.[38] The court in which a case was judged was determined more by the rank of the victim, as in the case of 1402 mentioned above, or by the rank of the aggressor, a clerk at the Parlement, than the type of crime. In collaboration with the Châtelet whose installations enabled the use of torture, Parlement assumed the prosecution of the poisoners of the wells in 1390, authors of a crime prejudicial to the royal majesty.[39] The poisoners sent by the King of Navarre against Charles V and Charles VI, and the poisoner Charles the Foolhardy (*le Téméraire*) sent to Louis XI appeared quite logically before the jurisdiction that is appropriate for this act of treason.[40]

In many cases, the acts of the court of Parlement were limited to requiring the bailiffs and seneschal to investigate, without revealing to us exactly how a lawsuit was brought before the royal judges.[41] The appeal of a decision,[42] or more often of a procedure (torture[43]), was a practice that is well attested but not frequent: the appeal of a capital sentence was even theoretically impossible, if the jurists remained faithful to Roman law.[44] Trial in Parlement was also requested by criminal subjects accused of the crime of poisoning before a subaltern jurisdiction and who registered a complaint against the accuser before the sovereign court on the grounds of defamation (1346).[45] There is even a record of an accuser who disputed before Parlement a complaint of defamation brought against him by those whom he accused of poisoning and who were finally dismissed from their complaint (1423).[46] But the weapon that was used was not a factor in these interventions by the court of the sovereign. When the crimes involved the aristocracy or members of the royal family, the jurisdiction that applied became a factor, but seldom left any trace. People loyal to the victims and palace officers were responsible for the investigation, and then the appropriate group pronounced a verdict.[47] The accusation against Pierre Gerbais and his defense were presented to the council of the Comte de Savoie.[48] A master of petitions in the ducal household was in charge of the information concerning the alleged poisoning of Michelle de France in 1422.[49] Within a poorly defined jurisdiction, the first chamberlain of the Comte de Charolais led an investigation of Jehan Coustain.[50] The Bon affair, which took place during the time of Louis XI, was entrusted to the provost of the royal household.[51] The handling of such cases depended entirely on how much publicity the ruler wanted to give them. A trial in Parlement had completely different repercussions in comparison with a hasty judgment given behind the closed door of an aristocratic household. We will return to this subject.

In the ecclesiastic sphere, the knowledge of *veneficia* unfolds between the spiritual dimension and the strictly judicial dimension. For the former, *veneficium,* or *veneni propinatio,* was the responsibility of the bishop, who was the only one authorized to excommunicate and to absolve. The ordinary priest did not have any such responsibility. This rule, enacted as early as the thirteenth century[52]—before that time, the low clergy seems to have been entitled to decide the spiritual fate of the *venefici*—did not make any exception for the crime of poison. It concerned homicides, as well as casters of spells, seers, and other criminals. Among the regular clergy, the knowledge of poisoning cases fell to the general annual chapter presided over by the *chef d'ordre*. The Cistercian archives show that various persons in authority, normally abbots of establishments located near the scene of the crime, conducted the investigation with the help of officers of the royal household, or even at their request.[53] Above the authority of an abbey, the *penitencerie apostolique* (a church tribunal) was supposed to intervene in accordance with the supreme *jus absolvendi* of the Pope. Philippe de Vigneulles reports that one of the three monks who poisoned their abbot in 1399 was absolved before the court of Rome after a flight of fifteen years.[54] His cause had probably been brought before this jurisdiction whose archives remain inaccessible. When cases implicated prelates, the papal justice system necessarily became involved. The *probatio infamiae* was entrusted by Clement V to the Franciscan Cardinal Bérenger Frédol or Frezouls in 1307[55]; John XXII commissioned the Bishop of Riez to conduct the investigation of the Bishop of Cahors.

The Inquisition intervened particularly when witchcraft and magic were used along with poison. The trial of Bernard Délicieux took place in this jurisdiction not because of the primary accusation, the *abbreviatio vitae papae* by poison, but because of the suspicion of witchcraft that was invoked against him, and more generally because of his adherence to an unorthodox Franciscan group.[56] In the trials in the area of

Lake Geneva in the second half of the fifteenth century, the Inquisition regained jurisdiction over *veneficium* by means of the investigation of witchcraft.

Since no jurisdiction had exclusive rights in cases of *toxicatio*, rival jurisdictions could argue for the right to pass a verdict on poisoners. In 1321, seigniorial or urban jurisdictions—such as the town council in Périgord—rapidly settled the fate of the lepers and Jews who were accused of the crime. But, on June 21, Philippe V proclaimed in an ordinance that it was the right of the king to prosecute and punish the guilty individuals. On August 16, he ordered their prosecution on the level of the *regnum* not without condemning the judicial lords who had seized the case wrongly and who had contested the point of view of the sovereign.[57] The king emphasized the form of the crime committed *ad injuriam publicam*—imperial law gave jurisdiction to public power[58]—and detrimental to the royal majesty, whereas his opponents maintained jurisdiction over the perpetrators, subject to trial by the ecclesiastic or urban authorities. In 1390, all hesitation between jurisdictions had disappeared. The justices of lower rank who had seized criminals such as the provost of Janville or ***juge ordinaire*** of Anjou and Maine[59] lost their jurisdiction to the Châtelet because "this case is a very bad example of a crime against the entire world and offending king's majesty" (*cas de tres-mauvais exemple contre l'universel monde, aïant regart a crime de les-majesté*). The *toxicatio* that was committed fell under the jurisdiction of the king,[60] hence the selection of the case by Aleaume Cachemarée. But ecclesiastic justice was on the same path as the king's justice.

Indeed, the crime of poisoning existed at some point between the Church and the State. Because it was linked to evil beliefs in the forces of nature or in spells, *veneficium* returned to the attention of the men of the Church who were concerned with the elimination of paganism in the early Middle Ages.[61] English legislation of the twelfth century stipulates that if the handing over of the poisoner to his victim's family is contested, then the bishop must deal with the case.[62] This pronouncement can probably be explained by the fact that poisoning was considered to belong to the same jurisdiction as evil spells, thus, the Church. The sources that we have consulted do not us lead to think that the ecclesiastic authorities subsequently argued systematically for the ancient relationship between *veneficium* and *maleficium* in order to demand exclusive jurisdiction. The reason is that at the end of the Middle Ages, most of the crimes of poisoning appear to lack any association with magic. But when magic is present, the case could be directed to the Inquisition. It appears that despite the displeasure of the royal agents, the leper Guillaume Agasse was referred in 1321 to the Inquisitor Jacques Fournier, who skillfully directed his confession toward the evil or heretical grounds controlled by the jurisdiction of the Inquisition,[63] which was also able to take charge of misdeeds associated with poison that were committed without any magic but by heretics like Mersende.[64]

Faced with such a situation, the king's people could claim that the area to which *toxicatio* was sometimes connected, that is, witchcraft and magic, also belonged to the jurisdiction of the prince. As early as the time of Constantine, magic was considered as a *crimen majestatis* and the Byzantine emperors logically assumed the right to prosecute *veneficium*.[65] The action of the Provost of Paris in the 1390s illustrates this prerogative, which, as an indirect consequence, resulted in the return of *toxicatio* to the royal courts.[66] Claude Tholossan, a zealous defender of the king's interests, believed that because Roman law entrusted the *venefici* to imperial power along with *malefici*, it was legitimate that the justice of the sovereign be involved in both types of cases. The trials conducted by the ***juge-mage*** of Briançon against Marguerite Daumas, Jubert de Ratisbonne, or John de Bari concern without question both witches and poisoners. To believe that the judge took advantage of the accusation of poisoning in order to take a case away from royal jurisdiction of a crime of witchcraft would be to misunderstand the situation. To him, all crimes that were damaging to divine and human majesty should be handled by the monarch.[67]

Another point of friction between the two jurisdictions, the question of clerks as poisoners is not presented in terms very different from those that concern other crimes committed by ecclesiastics. The case of Osbert is a good example of the clashes between the English monarchy and the Gregorian movement of the Church of England. In accordance with the atrocity of the murder of the Bishop of York attributed to the archdeacon, King Stephen intended to deal with the case, which was presented to him in September 1154. Faced with the fury of Stephen's successor Henry II, the Archbishop of Canterbury finally obtained the removal of the case from royal to ecclesiastic jurisdiction. This change of jurisdiction was also sought by the accused, who preferred to be judged by an assembly of English prelates or judges sent by the Pope.[68] In theory, ecclesiastic jurisdiction was familiar with this type of case in accordance with ***privilege de for***, but the transfer to a secular court did not necessarily take place at the last stage. The rapid delivery of the guilty party to a lay court after the determination of jurisdiction is suggested by Guillaume Durand for crimes committed *industriose et per insidias*.[69] Ecclesiastic assemblies at the end of the thirteenth century and the beginning of the following agreed with the views of this canon.[70] Probably because it may have seemed to favor lay jurisdiction, the stipulation was removed from the texts issued by the Council of Lavaur in 1368.[71] The transfer to Parlement of a priest accused of a poisoning surprised Jacques du Clerq in 1460: he saw in this situation manipulation in favor of the priest who had supporters in Parlement.[72]

When the power of the crown was challenged by a clerk who was a poisoner, a certain flexibility can be observed. Whatever John of Saint Victor says,[73] King Philippe le Bel respected the ***privilège de for*** of Guichard de Troyes even though the king had declared that he was entitled to deal with the case.[74] Clément V entrusted the investigation to the Archbishop of Sens, the legal seat of the province where Troyes is located, and to two bishops from the same province. Guichard appeared before the pontifical commission at Sainte-Geneviève. However, the bailiff of Sens, Guillaume de Hangest, before whom the bishop had been denounced, played the primary role with no reaction from the Pope, and the prelate was jailed at the Louvre, under the guard of the monarch.[75] The presumed poisoners of Charles of Guyenne, among whom there was an abbot, were first presented before the court of the Archbishop of Bordeaux. But the abbot was then transferred to the jurisdiction of the Duchy of Bretagne, because the Crown's seizing of Guyenne was considered a sign of impunity for a murderer who was considered by many as being inspired by Louis XI.[76] Politics controlled justice.

All jurisdictional scenarios were possible for *venenatio*. The *modus necandi* did not in any way determine the appropriate jurisdiction. The investigation and the judgment were decided depending on criteria that concerned the victim's rank or parameters more political than judicial. In the England of 1531, the *Act for poysoning* was passed for political reasons: the struggle against the courts of the Church.[77] Royal justice and the justice of the Inquisition were interested in *veneficium* only in precise circumstances that involved in some way human and divine majesties.

An Outburst of Repression?

In the Roman world, there were significant periods during which there were numerous attempts to repress *veneficium*. Titus-Livy talks about important trials that took place during the fourth century (332) and the second century (180) B.C.,[78] and the enforcement of the law of Sylla is itself linked to the desire to repress more effectively the upsurge in the number of poisonings. During the late Empire, similar outbreaks occurred with the probable purpose of suppressing practices tainted with magic and paganism. About 365, the prefect of Rome, Apronianus made the prosecution of *venefici* a priority even though at that time poisonings were becoming rarer.[79] Once the Roman judicial context disappeared and a penal order with different logic and means was put in place, the implementation of general principles was more difficult. The few glimmers concerning the continuation of the struggle against poisoning involve only the upper classes. The story that Grégoire de Tours relates about ineffective or injurious doctors, who were punished on the order of the wife of King Gontran about 575, makes us think more of an act of vengeance within the palace rather than an action emanating from a strictly judicial order.[80] In the middle of the seventh century, a Visigoth law from Chindaswinde mentions the confessions made during a trial by those who had tried to harm the king by sword or poison.[81] The judicial experience for ordinary people was quite different. The absence of major antipoisoning campaigns similar to those of the fourth century, in the writings of Grégoire de Tour, may betray a slow down in repressive operations. The Carolingian era brought back massive prosecutions. During a meeting in 850, the synod of Pavia reported actions taken against female enchanters and poisoners by the authorities.[82] But this is an isolated case.

A considerable increase in murders by poisoning coming to light is disputable, if not real, starting in the thirteenth century and especially in the fourteenth century. It would be tempting to establish a beginning point for the pursuit of poisoners parallel to that of the pursuit of witches, if the term "beginning" suited. But this is not the case when it is realized that there was nothing new about the repression. However, there are similarities in the chronology of the trials. Outbreaks of repression appeared during the years 1300 and 1320 and again from 1401 to 1410, but we have to wait for the last four decades of the fifteenth century for the attempts to repress poisoning to become significant. At the same time, or somewhat later, witchcraft trials became more and more numerous, first of individuals and then of groups. Yet, while the repression of poisoning temporarily slowed down after 1420, the repression of witchcraft literally exploded. The increase in the number of prosecutions brought against poisoners can therefore not be seen as some kind of corollary for the pursuit of witches. Different from the struggle against witchcraft, the struggle against poisoning did not live on its own dynamics.

There is no doubt that the repression of the despicable crime of poisoning constituted a priority for the powers of justice during the entire medieval period. Whether effective prosecutions became more numerous from the fourteenth century on or somewhat earlier does not have anything to do with any kind of "invention" or rediscovery of *veneficium*, but it can be explained by the development of judicial tools, as well as the general atmosphere of the struggle against clandestine crime. The increase in the number of trials reflects the growing suspicion on the part of plaintiffs who were perhaps more likely, during the last centuries of the Middle Ages, to see their accusations considered seriously by the authorities, who had earlier been less inclined to act despite the desire of the justices to hunt down *veneficium*. These justices do seem, however, to have paid attention to the least rumor of poison that floated in the air using the methods of the Inquisition (see *infra*).

THE POISONER ON TRIAL

It would be wrong to imagine that there was only one way of settling a conflict that involved victims of poisoning and those accused of the act.

Even at the end of the Middle Ages, the existence of a formal judicial system did not exclude other ways. How did a poisoning case come to court? What were the types of evidence that were used and what procedures were followed?

The Origins and Beginning of Prosecutions

The accusation of a criminal followed an established procedure for a long time, even if the Carolingian period was for a short time marked by the willingness of the authorities to take up cases with no accusers.[83] It would be useless to list all the examples. Let us limit ourselves to the action taken against Queen Gundeberga, the wife of the King of the Lombards, following a formal accusation by a certain Adalulf.[84] In 1154, it was the accusation of the chaplain of William of York against the Archdeacon Osbert before the royal court gathered in Winchester that launched a judicial action, in a country where the established procedure continued beyond the twelfth century.[85] After the introduction of another procedure, the original one managed to survive and to be combined with the new one.[86] Having fallen fatally ill and believing he had been poisoned, Domingo Spina de Manosque managed to summon the strength to warn the local authorities about his servant.[87] Here it is clear that there is a large support group of the victim's relatives who continued the case after his death. In 1379, four years after a death that he had always considered criminal, the brother of Hugues de Grammont formally accused Pierre Gerbais before the court of the Comte de Savoie.[88] Juvenal des Ursins attributed the origin of the proceedings brought in 1402 against a prosecutor's widow and her new husband to the parents of the late husband who "had [them] convene before the Provost of Paris [and] stated that she had a bad reputation and that she had poisoned her first husband" (*feirent adjourner ... par-devant le prevost de Paris ... proposerent qu'elle avoit mauvaise renomée de sa personne et qu'elle avoit empoisonné son premier mari*).[89] The victim's words, then his death, the youth of his too pretty widow, and her quick remarriage were the foundation of an accusation of poisoning that originated completely with an individual complaint.

The judicial procedure is very often hard to distinguish from the procedure of the inquisition *cum promovente*, which replaced the accuser by the denouncer. Despite the ambiguities in vocabulary,[90] the origin of a large number of cases lies, in reality, within the domain of denouncing, which exposed the accuser to fewer risks than a formal accusation.[91] The general hearsay following the death of Louis X encouraged the denunciations that two persons made against Mahaut d'Artois. Once this first procedure was complete, the king automatically ordered an investigation.[92] In 1404, the parents of Guiette Guillonne started proceedings in order to restore the honor of the family that had been tarnished by the *infamia* of the crime that was committed against one of its members. She was the one who served as the source of the denunciation.[93] In order to anticipate the suspicions easily turned toward domestics, to whom Roman law gave the obligation to take precautions against poisoning,[94] the servants of persons who were poisoned often served themselves as denouncers. Olivier de Bernezay's female servant warned the judicial authorities against two persons who were strongly suspected of killing him (1408).[95] A ***lettre de rémission***, granted in 1375, related that an inquiry was undertaken by the bailiff of Sens and Auxerre after the preventive intervention of a husband whose wife and father-in-law were threatened by suspicious powders.[96] Without doubt wanting to avoid all confusion and to conform strictly to the regulations, some providers of deadly substances turned over to the justice system the names of suspicious customers. In 1491, an apothecary from Saint-Nicolas-du-Port intrigued by the behavior of a buyer of **realgar**, informed the authorities about the client's visit, after suggesting pleasantly as he handed over the product that he purchase the rope that goes with it.[97] A gallant English merchant who heard indiscreet words about the poisoning of Jean de Bavière, crossed the sea to report what he had heard to authorities.[98] Finally, legal proceedings were sometimes the result of the actions of denouncers that disconnected them from a crime in which they were in some way implicated. Probably because some high authorities suggested that he do it (let us leave aside this aspect for the moment), the hermit of Saint-Flavy denounced Guichard de Troyes before the bailiff of Sens (February 1308).[99] Hoping he would be treated with leniency by the king, the apothecary, who was employed by the Prince of Orange to poison Louis XI, revealed the plot.[100] Seeking revenge, John de Vy exposed the sinister projects of Jehan Coustain to two lords of the household of Philippe le Bon despite the promises of reward for the crime that Coustain wanted him to commit.[101]

Not well informed about the exact conditions under which the Bishop of Troyes was sued in 1308, but knowledgeable about legal procedures especially within the Church, Jean de Saint-Victor reported the start of legal procedures based solely on a suspicion conceived by Louis, King of Navarre,[102] an example of a tradition of legal proceedings based on rumors. The crime of poisoning is well suited to the world of innuendo. Less obvious than a violent death with numerous witnesses who were also potential accusers, murder by poisoning gave public authority the opportunity to intervene without the necessity of an accuser making a public complaint, simply because a death can demand investigation. The investigation that followed the death of Amédée VII de Savoie was launched *fama publica referente* because of a "public rumour" that rumbled in all the States belonging to the count.[103] It was not only the death of important people that triggered such a reaction. In 1348, the lieutenant of the bailiff of the Vermandois region near Reims had launched an investigation after hearing a rumor about the poisoning of the wife of Miles le Barbier.[104] In 1402, an investigation was launched as a matter of course following the widowing and rapid remarriage of a certain Jehanne.[105] But even vaguer reasons could suffice. An act of Parlement in 1341 reveals the incarceration of a certain Guy Mauvoisin by the Comte de Blois because of a rumor that had spread about his poisonous activities.[106] A ***lettre de rémission*** in 1355 indicates that the bailiff of Troyes had jailed a suspect because of a scandal between two women about powders that seemed to be harmless. A proliferation of insults probably led to the assumption of criminal intent.[107]

The origin of legal proceedings did not necessarily result from the investigation of the crime itself. A significant portion (20 percent) of judicial actions were the result of proceedings instituted for other reasons. Some investigations accidentally uncovered cases reported by witnesses or accusers. Because of fear, a woman who was tortured about a serious accusation revealed, in addition, a case of poisoning (1423).[108] Some convicted criminals at the foot of the gallows relieved their conscience by confessing their participation in other crimes, or by revealing knowledge of them.[109] Thus, the supposed accomplice of Guichard de Troyes confessed that she had helped a woman poison two husbands in succession.[110]

It is evident that the principal path to the prosecution of *veneficium* was the inquisitory way starting from the moment that it competed with the accusatory one. In that matter, murder by poisoning is not in any way original, but it lent itself to new procedures.

Ways to Search for the Truth

In a *consilium* about the trial of a poisoner in Ferrara at the beginning of the fifteenth century, Andrea Barbazza wondered whether the judicial procedure had been respected. But the only issue in question was the statute of limitation.[111] In ancient times, the prosecution of poisoners followed a procedure determined in advance. During the sixteenth century, the *Constitutio carolina* indicates the rules that judges of the Empire were obligated to follow when dealing with a case of poisoning.[112] Books on the investigation and procedures to be followed when dealing with heretics and witches instructed medieval inquisitors; no general instructions existed concerning *veneficium*.[113] However, judges did not proceed blindly. A trial in Parlement in 1404 mentions the *Lex de questione familie*.[114] Let us see how it was brought to light.

Most of the extant data comes from the last part of the Middle Ages when, with some exceptions, cases resulted in investigations that were called "Roman-canonical" in an attempt to find a base in reason. But this way of proceeding was not always followed and other procedures were used even after its advent. In the area of *veneficium*, the custom of the ordeal was often followed at the beginning of the Middle Ages. The judgment of God was considered a dependable way to arrive at the truth. The legislation of the Thuringians stipulates that a woman accused of poisoning, and who does not have a champion to defend her, will have to walk on nine ploughshares heated white-hot.[115] Women accused of adultery also had to submit to this test. This fact confirms the relationship between the two crimes as we have already demonstrated. In 1154, the chaplain who accused Osbert de Bayeux of causing the death of Archbishop Guillaume volunteered to prove his statement by means of the ordeal of boiling water or the branding iron,[116] an ordeal that was still in use for alleged poisoners in Hungary during the first third of the thirteenth century.[117] The water ordeal was inflicted on the *venefice hominum* during the Vötting case in 1091.[118] Different from African cultures or societies in the South Sea Islands, and despite the example of the "cursed water" in the story of Joseph and Mary,[119] this ordeal never involved the taking of poison. In fact, in Africa, it is the resistance and not the vulnerability to the poison ordeal, that proves guilt, because it demonstrates a capacity to assimilate poison that is linked to the evil nature (poisonous and enchanted) of the suspect.[120] More than a shortage of suitable substances,[121] it is the attachment of the makers of poison to the world of magic that made it unthinkable to ask them for their help in discovering the judgment of God in the medieval West.[122] Contrary to what literature shows,[123] suspects being forced to take the substance they were about to give to their victims was not part of the ordeal. About 1360, the bailiff of Mâcon used this approach in his investigation in order to check the toxicity of the substance that was used and it was not used to establish the guiltiness of the accused. This person skillfully passed the test but even so did not avoid the scaffold.[124]

The judicial duel is a kind of bilateral ordeal that was used for a long time in dealing with cases of poisoning. About 630, King Charoald of the Lombards called upon God's judgment on behalf of the family of his wife who was accused of *veneficium*. The queen's champion killed the accuser to the satisfaction of Frédégaire who was delighted to see the Merovingian princess cleared of the accusation.[125] Lombardian legislation considered the reverse case of a poisoner *convictus per pugnam*.[126] Yet, the procedure had to be used with moderation. A duel risked the life and belongings of the person who wanted to prove that a man found dead in his bed had died because of poison.[127] In 1154, Osbert de Bayeux's accuser proposed single combat to his adversary, but he failed to convince those who supported him. In addition, the fact that the two parties were clerks prevented this solution.[128]

The establishment of a judicial procedure did not put an end to the *duellum*, despite the fact that it was rejected by the Church as *reprobata probatio* (1215).[129] In the case of *toxicatio*, the *modus necandi* partly explains its survival. In 1231, even though it was hostile in principle to the duel that it believed to be a sort of divination, the *Liber augustalis* stipulated that, because of its clandestine character, *veneficium* sometimes remained impenetrable to the investigation procedure and that consequently, the duel could be required as a last resort, under the strict control of the authorities.[130] Less restrictive, the English author of *Fleta* states at the end of the thirteenth century that the major proof of poisoning should be a duel instead of testimony because the known facts about such a crime were so vague that no one could prove or disprove it.[131] When at the end of the fourteenth century Honorat Bovet mentioned sixteen cases where a duel is permitted, he was indeed talking about the poisoning of the king or the king's spouse.[132]

After judicial dueling had been forbidden by Saint Louis in 1306[133] the desire to establish the truth led judges to accept a duel when the participants were both noble and if the guarantee of the duel was well defined within a judicial context, when it replaced torture that was in principle not used with nobles. In 1341, the Parlement required only a preliminary investigation in order to judge the validity of a demand originating with a relative of the victim. This case illustrates clearly the prescriptive texts. The accused party had disposed of all the witnesses to his crime. Therefore, the normal investigative methods were useless. Therefore, a duel was the only recourse.[134] In 1360, this principle was accepted: Robert Gui, who was summoned to fight before the seneschal of Ponthieu by his adversaries eager to prove the validity of their accusations, defaulted and made excuses.[135] In 1397, Othe de Grandson, who was accused by a young noble of being the instigator of the poisoning of Amédée, died during a duel that was meant to clarify a case that had been dealt with by an investigation.[136]

Literature has not been negligent in giving accounts of duels that are such a rich source of narrative potential. About 1230, *La Mort le roi Artu* gives thorough treatment to the episode in which Lancelot stands as the defender of Queen Guinevere, accused of treason (*appelée de traïson*) by the knight Mador who believes her responsible for his brother's poisoning. Mador is vanquished and the queen's innocence is acknowledged.[137] In the first half of the fourteenth century, *Li bastard de Bouillon* stages a duel that is clearly successful. Trancrède is suspected of having hastened the death of Godefroy de Bouillon with poison. In order to dissipate suspicion, the cunning and shameless Norman challenges to a duel the very person whom he had put in charge of performing the crime, a certain Eracle, who was positively guilty. He won the duel, but the relatives of the first sovereign of Jerusalem refused to believe that Tancrède was absolved by this victory, which had the appearance of trickery. This episode leads the author to make comments about duels that reveal his disenchantment.[138]

For clerks, the equivalent of the *purgatio vulgaris*, also called a duel,[139] is the purgatory sermon, a less brutal method. In 1154, Osbert de Bayeux decided to submit to it before an assembly of English prelates to whom he finally preferred pontifical judges.[140] The Englishman who was accused of poisoning the Bishop of Valence in 1239 brought the truth to light in that way.[141] Finally, another certainly controversial method of seeking the truth was judicial astrology that could also be a way to get at the truth if we believe the very untrustworthy Simon de Phares who wrote during the time of Charles VIII that a certain Nicolas de Paginca became famous during the fourteenth century by discovering in the stars the identities of poisoners who had acted against important people. They would have remained unknown without astrological science, which was useful in penetrating the deepest mysteries of what is to come as well of what has already happened.[142]

The vast majority of poisoners underwent a trial according to the rules of the Roman-Canonical investigation, which consisted in gathering evidence and testimony with or without the participation of the defendant or the suspect, whether he was jailed or free. A subpoena for an investigation from February 1318 orders the capture of all those suspected in the poisoning of the son of Gui de Sénanque.[143] Etienne *de Vallibus* was detained for two years in the dungeons of the Sénéchal of Toulouse. He points out that he was jailed even before the beginning of the investigation, a statement disputed by his adversaries. His protests finally led to his liberation.[144] There was nothing exceptional about his demand because the gravity of a suspected crime was not necessarily taken into account in the decision to free someone, accompanied by house arrest and the seizure of possessions as bail. On August 21, 1408, Parlement released a couple who had been detained on suspicion of a conjugal poisoning that was finally refuted sixteen months later.[145] Therefore, presumed *toxicatores* did not seem to represent a danger important enough for them to be incarcerated while evidence is collected.

Testimony was one of the cornerstones of an investigation. The accusatory procedure enabled two opposing parties to produce witnesses who could give evidence publicly, whereas the inquisitorial path delegated to the dispenser of justice the task of soliciting witnesses suggested by the involved parties.[146] In the case of John de Jaux, the dispenser of justice gathered the testimony. The bailiff of Senlis, listening to the *fama publica*, launched a "country investigation" aimed at establishing its basis, which corresponds to the *probatio infamiae* of the canonical procedure.[147] In the Gerbais case, it was the responsibility of the opposing party to provide the witnesses, a particularly difficult task for the defendant who was incarcerated.[148]

The number of witnesses varied considerably; it is not possible to determine whether an investigation of *venenatio* involved more because of the difficulty in proving the crime, or if, on the contrary, it relied on few testimonies because the *modus necandi* is secret. Only five persons gave evidence on the circumstances of the death of Louis X.[149] In the papal prison of Noves, the judges of Hugues Géraud heard twenty-four persons not including the bishop who was not able to call any witnesses in his favour.[150] The first investigation launched against Guichard de Troyes in 1308 heard eight witnesses on the death of Jeanne of Navarre as well as the poisoning plans of Charles de Valois and the sons of Philippe IV; seventy-one persons took part in the second investigation conducted after the queen's death. Thirty-three were examined concerning the death of the Prior of Saint-Ayoul that had taken place thirty-five years before; eighty-six gave evidence on the death of Queen Blanche who had died six years earlier; "only" twenty-seven for the less important death of Jeanne's squire.[151] The cases that shook Savoie at the end of the fourteenth century also involved a large number of witnesses. Pierre Gerbais produced ninety-one to compete with the hundred who gave evidence in favor of his accuser.[152] The cases that occurred among those from more modest classes also involved a large number of witnesses: in 1357, it was even an argument used by the adversaries of Etienne *de Vallibus*. They said that he (Etienne *de Vallibus*) had provided a multitude of witnesses who gave no useful information. Therefore, he should be tortured.[153] The testimonies of the victim's servants and relatives were the object of special attention. The crime of poisoning is a crime of intimacy. Those who lived *ex officio* in the intimacy of the victim were, therefore, supposed to have known or seen many things. Members of the entourage of Guichard, (his chamberlain, his barber) gave information for the first investigation. The investigation of Jehan de Grandville gathered depositions from Count Amédée's other doctors—among whom one was approached in his retirement in Melun!—his surgeon, his barber, his confessor, his chamberlain, a page, a groom, a baker, and squires.[154] The search for witnesses did not necessarily operate on a small scale. Even if a poisoning was confined to a narrow social stratum, news of it spread quickly and far. The collection of testimony on the death of Amédée VII was extended throughout Savoie: a man from Geneva asserted that the *fama* of the prince's poisoning in his castle at Ripaille had travelled across Lake Geneva.[155]

Is the role of extraordinary procedure in poisoning investigations remarkable? J.Chiffoleau has demonstrated the link that exists between supernatural crimes, secret information, and torture destined to reveal the clandestine and to have the inexpressible expressed. As far as the ignorance in which the suspect was kept concerning his or her case, there is nothing special to be noted except for the beneficial outcome of this way of proceeding that was used to confuse the two lovers, accused as poisoners in 1402.[156] The matter of torture is more interesting. *Venenatio* corresponds par excellence to *crimen clandestinum* that the torture must help to flush out, given the absence of clues that were left in other kinds of homicides. Logically following the same reasoning as for the duel, Balde thinks that poisoning required torture because often the guilty party is the only one who knows about it.[157] Yet, it is used in only one-third of the extant cases. The social rank of the defendant can explain its absence: Guichard de Troyes escaped torture even though it was used on his chamberlain and on a witch of his acquaintance.[158] Those who gave information often avoided torture. Quick to confess, Geoffroy de Salagny's servant does not seem to have been tortured, hence a jurist's question on the difference between the *servus* for whom the *Code* systematically prescribes torture and the *famulus* to which this servant belongs.[159] Despite his low status, it seems that Coustain was not tortured, probably because he confessed rapidly and because the Comte de Charolais did not want to draw out a "trial" of which his father did not approve.[160]

The use of torture was more a response to the desire to uncover the ramifications of the crime than to its importance. It seems that despite their status as clerics, Frederick II tortured the Sicilian prelates who had attacked him with poison in 1224. Full of his imperial prerogatives, he implemented Roman law.[161] Hugues Géraud was tortured in three out of seventeen interrogations.[162] In accordance with the royal act of June 21, 1321, torture was supposed to be used on male and female lepers above the age of 14.[163] At the end of the fourteenth century and the beginning of the fifteenth, the use of torture became more common, whatever procedure was being followed and whatever the level of jurisdiction.[164] Regnaut de Poilly, who was implicated in the affair of 1390, was first tortured at La Ferté-Bernard[165]; it was the jurisdiction of the cathedral chapter of Châlons that caused to be tortured the barber of the bishop, who had recently died, before transferring the suspect to the Châtelet.[166] This jurisdiction seems to have used torture with no hesitation on presumed poisoners. In 1355, a ***lettre de rémission*** presents the story of a presumed user of *pociones venenosas* against her husband and put to torture by the stubborn bishop, despite the negative result of a first investigation.[167] The Parisian jurisdiction used torture vigorously and generously on the poisoners of 1390.[168] A judge reckoned that an additional session would be useful to get more information on the poisons that were used: it turned out to be fatal. Jehan le Porchier also died during torture denying his involvement until the end.[169] Do these "blunders" indicate an intensification of the torturer's zeal because of the weapon that was used or the scale of the affair? Isn't it rather simply an ordinary case of excess that provoked appeals to the sovereign's court, which was in principle hostile to the unauthorized use of torture by lower jurisdictions?[170]

Partly involved in the trial of 1390, Parlement did not systematically reject the use of torture. Suspected of poisoning Le Charron, his widow and her new husband were both tortured at the Châtelet by the provost's lieutenant (1402). Perhaps alluding to civil law, Jean Juvénal des Ursins considered that there "was reason to torture them" (*y avoit matiere pour les questioner*),[171] which Parlement confirmed by rejecting the defendant's complaint against the procedure that was followed. In 1423, regarding Symon Anne and Jean Le Chat, the court indicated: "if it is necessary, the extraordinary procedure must be used" (*et se mestier est, que soit procedé contre eulx par voye extraordinaire*).[172] The so-called rank of squire of the latter did not impress the judges.

The use of torture was not very different outside the jurisdiction of the royal court. At the hands of the Duc de Berry who expected him to give very precise confessions, John de Grandville complained of having endured the rope torture during an entire day.[173] In the blurred jurisdictional context of the princely households, torture was common. The beguine suspected of wanting to poison Charles de Valois in 1304 had the soles of her feet burned.[174] The fake mute surprised when he was about to put poison in the food of Charles de Luxembourg in 1331 was severely and effectively tortured.[175] According to Monsterelet, the squire Dunot was "severely tortured, questioned, and interrogated" (*très durement jehiné, questionné et examiné*) about the attempted poisoning of Charles d'Orléans in 1440.[176] But is torture appropriate for the crime of poisoning? The extraordinary procedure had certainly every reason to be used for cases of poisoning, a hidden crime that had to be brought to light, but nothing shows that torture was used more for poisonings than for other kind of crimes. It seems simply that it was used unequally, since it depended on the whims of judicial authorities.

"Ferme prove e certa verità." The Consistency of Proof

In his famous book on the scapegoat, René Girard writes that, in ancient times, because the crime of poisoning was impossible to prove, it did not need to be proved.[177] Such a statement does not match the judicial reality. As stated during a trial in 1404, it was necessary to establish with evidence that the crime had been committed.[178] Pressed by public opinion to punish a presumed poisoner, Tuscan judges written about by the author of *Il pecorone* required the existence of "strong proof and absolute truth" before condemning the one implicated by appearances.[179] Investigations aimed precisely to gather evidence whose strength ranging from *plena probatio* to the simple *presumptio*[180] determined the sentence. Of what did this evidence consist?

"Witnesses are more important than letters," says a decree of Innocent III in 1208.[181] Recent research has proved that, far from being the spontaneous words of witnesses, the deposition followed a "system" conditioned both by the kind of interrogation that was used and left little leeway for the one in charge and by the transcription of the words that were shaped by judicial language. All testimonies did not have the same strength.

As for other methods of homicide, the criteria of admissibility did not lie in the plausibility of the words but the *fama* of the one who spoke them. The weight of the words of "those with a bad reputation" (*maus renomez*) (*Livre de jostice et de plet*) was nil. Canon law lists people who are said to be "vile" meaning that they could not be believed as witnesses. Among them there are the *venefici*.[182] Because of the social status of his accusers, Mahaut d'Artois denied their right to testify against him.[183] In 1423, Jouvenel who defended Symon Anne before Parlement considered invalid the words of the woman who revealed the poisoning because she was unknown and driven to extravagant confessions because of torture.[184] The objection to some witnesses can be based also on their "malicious intent." In the middle of the fourteenth century, John de Jeaux accepted the principle of the regional investigation provided that the testimony of three or four persons who had a grudge against him be excluded.[185] The money changer from Toulouse, Etienne *de Vallibus* reproached the seneschal of having sought information from people of ill-will.[186] It is certain that *toxicatio* was more likely than other crimes to invite erroneous testimony and denunciations that were difficult to verify.

Testimony concerning cases of *veneficium* excluded none of the paths of investigation used by those in charge of justice (the *scire*, the *videre*, the *audire*, the *audire dici*, and the *credere*)[187] but they privileged some. This crime can make use of specific questions that ancient books of judicial rhetoric recommend, either for a conviction of poisoning, or, on the contrary, to prove innocence.[188] Only the guilty party along with his or her accomplices in the preparation of the poison and its execution have direct knowledge of the crime. Otherwise, the only one to know the truth is the guilty person. Therefore, the testimony of Marguerite Bellevillette provided very strong proof of the two poisonings perpetrated by Emeline la Hanriotte with the help of powders provided by the witch.[189] Visual knowledge of *toxicatio* existed less from seeing the crime being committed than from seeing it being prepared in the dispensary of the Lombard apothecary who was Guichard de Troyes' provider[190] and from the spectacle of the victim during the last moments of life as well as his *post mortem* appearance. In the Grandville case, several witnesses provided information on these subjects.[191] The *videre* was sometimes only indirect and relied on the deductive reasoning (perhaps suggested to him) of the person being questioned. A witness saw Guichard de Troyes touch some plums before a knight ate them and died soon afterwards.[192] In 1423, Symon Anne's adversaries said that it was a "damaging assumption" (*mauvaise presumpcion*) that one of her friends was seen secretly throwing away the remaining liquid in the goblet that had been given to their victim.[193] The testimony concerning the suspect's flight or hasty departure is another indirect proof that the *Tractatus de fama* of Thomas de Piperata gives as an example.[194]

The invisible crime has above all auditory witnesses who report what they have heard from the mouth of the accused or the victim. Queen Jeanne de Navarre said that she feared following in her mother's path.[195] In the case of 1423, the victim "often said during his illness that Le Chat had poisoned him" (*souvent dit en sa maladie que le Chat l'avoit empoisonné*).[196] The foolish or threatening words of the suspected poisoner were also reported. Based on both divination and threats, the words that Bernard Délicieux held against Benedict XI weighed heavily against him.[197] The *audire* did not always directly concern the protagonists in a given case. A witness related that he heard a monk call out to a cousin of Buretel de Saint-Ayoul telling him that he should hate the one responsible (Guichard of Troyes) for the death of the person they were burying.[198] The weight of such testimony was diminished but not totally invalidated. It was an investigative method that was authorized and convenient to use. The most indirect knowledge of a fact *de auditu* came from the listening to the *fama*. At the end of the Middle Ages, the death of powerful people naturally elicited rumors about crime more or less amplified by conjecture.[199] The most credible *fama* came from the consensus of those who reported it.[200] Yet, it should be said that even if it was unanimous, the "public voice" did not guarantee the truth of what it reported. At the death of Michelle de France, Chastellain wrote with skepticism tainted with disdain "there was no proven truth only the voice of the people" (*il n'y avoit nulle verité prouvée sinon voix de peuple*).[201] During the Cuisel affair, the public furor raised by the accused party during the victim's funeral was not considered very convincing: "reputation does not provide sufficient proof" (*renomée ne seroit pas preuve souffisant*) because it "is not based on true knowledge" (*ne prent pas sa naissance de vraye science*).[202] Nevertheless, those in charge of justice listened to the witnesses who confined themselves to relating during the investigation the opinion of the "public voice." Michel de l'Ausmone testified that the streets of Albi were full of the rumor that the local bishop, Bernard Castanet, could poison whomever he wanted.[203] Some of the testimony gathered for the Grandville case consisted in statements that all Savoie was resounding with the news of its count's poisoning.[204] Half a century after the fact, the persistence of the rumor of the clandestine crime committed against the brother of the Duc de Bretagne shows the importance, if not the truth of the *fama*, because, according to Aristotle, *Fama quam omnes famant, de toto non perit*.[205]

The field of testimony was vast, from the suspicious substance and its provider to the words and attitudes of the victim and the suspect, to which the suspect's reputation could sometimes be added; the social *fama* had to be contrasted to the rumors in the street,[206] unless they were alike. The local tyranny of the Provost of Compiègne matched well with the charge of poisoning of which he was accused.[207]

Next to the evidence from witnesses, material proof may have played a somewhat more important role than for other kinds of homicide. The first proof of a poisoning was the substance that was administered, the object of the offense. Its discovery on an individual weighed heavily against him. The substance carried by Robert Wourdreton, the herbs found on one of the accused in 1390, the powders carried by Bernard de la Roche,[208] or the items recovered at the home of a suspect or an accomplice (the Jews in 1348, the women in 1482)[209] were important pieces of evidence. Philippe V ordered an assessment of the poison spread by the lepers in 1321. Its form was not indicated but its result demonstrated the great danger of the substance.[210] The judges, who were in charge of investigating the attempt to poison Robert in 1385, subjected the substance they found on him to an examination by five surgeons and as many apothecaries who identified it as arsenic. For the poisoners of the wells in 1390, the officials investigated the nature and composition of the powders that were cast into the water. A herb specialist, probably required by the Châtelet, declared that the herbs carried by the hermit Jehan le Porchier were toxic.[211] More rudimentary assessments also had their place in the investigations. English authorities tested the poison they found in 1258 on animals.[212] The decision to give to a dog and then to the servant suspected of the crime against Geoffroy de Salagny some of the powder supposed to be the weapon was obviously made by the bailiff of Mâcon.[213] When the substances themselves were not available, their recipe written in the hand of Jehan de Grandville was subjected to examination by doctors in order to determine if they were likely to be the cause of the death of the Comte de Savoie.[214] But we should not overrate the curiosity of the justice authorities. The notary who transcribed Marguerite of Bellevillette's answers in 1319 indicates that she was not questioned on the exact nature of the substances given to a poisoned spouse.[215]

In Italy, as early as the end of the thirteenth century, and then from the second half of the fourteenth century in France,[216] judicial procedure included the examination of the dead victims by means of external and internal assessments specifically intended to corroborate or invalidate the hypothesis of *toxicatio*.[217] Doctors under oath and their auxiliaries, surgeons or more often barbers, performed the operations and their opinion was not without value: "we can say that greater faith must be placed in the medical profession than in the masters of theology" (*nous povons dire que le plus grant foy doist estre adjoustée a la faculté de medecine qu'audit maistre en theologie*) clearly asserts the opponent of Jean le Petit in 1408.[218] It is not always easy to distinguish an expertise in legal medicine from the retrospective testimony of physicians present during the last moments of a victim's life, nor from an examination performed, for example, during an embalming.[219] In 1308, the "doctors' assessment" determined that a woman had been poisoned, but Jean de Saint-Victor does not specify the kind of examination nor if the assessment was done at the request of the justice system.[220] The adversaries of Chevrier who was taken before the Parlement of Paris in 1404, say with no further specifications that two doctors examined the corpse of the victim without being able to give an opinion.[221] The records from the trial in 1423 talk about the "signs of poisoning according to the doctrine given by the doctors" (*signes d'empoisonnement selon la doctrine que avoient baillée les medecins*) but we do not really understand whether it was a general "doctrine" drawn from books, or a report made at the time of the death or a deposition done after the assessment required by the justice system.[222] Some other cases are more transparent. The man from Manosque who was convinced in 1300 that he had been poisoned by his servant and mistress was assuredly examined within a judicial framework.[223] On October 4, 1302, the important master from Bologne Bartolomeo de Varignana proceeded upon the request of the justice system to invalidate the suspicion of poisoning or witchcraft, which hung over a wife.[224] In 1380, seven doctors and a barber had to reach a verdict, from a distance and based only on simple descriptions of the victim's state, on the possible poisoning of the Sire de Grammont.[225] In 1394, believing himself poisoned by a man, Arnaud Guihom asked for and obtained approval from Parlement for an analysis of his blood supervised by the court of justice and by skeptical practitioners.[226]

The quest for well-hidden truth sometimes led judges to order autopsies, the first known autopsy dating from 1302.[227] J. Shatzmiller reports several stomach examinations done in Bologna in the years 1310–1330.[228] In 1430, the Duc de Brabant was examined "according to the custom" (inspection of heart, liver, lungs, stomach, spleen, and intestines) by doctors from the new University of Louvain after conducting first an external examination that was not conclusive. The experts revealed their results under oath.[229] Nevertheless, it is doubtful that that kind of proof, which was difficult to establish for all kinds of reasons (insufficient information, ambiguous observations, impossibility of exhumation), played a determining role in those prescientific times. The examination of bodies was less convincing than revealing the depths of hearts and minds.

In the hierarchy of evidence, confession comes first. It is all the more important because the crime of poisoning had by definition neither the notoriety nor the factual evidence that did not need to be proved, unless, in extremely rare circumstances where the poisoner was caught in the act, as during the peacock banquet of Charles de Luxembourg in 1331.[230] Whether it was obtained with or without torture, the confession of *veneficium* cannot be considered as true as the free expression of the guilty party. Its content was sometimes suggested by the interrogators, who were quite ready to furnish a version of the facts to Jean de Grandville or Bernard de la Roche.[231] Even in more normal cases, the transcript of the confession was never written on the spot; it was reorganized by the judicial authorities, sometimes long after the trial.[232] The transcript of Hugues Géraud's confession was not put in its definitive written form until 1322.[233]

Confessions reveal what the judicial authorities expected from the accused: information about himself—Jean de Grandville's confession relates his studies and "professional" itinerary,[234]—the reasons for his act, the identity and the motivations of those who participated in it, the nature of the poisonous substance, the way that it was administered, and sometimes its effects. After the traditional presentation of his identity, Wourdreton related the origin of his mission by relating in a direct style the words of *le Mauvais*. The name and address of the provider of the poison in Bayonne escaped his mind but not the apothecary's reaction to his request.[235] Regnault de Poilly, who was arrested with other poisoners of the wells in 1390, revealed the motivation for his act, his partners' words, the places, and the instructions on how to cast the powders. He was also asked about the reason for the itinerary they took. The accused were also questioned about the objective of their act, but few of them were capable of answering this question. The consistency and the effects of the powders, the size of the infected fountains also interested the questioners. To all this is added the description of the act that accompanied throwing the bags of powder into the water: a gesture that was revealed under the pressure of the judges who had a preconceived idea.[236] Nevertheless, the judges did not try to prove that those who confessed *toxicationes* were also guilty of witchcraft. The profile of someone accused of poisoning did not automatically match the profile of a witch. The judicial authorities did not systematically strive to make suspects confess preceding poisonings either, except in a few cases, which are more political than judicial, such as the case of Guichard de Troyes, and with doctors suspected *ex officio* of having committed many murders. To the crime, which was the center of Jean de Bari's case, other poisonings were added among which, one was committed far from the man from Briançon, in the Apulia where the doctor had come from.[237] But normally, the confession did not go beyond the limits of the precise crime for which the accused had been arrested. In this way, the trial for poisoning can be distinguished from a trial for witchcraft during which the confession revealed many other crimes.

The judges were not always successful in achieving their goals. Jehan Le Porchier, examined at the Châtelet in 1390, confessed several crimes, but even torture could not make him admit his involvement in the poisoning of the wells.[238] A confession was not always definitive. Jean de Grandville recanted his confession of March 1393 in September 1395.[239] However, it was from the mouth of the poisoner that came the most reliable *probatio* of a crime that was so well concealed.

The poisoning trials do not show any real jurisdictional or procedural specificity. Even the recourse to inquiries is not surprising. As early as the thirteenth century, doctors were appointed by judicial authorities to examine wounds. The slowness of the trials is not unique in these cases. In cases that involved aristocratic households, they could be very quick: only five days elapsed between Jehan Coustain's arrest and his sentence, which was performed immediately.[240] But when the affairs go before local jurisdictions, they were delayed indefinitely by appeals, further investigations, and counterappeals. If the fate of Hugues Géraud was decided within a few months, his accomplices' case were lost in the sands of time: in 1322, several defendants were still rotting in the papal jails.[241] The case of Etienne *de Vallibus* was completed three investigations and seven years after the accusation brought in 1355 before the sénéchal of Toulouse, who forgot about the dossier and left the accused in jail.[242] Nine years passed between the beginning of the Cordeilly affair and the act of Parlement that discusses it.[243] The wheels of justice moved slowly. But could they be appeased?

SENTENCES AND SANCTIONS

In an order of prosecution issued by Parlement in 1318, it is stated that the punishment to be inflicted on poisoners who have fled should be implemented *juxta qualitatem delicti*.[244] The horrifying perception of criminal poisoning and the intense fear of *toxicatores* required a severity of punishment that might deter other such crimes. This type of punishment could be considered a compensation for the large number of cases that managed to avoid being brought to justice and thus avoided the courts. In the eyes of a judge in 1390, the particular seriousness of *toxicatio* engendered the necessity to deal with it with zeal and severity.[245] The clerk of Parlement's sessions in April 1402 and December 1404 wrote, concerning two cases of poisoning, that "[t]he act is by nature criminal and deserves the death penalty" (*Le fait est criminel et capital de sa nature*).[246] Because of the nature of his crime, does the poisoner get a particularly severe punishment? As important as it is, can his crime be pardoned? Such questions need to be addressed despite the imprecision of the sources, which means that 30 percent of the cases presented before the courts have an unknown outcome and that many chroniclers do not bother to indicate what became of suspects who were arrested.[247]

When Doubt or Mercy Benefits the Defendant

The trials of people suspected of poisoning did not inevitably lead to the death penalty. Besides the abandonment of prosecution in favor of protection, or because of a lack of accusation,[248] two phenomena contradicted the idea of a blind and implacable medieval justice: the acknowledgement of innocence and the pardoning of the crime.

In fewer than 10 percent of the cases for individuals suspected of poisoning, in fewer than 4 percent for the presumed killers, the investigation culminated in exoneration. The percentages may seem low and their disparity undoubtedly reveals the unequal capability of the defendants to prove their innocence according to their social rank on which their reputation may have been based. But these figures show, nevertheless, that doubt could sometimes benefit the person who was being prosecuted. Even in the harsh world that surrounded Frederick II, a suspect was not automatically considered guilty: a Swabian count was recognized as being innocent of a poisoning from a cup into which a toad had accidentally fallen.[249] In Manosque, at the beginning of the fourteenth century, the judicial authorities absolved the Jewish baker who was reputed to have cast toxic substances into the bread oven.[250] The exoneration of defendants resulted, first of all, from the lack of sufficient evidence: it enabled Bernard Délicieux to be cleared of the crime of poison against Benedict XI.[251] It benefited Bernard of Castanet, whose good reputation was restored thanks to the letter of absolution, indulgence, and mercy written by Clement V.[252] Jean de Saint-Victor wrote that Guichard de Troyes was finally freed in 1313 because nothing could be proved against him.[253] In a matter of *veneficium*, proof, even if it was fabricated, was as essential as it was for other kinds of crime.

Innocence was also recognized when the accusers were proved guilty of lying, as was the case for Mahaut d'Artois, who was formally cleared of all the accusations that had been brought against him by a ruling of Parlement on October 9, 1317.[254] In 1409, after receiving an appeal about a sentence given by the court of the Duc d'Anjou, Parlement exonerated the condemned man and ordered that his false accusers be put in the stocks.[255] The *fama* of the suspects played an important role in their fate. In 1355, the good reputation of an accused woman enabled her to be acquitted after confessions proved to be invalid.[256] Finally set free, Etienne *de Vallibus* probably made use of his reputation as an honest merchant *pacificus et non rixosus*, which was totally incompatible with the crime of which he was accused.[257] Other defendants whose fates remain unknown tried to prove their innocence based on their honor as soldiers.[258] Finally, the balance of power could also play a role: the canons of Avignon, who were the instigators of the poisoning of Bertrand Aimini, the poor isolated bishop, united and remained unscathed. Their social base in the city protected them. In 1310, the prelate who was the injured party was even obliged to resign his position for one in Fréjus.[259]

Therefore, the individual who was accused of poisoning was not always hopelessly trapped. Unless his trial sought a goal other than the establishment of the truth, it was possible for him to have his innocence acknowledged, even when there were other sound and related charges. For example, Ysabeau de Cambray, a proven adulteress and thief, was exonerated in 1466 of her husband's accusation that she was making preparations to poison him.[260]

Besides the accused who were exonerated, there were some people who were, in fact, truly guilty, but they eluded the rigors of the punishment they deserved by making peace with the offended party, or by seeking pardon or forgiveness. The documentation, which has been scrutinized, does not reveal if the peace agreements between parties, still current during the fourteenth century and still possible afterwards,[261] were a factor in cases of poisoning. This kind of arrangement was surely the desire of Adam Bargon, who would have preferred this discrete solution to the disturbance leading to dishonor created by the lawsuit his relatives secretly instituted against him (1375).[262] According to Juvénal des Ursins, it was sufficient for the Cardinal de Laon to pardon his anonymous poisoner *in articulo mortis*, in order to prevent the start of an investigation.[263] That gesture, made privately by the victim to the aggressor, demonstrates that the horror of *toxicatio* did not prevent forgiveness in individual cases.

On the other hand, forgiveness by a prince was in theory impossible, in accordance with an old tradition. Roman law excluded *veneficus* from the Easter indulgence.[264] The English laws, also called the laws of Henry I, declare that it was impossible to pardon the crime of poisoning as well as the crimes of bewitchment, enchantment, and casting spells.[265] In reality, the crime of poisoning, like any other crime, and despite periodic resolutions made by those in power,[266] could be exonerated after prosecution. In practice, at least until the end of the fifteenth century, no homicide was excluded from exoneration.[267] In 1375, a pardon was obtained for a woman, who was suspected of having tried to harm her husband and his daughter from a first marriage. Four factors seem to have motivated this decision: the exact nature of the substance to be administered that was closer to a potion of reconciliation than to poison (but the records of the investigation have not survived), the murderous plot was not carried out, the good reputation of the accused, and last, but not least, it was the husband who requested the pardon for his wife because he wanted to prevent the dishonor that his wife's incarceration would bring to his lineage.[268] In another case a few years later, the uncertainty concerning the nature of the product could no longer be invoked because it was **realgar**. On the other hand, this request came also from the husband, the victim, whose leniency can be explained partly by the fact that the complaint was lodged without his knowledge, and before the accomplishment of the crime, and was probably considered detrimental to his honor.[269] In 1408, a pardon was granted to Richard Martin on the grounds that the crime had not been committed. The evil intention of the person behind the crime did not matter.[270] In 1501, a pardon was justified by the bad treatment a woman received from her husband, who was, moreover, not harmed by the poison.[271] Even though essential, the fact that the crime was not carried out is not self-evident.

Medieval jurists lost sight of the dimension of the attempted act of *veneficium* that was still important in Visigoth Spain.[272] When Bartole reflects on *animus occidendi*, he notes that if the *Lex Cornelia* considered the intention more than the act, on the contrary, the *Lex Aquilia* gave consideration to the accomplished act as the only criterion for sanction. The Italian penal practice, in general, is based on the *Lex Aquilia*.[273] Using the example of the son who bought poison to kill his father, Placentin asserts that this act cannot be considered as a parricide because, contrary to divine law that considers the will and the outcome (*voluntas* and *exitus*), human law only considers the accomplishment of an act.[274] Can the fact that in Ferrara in 1465, the accomplice of a poisoning, which was not carried out, was executed be considered a return to the severity of ancient legislation?[275] Such a conclusion would be rather hasty. Other princes besides the King of France showed such mercy under the same conditions. In Lorraine, at the end of the fifteenth century, two poisoners who had been prosecuted received a ducal pardon because their criminal project was never carried out.[276] The same situation occurred in the States governed by Philippe le Bon, in 1459, when he pardoned a crime, so that the convicted woman who had been banished by the court from Aire would not fall into the debauchery that could result from exile.[277]

A prince's pardon was not limited to the would-be poisoner. In 1469, Guillemette, a partner in a poisonous plot, was pardoned for a murder that was carried out because she had been influenced by her lover. An act committed under duress or the influence of a third party was a reason for a pardon because the responsibility for the act was transferred to another. Moreover, the question of restored honor played a role in Guillemette's pardon since her second husband, a notary, insisted that no infamy should tarnish his name (1469).[278] Therefore, during the fifteenth century, a premeditated, secret, and perfidious murder was forgivable through an act of mercy, whose mystery is similar to the priest's *jus absolvendi*.[279] We can see how criminal casuistry has evolved since the time where the simple fact of giving poison, accidentally or without knowing it, was considered a capital crime.[280]

Providential, Symbolic, or Informal Punishments

Approximately 10 percent of the cases that can be used as evidence resulted in a sanction foreign to institutional justice. Even if it was concealed from the knowledge of men, the most supernatural crime could not escape from God's omniscience, which would punish its perpetrator, either on earth or in the beyond.[281] We should not be surprised that in the early Middle Ages, when powerful judicial bodies did not exist, three-quarters of the providential sentences are found. According to the hagiographic model, Heaven punished the guilty and helped the victims.[282] Marcatrude lost her child because she had her stepson poisoned and died herself soon afterwards.[283] Florent de Subiaco perished in the collapse of a building in which he was rejoicing in the success of his crime against Benoît de Nursie.[284] The murderer of Bishop Marachaire d'Angoulême spent very little time on the Episcopal throne.[285]

A proverb from the end of the Middle Ages says "he who prepares the poison must drink it" (*quy brasse le puison, il le doibt boire*).[286] The punishments given by Providence were sometimes linked to the *modus necandi.* The death of Robert de Normandie, who was poisoned during his pilgrimage to the Holy Land for the expiation of his brother's poisoning in 1028, punished the guilty party with the weapon with which he had committed murder.[287] More metaphorically, the venom of his mischievousness killed Sabin of Canossa's aggressor at the precise moment the bishop was drinking the poisoned cup.[288] The invisible power of poison was counterbalanced by the incomparable power of the Invisible. The same pattern can be seen during the fourteenth and fifteenth centuries. However, in these times, God intervened only indirectly, through events such as a poisoned cup or dish being served to one of the murderer's relatives or even to the murderer himself or herself instead of the planned victim. In front of the corpse of her child who died after eating the apple meant for the Dauphin, Valentine Visconti exclaimed: "God, how just you are! You know how to punish your people!" (*vray Dieu, que tu es juste! Comment tu sces bien tes gens payer*). That is how the justice of Heaven operated according to the imaginative propaganda from Bourgogne.[289]

Like other crimes, poisoning was also sanctioned outside a judicial framework or afterwards. During the early Middle Ages, the chroniclers like to tell stories in which the murderer was compelled to drink from the same cup that was offered to the victim, as was the case for Rosamund la Lombarde or Ava la Castillane.[290] Driven by a nameless fury, Robert de Béthune killed his venomous spouse with his own hands.[291] Sometimes, the source of the poisoner's punishment was the person whom the crime benefited the most: King Avar Cacanus chastised Romilde, the *basileus* Alexis sent Sichelgaïte to execution,[292] as if the accomplishment of a treacherous act such as *venenatio* made its author forever unworthy of trust. The horror of poisoning also triggered violence in mobs that vowed to lynch criminals made heinous because of the seriousness of their act and their personality. Some of the people who requested ***lettres de rémission*** had killed impulsively or involuntarily a poisoner who was also often a witch.[293] In 1276, after the suspicious death of Prince Louis, the women from the household of Marie de Brabant hide "for fear that the people would attack with stones" (*par poeur de ce que li people ne leur corust sus les lapidas*).[294] The same danger threatened Valentine Visconti: "the rumor circulated in Paris that if she was not removed from the king's household, they would go to get her and kill her for they said that she wanted to poison the king and his children" (*Commune renomee couroit a Paris que si on ne l'ostoit de de-lez le roi, on l'iroit querir de fait et seroit morte; car on disoit qu'elle vouloit empoisonner le roi et ses enfans*).[295] The love of subjects for their sovereign was demonstrated by the people's public condemnation of his enemies. In 1321, the population attacked fiercely and unrelentingly the poisoners of the wells. A Flemish chronicle says that the Jews and the lepers were punished more because of the will of the people than by the decisions of the court.[296] An impulsive and disorganized repression responded to the crime against the masses showing the limits of royal authority, whatever the laws said. As far as the massacres of 1348 are concerned, they followed the same model in many places: the justices of the princes (particularly in Dauphiné and Savoie) acted under the pressure of the crowd or the flagellants.[297] Despite all that, can we say that the horror of the crime of poisoning alone set in motion the extrajudicial retaliation? Once again it is doubtful. It was the character of the poisoners and that of their victims, more than the act that provoked the outburst of punitive violence.

Sentences and Punishments within the Judicial System

An ordinance in 1682 provides for punishment with fire for people convicted of poisoning,[298] a remnant of the association of *crimen veneficii* with magic and witchcraft that were traditionally punished that way. Before the crime of poisoning was separated from the others, was the sentence reserved for poisoners equal to the seriousness of the act?

Even if they are close, the nature of poisoning and the nature of sin do not overlap. As Bernard of Pavia said about 1200, the law of man punishes with death those who are guilty of serious misdeeds; God who seeks the improvement of the sinners prefers penance.[299] Poisoning is assuredly a sin, and one of the most serious. Bernardin of Siena wondered during a Lenten sermon, "Who would be crazy enough to think that preparing a poison in order to kill is not a sin?"[300] Such a sin requires an appropriate punishment. The canons of Saint Grégoire put the spiritual sanction of the *veneficium* at the top of the scale of penances.[301] At the end of the ninth century, the Council of Tribur ordered double penance for the worst homicides including poisonings.[302] About 1200, Alain de Lille imposed seven years of fasting on a poisoner, in addition to perpetual penance.[303] The figure of seven is high: infanticide is the only crime with a more severe punishment; since ancient times, it had concerned premeditated crimes.[304] But seven is not a maximum. Reginon of Prüm imposed a decade of penance for a woman who poisoned her husband because she dared to attack her lord and master.[305] During the thirteenth century, Barthélémy of Exeter went further by imposing perpetual reclusion in a monastery on a man who poisoned his wife.[306] Was it with this logic that on July 4, 1322, a year after his questioning, the leper Agasse was sentenced to the wall punishment? It is difficult to say, all the more because this sentence was used to punish heresy more often than the *veneficium* of 1321.[307] However severe they are, these penances were flexible. The texts indicate a varying degree of punishment according to how well the crime was committed. Despite the importance of the intention in canon law, the penances inflicted on the poisoner also take into account the completion of the act. Only one year is required for someone who has planned a crime without carrying it out.[308]

Roman justice was extremely harsh in the punishment of poisoners. Galba ordered that a tutor be crucified, even though he was a Roman citizen, because he had poisoned his pupil in order to get his inheritance.[309] The texts of the Late Empire provided for putting the *veneficus* in a sack with beasts that would bite him and tear him to shreds, or for simply exiling him to an island if he was of high rank.[310] What was left of those sanctions in the Medieval West?

In 873, quoting a formula from Saint Cyprien, the capitular of Quierzy asserted that royal law forbad that evil people and poisoners be permitted to live.[311] Yet, we note that capital punishment appears only in somewhat less than 18 percent of the extant cases, and six out of ten occurred during the fourteenth and fifteenth centuries. The convicted poisoners from the lower classes were punished with death in more than half of the cases. Thus, capital punishment was far from being systematic and universal. Other sanctions existed. The *Lex romana Burgundionum* made provision for the repudiation of the *veneficus* or the *venefica*.[312] An illustration of this principle is given by Jordanès about an affair that took place during the fifth century. A Visigoth princess held responsible for an attempted poisoning was sent back to her father with her nose and ears cut off by the King of the Vandals, her husband.[313] The shame was certainly worse than death and no one knows what happened to the mutilated poisoner. The use of poison was mainly sanctioned by a fine whose purpose was to assuage the victim's relatives. Salic law determines the amount of the fine according to whether the poisoning led to the death of the victim or not.[314] The Alamans and the Bavarians did the same.[315] The amount—12 *sous* in the Alamans' law, 200 in Riparian and Salic law—is the same as the one set for serious cases such as fire. The dissimulation inherent to *veneficium* is an aggravating circumstance, which increased the amount.[316]

Noncapital punishments were always substituted for the death sentence at the end of the Middle Ages. Bolognese justice punished attempted *venenatio* only with a fine that was increased in 1455.[317] Do the few banishments that are reported have something to do with the Roman exile reserved for nobles and still mentioned in twelfth-century England?[318] The condemnation of the seigneur d'Ormoy, banished for perpetuity, could lead us to think so,[319] but other banishments from lower social ranks indicate a break in the ancient bond between a person's status and forced exile.[320] The arbitrariness of power plays fully in the case of Jehan Bon, who was accused of poisoning the heir of Louis XI. He had the choice between two rather problematic possibilities, beheading or blindness. The services that he had rendered to the sovereign may explain the so-called softening of the penalty.[321] The same goes for the financier Pierre Gerbais, whose death sentence, after an appeal and a second trial, had been commuted to perpetual detention, which he did not serve.[322]

"The case is so bad that it should lead to a death penalty" (*est le cas si mauvais que paine de mort s'en doit ensuivre*) exclaimed a plaintiff during a case of poison that came before Parlement in 1402.[323] From the beginning of the Middle Ages, the death penalty was used to punish different kinds of crime. Visigoth legislation condemned to death free people or slaves who prepared lethal poison and handed over to the victim the perpetrators of crimes.[324] The law of the Lombard king, Rothari, condemned all poisoners, who were slaves, to death, whatever the outcome of the act.[325] During the eleventh century, imperial legislation in force in Lombardy required death for free people and the confiscation of their goods, which were used to compensate the wronged party.[326] Capital punishment became once again the common fate of the *venefici*. During the thirteenth century, the *Siete partidas* indicate once again the bag punishment, but it is only a formal reference to the law of Rome: a gloss explains that it is no longer used.[327] Instead, there were diverse forms of torture that were closely linked to the *modus necandi*.[328] *Gaydon* enumerates the sentences promised to the eponym hero accused of treason by poisoning: "I will have all his members cut off / Burnt in fire and the powder thrown to the wind" (*Cui je ferai touz les membres coper / Ardoir en feu et la poudre venter*).[329] A vast range of tortures awaited the poisoner because no text set the exact kind of punishment they should receive.[330]

It is hard to create a connection between the seriousness of the crime and the mode of execution considering that we cannot see what was considered the highest point on the scale of capital sentences, even if the stake seems to have particularly frightened those condemned to it, for multiple corporal and spiritual reasons.[331] Commenting on the formula *plus est . . .*, Azon writes that its superior atrocity should be sanctioned by the major sentence, the one of fire.[332] And in fact, the stake often awaited the *toxicatores*. "To the fire he was condemned, a just decision" (*A ardoir fu jugié, et par droit jugement*). In that way, Adenet Le Roy portrays the sentence given to an old witch, also a poisoner in the thirteenth century.[333] The sentence of fire was certainly given to poisoners with reference to the torture reserved for sorcerers and witches with whom judicial tradition often associated them. But there is no proof that the judicial authorities were aware of this tradition. In June 1390, the mayor of Dartmouth condemned the poisoner Denys Beaumont to die in live charcoal without the express authorization of the monarchy.[334] Therefore, the mayor had spontaneously chosen the stake. The situation is analogous on the continent. The women who poisoned Eleonore de Trie on behalf of her husband were burned or buried alive,[335] like the *veneficae* of the Bishop of Châlons in 1315.[336] The Bishop of Cahors, as much a witch as a poisoner, was burned alive in 1317, and not flayed alive, as it was first thought because of an incorrect interpretation of the rite of degradation, which preceded the execution.[337] The flames were also chosen for the lepers in 1321 because of the sacrilegious dimension of their crime and because this method was useful for mass executions. We find lepers hanged in Saint-Omer, but only in smaller numbers.[338] In 1390, some of the poisoners of the wells were burned, starting with the woman, who was implicated in this affair.[339] In a first sentence, the ***juge ordinaire*** of Anjou and Maine had also condemned Pierre of Thoulouse to the stake. But the redefinition of his acts into a crime of treason brought about a change in the way he was to be executed: he and his accomplices were beheaded and/or hanged.[340]

The *crimen majestatis* as well as treason, present in 1390—the criminals worked for the English enemy or their Flemish allies—effectively brought about, at the end of the Middle Ages, particular methods of execution, whatever sort of crime was committed or planned since the difference between what was planned and what was accomplished was abolished.[341] It was treason, and not the use of poison, that justified the exemplary punishment of Pierre du Tertre and Jacquet de Rue in 1378[342] that of John Delstein, the King of Navarre's henchman who was beheaded, quartered, and displayed at the gates of Paris in 1385[343] or, the atrocious torture of the poisoner of Louis XI, Jehan Hardy.[344] Desirous of affirming their majesty, if not their sovereignty, the princely powers acted in the same way. John of Vliet's squire was quartered after being beheaded for treason (1425), his head was mounted on a pike at a gate of La Haye, and the four parts of his body were displayed on four important squares of the county of Holland.[345] On the other hand, the kind of torture Jehan Coustain received toned down this violent dimension[346]: Jacques du Clercq indicates that the accused requested and received the right to be beheaded behind closed doors without being dismembered and to be buried in Christian ground.[347] On a much lower level, the crime of the servant who poisoned Geoffroy de Salagny was punished by decapitation, but his powders were burned on a public square of Mâcon, on order of the bailiff,[348] whereas in other cases, the condemned person and the fatal substance were burned together.[349] Decapitation punished fatal poisonings in the fifteenth century in Ferrara.[350]

Other methods of execution were also in use. Scalding evoked in a thirteenth-century literary work[351] was used in England under Henry VIII. The *Act for poysoning* of 1531 considered that the crime of poisoning was so horrible that it had to be punished appropriately.[352] Should we look for the reason for this choice in a relationship between counterfeiting—also punished in this way—and *toxicatio*, since both crimes were founded on falsification, deceit, and even the manipulation of material with the aid of occult knowledge? Nothing explicitly indicates such a comparison. Drowning appears as a punishment in the case of the squire Dunot for the failed attempt to poison the Duc d'Orléans (1440).[353] Frequently encountered as a punishment during the thirteenth century, hanging, the punishment for people of low rank is required for providers of poison by the *Liber augustalis*.[354] Those who carried out the plans of the Sicilian prelates to poison Frederick II and Thibaud de Champagne were condemned to the gallows,[355] as was the scoundrel, who helped the Comtesse de la Marche in 1242 or Gautier of Scotenny in May 1259.[356] In 1402, in accordance with the customary distinction between the sexes, the man of the couple of lovers was hanged while the woman was burned.[357] But the justice system in Metz did not hesitate to send to the gallows a female poisoner, who had repeated her crime in 1493[358] and the female servant of the Duchess of Clarence, treated like a traitor, died at the end of a rope.[359] Such diversity comes from the fact that other criteria, besides the type of the crime, determined the kind of punishment. To find a correlation between *modus necandi* and *modus suplicii* is a hazardous task. What is certain is that the horror of *veneficium* favored a severe punishment. Finally, let us note that no poisoner died from poison as punishment, a penalty as foreign to medieval civilization as the test by poison.

The prosecution and repression of the medieval crime of poisoning reflects more the evolution of political and judicial coordination than a particular desire to punish a form of heinous homicide. The creation of a procedure for the pursuit of *toxicatores* similar to the one used for those who practiced witchcraft cannot be clearly established. Nevertheless, the similarity between the repression of witchcraft and the increased repression of poisoning starting in the thirteenth century is not by chance. It results from the assertion of judicial structures, as well as the spiritual and political will to drive out Evil. Demanded by the highest authorities of both the Church and the State, it was applied to *toxicatio*. It used the inquisitorial and extraordinary procedure (torture), which is linked to the uncovering of the crime. But the act sought other ways to find the truth that preceded the investigative procedure. Since making someone say the unsayable is, in the final analysis, easier than seeing what is invisible, the confessions of the accused took on a crucial importance. Usually, they doomed the guilty party to capital punishment, which was carried out in various ways because of the intrusion of other charges made against the poisoners: the crime of casting evil spells led to the stake, treason to the axe. But the "outburst of torture" should not fool us. Even if it was probably compensatory, revealing in broad daylight the loathsome deeds of the murderer that were hidden away in secret, we should forget neither those who were exonerated nor the forgiven *potionatores*, in a time of both harshness and mercy.

NOTES

1. Use of stereotyped formulas in the ordinances of Philippe V concerning the poisonous lepers: *ne tanti scelus maleficii impunitum, prout nec decet, remaneat*... (21 juin, Duplès, pp. 270–272).
2. *Fontes juris romani antiqui*..., p. 93. S. N. Toianos, Zauberei und Giftmischerei..., pp. 37–38 and p. 47.
3. *Lex salica*, pp. 81–82. *Lex Alammanorum*, IV, 21 and 22, p. 330.
4. *Leges Wisigothorum*, VI, 1, 5, p. 255, Code de Chindasvinde.
5. *Capitularia regum Francorum*, n°196, *Episcoporum ad Ludovicum relatio*, 829, t. 2, p. 44.
6. Id., n°278 (Quierzy, 873), chap. 7, t. 2, p. 345.
7. Id., n°252, *Concilium triburiense*, 895, chap. 50, t. 2, p. 241.
8. Reginon de Prüm, *Ordo ad dandam poenitentiam*, ed. Migne, *PL* 132, I, 300, col. 250.
9. *Constitutiones regni Siciliae*, t. 4-1, titres 47, p. 151 and 69 to 72, p. 166 and sq.; *Lois de Guillaume le Conquérant*, art. 36 and *Lois d'Henri Ier*, p. 251.
10. *Siete partidas*, Partie 5, titre 5, loi 17, t. 3, p. 302 et Partie 7, titre 8, loi 7, t. 4, p. 495.
11. *Li livre de jostice et de plet*, p. 83; repeats the *Digeste*, XLVIII, 8.
12. Exemple Rogerius, *Summa codicis*, t. 1, p. 166.
13. J. Chiffoleau, *Les justices du pape*, p. 277: "A new attempt to create a structure for, to watch over, protect, and pacify all members of society."
14. *Parlement criminel*, X2a 14, f. 411 v.
15. Vigneulles, t. 2, p. 26: reference to a "Bohemian" woman who was sleeping peacefully on the gallows in Metz, about 1440.
16. Cf. J.-N. Biraben, *Les hommes et la peste*, t. 1, pp. 58–59, letter from a magistrate from Narbonne, April 17, 1348.
17. *Registre criminel du Châtelet*, t. 1 p. 312.
18. Carbonelli, p. 349.
19. Orderic Vital, t. 2, p. 80, and Carbonelli, *passim*. See also the accusations brought against a Jewish physician by patients who were treated badly before (*Actes du Parlement de Paris, 1254–1328*, n°5023, 1317) and after the plague (*Registres du trésor des Chartes*, JJ 81, f. 258 v, 1352).
20. Honorat Bovet, *L'apparicion de Jehan de Meun*, p. 11.
21. Valère Maxime, *Faits et dits mémorables*, ed.-tr. R. Combès, Paris, 2 vol., 1997, VI, 3, 8, t. 2, p. 163.
22. Jean de Salisbury, *Policraticus*, IV, 11, p. 79 of Brucker's edition.
23. *Lois d'Henri Ier*, p. 251: *Reddatur utique qui fuerit reus hujusmodi parentibus et amicis interfecti ut eorum misericordiam aut judicium sentiat quibus ipse non pepercit*...
24. Carbonelli, Come vissero..., pp. 203–208.
25. *Fontes juris romani antiqui*, p. 93.
26. A. Laingui, A. Lebigre, *Histoire du droit pénal*, t. 2, p. 18.
27. J.-M. Carbasse, *Introduction historique au droit pénal*, p. 31.

28. F. Cardini, *Magia, stregoneria, superstizioni nell'Occidente medievale*, Florence, 1979, p. 72. In 1330, the pope entrusted the prosecution of witches to special commissions appointed by him.

29. *Actes du Parlement de Paris, 1254–1328*, n°4767: *quando et quociens per dictam Marguerітam vel procuratorem suum fueritis requisiti, ipsos ad jura nostra regia sollempniter evocetis....* Does the word *ipsos* refer to the criminals or to the plaintiffs?

30. *Actes du Parlement de Paris, 1254–1328*, n°2323.

31. Shatzmiller, pp. 88–89, 233, 298.

32. J. G. Bellamy, *Crime and public order in England in the Late Middle Ages*, Londres, 1973, p. 57.

33. *Parlement criminel*, X2a 6, f. 368 v–369 et X2a 7, f. 33–34, 1357–1361.

34. Geoffroy de Salagny, p. 107 v.

35. Jean de Saint-Victor, p. 651: a nobleman from the surrounding area of Corbeil is implicated; *Registres du trésor des Chartes*, JJ 84, f. 145.

36. *Choix de pièces inédites relatives au règne de Charles VI*, n°106, t. 1, p. 245.

37. *Select cases; Richard II, etc.*, pp. 113 and 251.

38. Godefroy Ménilglaise, p. 201: Philippe V granted on July 10, 1317 letters to the woman involved in the case that indicated that she was not to be accused. She accepted the procedure after having protested it. She appeared *personaliter*.

39. *Registre criminel du Châtelet*, t. 1, p. 469: the provost gave his verdict against Julien Bernier with the advice and in the presence of the members of Parlement.

40. Secousse, p. 373 and sq., 494 and sq.: Vitu, pp. 58–59.

41. *Actes du Parlement de Paris, 1254–1328*, n°5048, 4767, 4826.

42. *Parlement criminel*, X2a 15, f. 160: an appeal to Parlement concerning a decision handed down from the court of the Duc d'Anjou, 1407; X2a 6, f. 178–181: appeal from a man accused of poisoning concerning the suspension of his official duties as provost.

43. *Choix de pièces inédites relatives au règne de Charles VI*, n°106, t. 1, p. 245. Most of the appeals concern appeals made before the sentence was given, not definitive sentences, which were permitted to be the object of an appeal in France only in 1454.

44. Pierre de Fontaine, *Conseil à un ami*, XXII, 28, p. 308. The jurist limits this impossibility to criminals who have acknowledged their crime or who have been convicted through proof, testimony, or arguments. Balde, *Consilia*, n°221, p. 44, stipulates that this impossibility concerns also the accomplice in a poisoning.

45. *Parlement criminel*, X2a 5, f. 13, then 70; same format X2a 15, f. 224 v et X2a 16, f. 35 v–36, 1408–1409.

46. *Parlement criminel*, X2a 18, f. 11 v–14.

47. A. Esmein, *Histoire de la procédure criminelle en France*, p. 40: crimes committed at court were judged jointly by the provost, the *Grand Conseil* and the officials in charge of petitions of his choice.

48. A.-M. Courtray, p. 42.

49. Pierre de Fénin, *Mémoires*, ed. Dupont, Paris, 1837, p. 182, note.

50. Du Clercq, pp. 636–638.

51. Jean de Roye, t. 2, p. 30. S. Cuttler, *The Law of Treason and Treason Trials in Later Medieval France*, Cambridge, 1981, p. 62, indicates the frequent seizure of this jurisdiction by Louis XI.

52. *Sacrorum conciliorum amplissima collectio*, XXXII, Council of Freising, 1440, canon 24, col. 18. See also *Statuts synodaux français du xiiie siècle. IV*, statutes of Cambrai (1277), titre X, p. 102, repeating the statutes of Guiard de Laon, about 1238–1248; statutes of Tournai (1300), p. 327.

53. *Statuta capitulorum generalium ordinis cisterciensis*, t. 5, pp. 588–589. At the end of the fifteenth century the following formula is seen again: *Capitulum generale... quasdam informationes a quibusdam regiis officiariis virtute quorundam mandatorum secundum formam juris factas audiens...*

54. Vigneulles, t. 2, p. 122: "since then, his friends have made peace with him and also he was absolved by our Holy Father the Pope" (*depuis, ses amis luy refirent sa paix et aucy il fut absoul de nostre sainct perre le pappe*).

55. J. Théry, p. 35; L. de Lacger, Bernard de Castanet, Bishop of Albi (1276–1308), *Bulletin de littérature ecclésiastique*, 1954, pp. 193–220.

56. However, S. Cuttler, *The Law of Treason*, p. 71, points out the presence of the *sénéchaux* of Toulouse et Carcassonne as well as the Comte de Forez. Charges of treason against the King of France in favor of the King of Majorca weighed heavily indeed against Délicieux.

57. Duplès-Agier, pp. 270–272: *cognitio et pugnitio prelibati criminis ad nos et non ad alium de jure pertinere noscantur*; in letters of August 18, 1321, the king recognizes the jurisdiction of justices outside the royal system (that of the Bishop of Albi in this case), while calling it exceptional (*Ordonnances des rois de France*, XI, 482).

58. *Digeste*, XLVII, 11.

59. *Registre criminel du Châtelet*, t. 1, pp. 449, 474, and 430.

60. Id., p. 469.

61. *Capitularia regum Francorum*, t. 2, n° 196, *Episcoporum ad Ludovicum relatio*, 829, p. 44.

62. *Lois d'Henri Ier*, LXXI, p. 251: *Si res in compellacione sit et emundacione misseveniat, episcopi judicio reservetur.*

63. C. Ginzburg, *Le sabbat des sorcières*, p. 69; Jacques Fournier, p. 143. Lepers interrogated at other times also confessed magical and heretical practices such as the profanation of the host. (Nangis, continuation, t. 2, p. 31 and sq.). La *Chronique parisienne anonyme* gives to the episode the name "the work of the devil" (pp. 57–59).

64. Jacques Fournier, t. 2, p. 56.

65. S. Troianos, Zauberei und Giftmischerei..., p. 42: it was during the seventh century that the emperors assumed the repression of *veneficium* which up to that time had been shared with the Church.

66. C. Gauvard, Les sources judiciaires de la fin du Moyen Âge..., edits in an appendix the table of contents of the *Registre criminel du Châtelet* drawn up by Aleaume Cachemarée; concerning two witches of whom one is also accused of using poisons, he indicates: "Note that however often *Monseigneur de Paris* required them to be held and questioned, it was said, nevertheless, that the Provost of Paris had jurisdiction (*Noter que combien que Monseigneur de Paris les eust requises a bailler et questionner en Parlement, neanmoins fut dit que le prevost de Paris en avoit la cognoissance*).

67. P. Paravy, À propos de la genèse médiévale de la chasse au sorcière..., et J. Chiffoleau, Sur la pratique et la conjoncture..., p. 369.

68. Jean de Salisbury, *Epistolae*, n° 16.

69. R. Génestal, *Le Privilegium fori en France du* Décret *de Gratien à la fin du xiv*[e] *siècle*, Paris, 2 vol., 1921 et 1924, t. 2, p. 154. The justification, found in the *De modo celebrandi generalis concilii* where the canon raises questions, is probably the extreme seriousness of the crimes whose perpetrators do not deserve any protection from the Church.

70. Id., t. 2, p. 156, Council of Riez (1285), canon 14: *quicumque herbas mortiferas in mortem vel abortivum cuiquam dederit, eo ipso excommunicationem incurrat, a qua non nisi per sedem apostolicam absolvatur. Et si clericus beneficiatus fuerit, ille sit privatus beneficiis ipso facto et ab ordine quem susceperat degradetur, tradendus curiae saeculari*; *Sacrorum conciliorum amplissima collectio*, XXV, Concile d'Avignon (1326), col. 755.

71. R. Génestal, *Le* Privilegium fori *en France...*, t. 2, p. 158.

72. Du Clercq, p. 668 in Buchon's edition.

73. Jean de Saint-Victor, p. 652.

74. Cf. A. Provost, *L'imagination au pouvoir...*, p. 51.

75. Guillaume de Nangis' continuator is indignant about this situation: *sub carceris arcta custodia etiam de voluntate summi pontificis... detinetur* (t. 1, p. 369).

76. Basin, t. 2, p. 130 and sq. H. Stein, *Charles de France*, chap. 10.

77. K. J. Kesselring, A Draft of the 1531 " Acte for Poysoning," p. 895 and sq.

78. Tite-Live, *Histoire romaine*, 8, 18; 40, 37, 4; 40, 43, 2 et 40, 44, 6.

79. Ammien Marcellin, *Histoires*, XXVI, 3, t. 2, pp. 6–7 in the Seyfarth ed., Leipzig, 1978: *inter curarum praecipua (...) id primum opera curabat enixa, ut veneficos, qui tunc rarescebant (...) morte mulctaret.*

80. Grégoire de Tours, V, 35, t. 1, p. 298 from R. Latouche's translation.

81. *Leges Wisigothorum*, II, 5, 19, p. 119.

82. *Capitularia regum Francorum*, n°228, t. 2, p. 122: *hujusmodi diaboli ministras [venenarias] diligenti examinatione proditas sub accerrima penitentia redigendas statuimus...*

83. J-M. Carbasse, La peine en droit français des origines au xviie siècle, *Recueil de la Société Jean Bodin*, t. LVI, *La peine*, 2e partie, Bruxelles, 1991, pp. 157–172, p. 159.

84. Frédégaire, p. 145; Adalulf presents these words to the king: "*Regina Gundeberga apud Tasonem ducem secrecius tribus diebus locuta est ut te venino interficerit, ipsum congugatum sublimarit in regnum.*"

85. Jean de Salisbury, *Epistolae*, n°16.

86. A. Esmein, *Histoire de la procédure criminelle en France*, p. 108: two cases of formal accusation survive in the register of Saint-Martin-des-Champs. A. Laingui, A. Lebigre, *Histoire du droit pénal*, t. 2, p. 68, on establishing the source of the *fama* before the appearance of an accusor.

87. *Actes du Parlement de Paris, 1254–1328*, n°4767: the victim who is accusing had not been affected; n°5187: victim wrongly left for dead.

88. Carbonelli, *Come vissero...*, pp. 203–208.

89. Juvénal des Ursins, p. 187 in the edition of 1614.

90. A. Esmein, *Histoire de la procédure criminelle en France*, p. 76 and sq. The author observes that the word "accusation" occurs in the criminal register of the Châtelet without any accusatory proceedings (p. 124).

91. A. Laingui, A. Lebigre, *Histoire du droit pénal*, t. 2, p. 46 et 58.

92. Godefroy Ménilglaise, p. 189, then 214.

93. *Parlement criminel,* X2a 14, f. 214 v–217 v.

94. *Digeste,* XXIX, 1, 17 p. 411.

95. *Parlement criminel,* X2a 15, f. 224 v and X2a 16, f. 35 v–36.

96. *Registres du trésor des Chartes,* JJ 106, f. 191 v–192.

97. Des Godins de Souhesmes, p. 134.

98. Dynter, t. 3, p. 441, and Zantfliet, col. 417.

99. A. Provost, *L'imagination au pouvoir...,* p. 41. Edition of deposition p. 535 and sq.

100. *Lettres de Louis XI,* n°1164.

101. Du Clercq, p. 636: judging Coustain to be full of "pompous, spiteful talk" (*hautains parlers despiteux*), he exposed the affair.

102. Jean de Saint Victor, p. 652: *ob suspicionem exortam et inquisitionem postmodum rite factam.*

103. Carbonelli, p. 220 and p. 233.

104. *Archives administratives de la ville de Reims,* t. 2-2, p. 1186: poisoning "as the said lieutenant claimed that he had become aware of it" (*si comme lidis lieutenens disoit estre venu à sa cognoissance*).

105. *Parlement criminel,* X2a 14, f. 93 v.

106. *Actes du Parlement de Paris, 1328–1350,* n°4205.

107. *Registres du trésor des Chartes,* JJ 84, 7 août 1355, n°205, f. 116 v: ... *baillivus trecensis habita horum noticia dictam Johannam capi fecit*... See *Registre criminel de Saint-Martin-des-Champs,* p. 105, insults exchanged by two women accusing each other of being poisoners (1337).

108. *Parlement criminel,* X2a 18, f. 11 v–14.

109. *Registres du trésor des Chartes,* JJ 84, f. 145 ou JJ 120, f. 85–85 v or *Parlement criminel,* X2a 18, f. 11 v–14.

110. Confessions et jugements, p. 30.

111. Andrea Barbazza, *Consilia,* t. 4, f. 150 v: *debitus ordo judiciarius fuit perversus.* The author indicates that the statues of Ferrara (that we were not able to consult) prescribed homicide by poisoning at the end of two years. The object of *consilium* is to show that this prescription is null and void in case of a crime of *lèse-majesté.*

112. *Constitutio criminalis carolina,* articles 37 et 50, p. 27 et 34: evidence to gather, questions to ask.

113. Le *Speculum juris* by Guillaume Durand treats briefly the investigation to be carried out in the *familia* of a poison victim without going further (III, 2, 1, Frankfort edition, 1592, fol. 17).

114. *Parlement criminel,* X2a 14, f. 214 v–217 v. Reference to Code, IX, 41, 3, *De quaestionibus.*

115. *Lex Thuringorum,* ed. K. F. von Richthoffen, in *MGH, Leges,* t. 5, Hanover, 1872, article 55: *Si mulier maritum veneficio dicatur occidisse, vel dolo malo ad occidendum prodidisse, proximus mulieris campio innocentem eam efficiat; aut, si campionem non habuerit, ipsa ad novem vomeres ignitos examinanda mittatur.*

116. Jean de Salisbury, *Epistolae,* n°16. Voir D. Knowles, The case of Saint William of York.

117. R. Van Caeneghem, La preuve dans le droit du Moyen Âge occidental, *Recueil de la Société Jean Bodin,* 17, *La preuve,* Bruxelles, 1965, pp. 691–753, p. 699.

118. Cohn, p. 191. The author believes that the crime was essentially one of witchcraft.

119. *Ci nous dit*, chap. 25 p. 50: the Virgin and Joseph were forced to swallow "cursed water" because of the suspected pregnancy of Mary: "And whoever drank it would die within an hour of drinking if he were guilty of what he was accused. And when they saw that the water did them no harm, they believed that she had conceived by the Holy Spirit" (*Et quiconques en buvoit il mouroit en l'eure qu'il en avoit beu c'il eistoit coulpables de ce qu'en li metoit sus. Et quant il virent qu'elle ne leur fist nul mal, si crurent qu'elle avoit conceu dou Saint Esperit*).

120. See P. de Félice, *Poisons sacrés, ivresses divines*, Paris, 1936, reed. 1970, pp. 91–125; E. Vogt, E. Perrot, *Poisons de flèches et poisons d'épreuve*, Paris, 1913, point out, p. 53 then 143, that the ordeal by poison is effective for accusations of witchcraft, but also for accusations of poisoning (Madagascar). A. Retel-Laurentin, p. 14 and 181, detects in an idiomatic German expression ("on this point, I would drink poison") the vestiges of an ordeal of poison in the pre-Christian Anglo-Saxon world.

121. J. de Maleyssie, *Histoire du poison*, p. 106.

122. These considerations would perhaps be corrected by reading the work of L. Lewin, *Gottesurteile durch Gifte und andere Verfahren*, Berlin, 1929, to which we could not have access.

123. See for example *Li romans de Dolopathos*, v. 1720 and sq.; *Ciperis de Vignevaux*, p. 116: an order is given to an alleged poisoner to "free himself" from the accusation by drinking the cup intended for his victim. If he remains alive, then his accuser will die.

124. Geoffroy de Salagny, p. 107 v.

125. Frédégaire, p. 145 of the Krusch ed. See A. Esmein, *Histoire de la procédure criminelle*, p. 47, on the recourse to a duel after an accusation by witnesses. In this case, it is the accused party who demands a duel.

126. *Leges Langobardorum*, p. 312 then p. 584, text of Emperor Henry II.

127. Text published in *RIS* I-2, Milan, 1725, p. 74:*... dum repeterent singuli homines, quos forte aliqua duritia detinebat, quod parens illorum, qui in lectulo mortuus fuerit, per venenum occisus fuerit. Et dum per pugnam ipsam causam ... quaerere disponebant, gravis causa nobis esse comparuit, ut sub uno scuto per unam pugnam omnem suam substanciam homo amittat ...*

128. Jean de Salisbury, *Epistolae*, n°16.

129. J.-Ph. Lévy, *La hiérarchie des preuves dans le droit savant du Moyen Âge*, Paris, 1939, p. 149.

130. *Liber augustalis*, II, 33, pp. 105–106: *Ab hujus autem sanctionis humanitate precludimus homicidas qui veneficio vel quolibet genere furtive mortis aliquem alium extinxisse dicuntur; in quibus etiam a pugne probatione non permittimus inchoari, sed per probationes ordinarias, si supersint alique, procedi primo debere jubemus, et denique officio curie subtili prius inquisitione premissa, si per probationes aliquas vel per inquisitionem plene non poterit facinus comprobari, tunc demum ad pugne judicium indiciis precedentibus descendatur: que omnia per officium judicis provide cognoscentis volumus explicari ...*

131. *Fleta*, I, 31, p. 79: *item nec per patriam se defendere debet quis in appello dato de veneno set tantum per corpus suum, eo quod inicium facti non fuit tam publicum quod sciri poterit a patria ...*

132. Honorat Bovet, *L'arbre des batailles*, ed. E. Nys, Bruxelles, 1883, IV, 112, pp. 224–225.

133. A. Esmein, *Histoire de la procédure criminelle*, p. 92. In the edict of Philippe le Bel who reports the abolition of the duel of 1260, it is a question only of crimes committed so secretly that there are no possible witnesses (*Ordonnances des rois de France*, I, 437).

134. *Parlement criminel*, X2a 4, f. 143; X2a 14, f. 173–177 v: the affair goes back to the Exchequer of Normandie in Parlement who examines the demand for a duel made by the accused party who wished to reestablish his honor.

135. *Parlement criminel*, X2a 6, f. 442–443. Robert Gui explains this default by his loyalty to the king who, he claims was his advisor in this affair, and by his poverty that prevented him from assembling the sum necessary for a forfeit for the duel.

136. Carbonelli, p. 189. B. Demotz, *Le comté de Savoie du xi*[e] *au xv*[e] *siècle*, Genève, Slatkine, 2000, p. 265, points out that Amédée VIII decided to forbid this kind of duel following the defeat of Othe, who was aged and weak, faced with a young and fiery adversary. The inequality of strength between the combatants was already an argument for the rejection of a duel in le *Liber augustalis*, II, 33.

137. *La mort le roi Artu*, p. 83 and sq. Another account of a duel that follows an accusation of poisoning against a princess in *Parise la Duchesse*, p. 6 and sq.

138. *Li bastard de Bouillon*, v. 6499 and sq. then v. 6510 and sq. *Godefroid de Bouillon* gives an account of the duel but believes it to be real (pp. 321–330).

139. *Parlement criminel*, X2a 18, f. 12 v. Duel demanded by Symon Anne in response to Pierre de Vendosme's accusation, 1423. On *purgatio vulgaris* reserved for lay people, see J.-M. Carbasse, *Introduction au droit pénal...*, p. 75, and J. Chiffoleau, Sur la pratique et la conjoncture..., p. 344.

140. Jean de Salisbury, *Epistolae*, n°16. *Pugatio* probably completed about 1175, before judges delegated by Alexandre III (A. Morey, Canonist evidence in the case of Saint William of York, *Cambridge historical Journal*, 1952, n°10, pp. 352–353).

141. Matthieu Paris, t. 3, p. 623. A. Esmein, *Histoire de la procédure criminelle*, p. 69 and sq. on *purgatio canonica*.

142. Simon de Phares, *Recueil des plus célèbres astrologues*, ed. J.- P. Boudet, Paris, 1997, X, 83, p. 508.

143. *Actes du Parlement de Paris, 1254–1328*, n°5221.

144. *Parlement criminel*, X2a 6, f. 369.

145. *Parlement criminel*, X2a 15, f. 224 v and X2a 16, f. 35 v–36.

146. It was possible for the accused party subjected to torture to produce witnesses. (A. Esmein, *Histoire de la procédure criminelle*, p. 129.)

147. *Parlement criminel*, X2a 6, f. 178–181. See A. Porteau-Bitker and A. Talazac-Laurent, La renommée dans le droit pénal laïque du xiiie au xve siècle, in *La renommée, Médiévales*, 1993, n°24, pp. 67–80.

148. A.-M. Courtray, p. 41.

149. Godefroy Ménilglaise, pp. 195–208.

150. A. Laingui, A. Lebigre, *Histoire du droit pénal...*, p. 50.

151. Rigault, chap. 3.

152. A.-M. Courtray, p. 42 et 48.

153. *Parlement criminel*, X2a 6, f. 369.

154. Carbonelli, PJ.

155. Id., p. 254. At Annecy and Evian, the same thing is said.

156. *Choix de pièces inédites relatives au règne de Charles VI*, n°106, t. 1, p. 245: one of the accused was made to believe that the other had confessed, which brought out his confession.

157. Balde, *Commentaria*, f. 124. One of the origins given for the Latin word meaning torture is precisely the forced exploration of the mind: *tormentum est torquere mentem.*

158. A. Provost, *L'imagination au pouvoir*, p. 83.

159. Geoffroy de Salagny, p. 107 v: *sine quibuscumque tortementis seu questionibus sponte et libere confessus*. The author points out that the *Siete partidas* puts those closely associated with the household into the same category as the slave of antiquity.

160. Du Clercq, p. 636.

161. *Chronicon turonense*, p. 470. Kantorowicz does not mention the case in his passage on the emperor's regaining control of the Church of Sicily. The *Liber augustalis* makes no stipulations in the material concerning poisoners.

162. Albe, *passim.*

163. Duplès-Agier, pp. 270–272.

164. C. Gauvard, "*De grace especial . . .* ," p. 149. A certain discrepancy exists between the principles, which exclude the use of torture during the discovery process, and the practice.

165. *Registre criminel du Châtelet*, p. 420.

166. *Parlement criminel*, X2a 14, f. 257 v.

167. *Registres du trésor des Chartes*, JJ 84, f. 145: *vi, timore ac cohercicione gehine.*

168. *Registre criminel du Châtelet*, p. 463.

169. Id., p. 546 and pp. 321–322.

170. C. Gauvard, "*De grace especial . . .* ," p. 153 and sq. Illustration of this position: when his enemies demanded the torture of Étienne *de Vallibus*, Parlement rejected the demand (*Parlement criminel*, X2a 6, f. 368 v–369 et X2a 7, f. 33–34, 1357–1362).

171. Juvénal des Ursins, p. 187 in the ed. of 1614. Cf. *Codex justinianus*, IX, 41, 3, p. 388: *ipsa quoque mulier torquebitur: neque enim aegre feret si torqueatur, quae venenis viscera hominis extinxit.*

172. *Parlement criminel*, X2a 18, f. 12.

173. Carbonelli, p. 327.

174. Géraud de Frachet, continuation, p. 23.

175. *Charles IV*, p. 37.

176. Monstrelet, t. 5, p. 470.

177. R. Girard, *Le bouc-émissaire*, Paris, 1982, p. 71.

178. *Parlement criminel*, X2a 14, f. 216 v: *liquere opportet evidenter crimen esse commissum.*

179. Ser Giovanni Fiorentino, *Il pecorone*, II, 23, p. 214.

180. G. A. Palazzolo, *Prova legale e pena. La crisi del sistema tra medio evo e moderno*, Naples, 1979, p. 43 and sq.

181. J.-Ph. Lévy, *La hiérarchie des preuves . . .* , p. 86.

182. *Corpus juris canonici*, II, 3, 5, 9, and II, 6, 1, 18: *Que personae infames habeantur.*

183. Godefroy Ménilglaise, p. 208: *viles personnae, pauperes tales in quibus non erat credendum in aliquo.*

184. *Parlement criminel*, X2a 18, f. 12 v–13.
185. *Parlement criminel*, X2a 6, f. 178–181.
186. *Parlement criminel*, X2a 6, f. 369 v.
187. J.-Ph. Lévy, La preuve dans les droits savants au Moyen Âge, in *La preuve...*, pp. 137–167.
188. Quintilien, *Institution oratoire*, V, 7 p. 120.
189. *Confessions et jugements*, p. 30.
190. A. Provost, p. 198.
191. Carbonelli, p. 258.
192. A. Provost, p. 277.
193. *Parlement criminel*, X2a 18, f. 11 v.
194. G. A. Palazzolo, *Prova legale e pena...*, p. 57. We were unable to consult this treatise.
195. Rigault, p. 95 and sq., articles 22 and 25 of the articles of the ecclesiastic investigation.
196. *Parlement criminel*, X2a 18, f. 11 v.
197. *Processus Bernardi Delitiosi*, p. 62, article 31 of the first series of articles on accusation: *dictus frater B. dixit quibusdam hominibus de Albia... quod ipse faceret abbreviare vitam dicti Benedicti papae.*
198. Provost, p. 246, deposition of Etienne, prior of Saint-Ayoul.
199. *Parlement criminel*, X2a 14, f. 257 v.: "It is rumored that Chalon was poisoned" (*On murmure que Chalon a esté empoisonné*).
200. F. Migliorino, *Fama e infamia...*, p. 71, gives this definition of *fama* from the Modénate Gabriele de Oseletti, second half of the thirteenth century, which insists on consensus: *opinio sive aestimatio omnium, vel maioris partis hominum alicuius civitatis, regionis, castri, villae, vicinae, loci circa aliquam rem seu aliquod factum in idem consentiens, sermonis ministerio potissime generata, ex incerto seu certo authore proveniens.*
201. Chastellain, t. 1, p. 341.
202. *Parlement criminel*, X2a 14, f. 217.
203. A. Friedlander, *The Hammer of the Inquisitors...*, p. 275.
204. Carbonelli, p. 254.
205. Formula taken from the *Ethics* and reproduced in the *Annales Maatsenses*, ed. *MGH SS*, IX, Hanover, 1851, p. 829.
206. C. Gauvard, La *Fama*, a basic speech, p. 9.
207. *Parlement criminel*, X2a 6, f. 178–181.
208. Secousse, p. 494 and sq.; *Registre criminel du Châtelet*, t. 1, p. 312; Carbonelli, PJ XXXIV.
209. F. Graus, *Pest-Geissler-Judenmorde*, p. 318. *Registres du trésor des Chartes*, JJ 209, f. 119 v: "found and brought to justice" (*trouvées et mises en justice*).
210. Nangis, t. 2, p. 32: *quod totum in ignem copiosum propter hoc accensum projectum, nullo modo comburi potuit, habito manifesto experimento et hoc itidem esse venenum fortissimum.*
211. *Registre criminel du Châtelet*, t. 1, p. 315.
212. Matthieu Paris, t. 5, p. 702 and sq.
213. Geoffroy de Salagny, f. 107 v, col. b.
214. Carbonelli, p. 225: *producuntur recepte..., super quibus requirunt pro parte curie proborum ferenda testimonia medicorum.*

215. G. Mollat, Guichard de Troyes et les révélations de la sorcière de Bourdenay, *Le Moyen Âge*, 1908, n°21, p. 316: *nec requisita fuit super hoc per me tamen notarium...*

216. D. Jacquart, *Le milieu médical en France du xiie au xve siècles*, Paris, 1981, pp. 291–293.

217. J. Shatzmiller, The jurisprudence of the dead body. Medical practice at the service of civic and legal authorities, in *Il cadavere, Micrologus*, 1999, n°7, pp. 223–230.

218. Monstrelet, t. 1, p. 320.

219. Concerning the *dauphins* of Charles VI, who died in 1415 and 1417, it is said: "the said *seigneurs...* were opened in the presence of physicians and others, and there was no sign of poisoning" (*lesdiz seigneurs...furent ouvers en presence de medicins et aultres, et n'y avoit quelque signe d'empoisonnement*) (Clément de Fauquembergue, *Journal*, ed. A. Tuetey, Paris, 2 vol., 1903–1910, t. 1, p. 32).

220. Jean de Saint-Victor, p. 651.

221. *Parlement criminel*, X2a 14, f. 215.

222. *Parlement criminel*, X2a 18, f. 11 v. The last hypothesis is doubtful because the death occurred much earlier.

223. Shatzmiller, pp. 88–89.

224. E. Dall'Osso, *L'organizzatione medico-legale...*, pp. 39–40.

225. The list of the concerned physicians is given in E. Wickersheimer, *Dictionnaire biographique des médecins en France au Moyen Âge*, Paris, 1936, reed. Genève, 1979.

226. *Parlement criminel*, X2a 12, f. 213 v: A physician confesses: "it is not treated in books of medicine how one can recognize for certain by only an examination of his blood if someone has been poisoned" (*il n'est pas a plain traictié es livres de medecine comment on peust certainement congnoistre s'aucune personne est empoisonnée par l'inspection de son sang seulement*).

227. G. Wolff, Leichen-besichtigung und -untersuchung bis zur *Karolina* als Vorstufe Gerichtlicher Sektion, *Janus*, 1938, n°42, pp. 225–286, p. 254.

228. Shatzmiller, The jurisprudence of dead body, p. 229.

229. Dynter, t. 3, pp. 497–498: *tres status brabancie, volentes de hiis fieri certiores, fecerunt coram nonnullis deputatis ipsorum in predicto castro Lovaniensi in multitudine copiosa ad hoc congregata, corpus ipsius anathomizari per medicos et chirurgicos quos habere potuerunt, numero septem, notabiles et expertos.* The successor of the late duke, Philippe le Bon, probably maneuvered in the shadows because he wanted to give the impression that his cousin died a natural death. Also, his origin in Brabant, which was challenged by those who were quick to point out the bad relationship that existed between the two men, brought his behavior into question. (See A. Uyttebrouck, *Le gouvernement du duché de Brabant au bas Moyen Âge (1355–1430)*, Bruxelles, 2 vol., 1975).

230. *Charles IV*, p. 37.

231. Carbonelli, p. 327 and 350.

232. A. Provost, 1re partie, chap. 2.

233. Ch.-V. Langlois, La fin d'Hugues Géraud, p. 535.

234. Carbonelli, p. 327.

235. Secousse, p. 494 and sq.

236. *Registre criminel du Châtelet*, confession of Julien Bernier, September 7, 1390, pp. 457–469.

237. Marx, PJ XI, pp. 226–227.

238. *Registre criminel du Châtelet*, t. 1, p. 321: "he did not admit anything about the said poisons and herbs that were found on him" (*il ne voult autre chose cognoistre des dites poisons et herbes sur lui trouvées*).

239. Carbonelli, document XXXIII.

240. Du Clercq, p. 637.

241. Ch.-V. Langlois, La fin d'Hugues Géraud, p. 546.

242. *Parlement criminel*, X2a 6, f. 442–443.

243. *Parlement criminel*, X2a 14, f. 173 and sq.

244. *Actes du Parlement de Paris, 1254–1328*, n 5221.

245. He introduces and justifies the verdict by *quia pejus est hominem veneno interficere...* (*Spicilegium brivatense*, p. 438 and sq.).

246. *Parlement criminel*, X2a 14, f. 174 and n°252, f. 215 v.

247. Nangis, Continuation, t. 2, p. 159: *quid de eis* [the people arrested at the Palace in 1337] *postea factum sit ignoratum est.*

248. *Parlement criminel*, X2a 7, f. 33–34: Because the pertinent witnesses were not gathered promptly, the complaint of the enemies of a money changer in Toulouse was dismissed from court in 1362.

249. Jean de Winterthur, p. 11.

250. Shatzmiller, p. 131.

251. *Processus Bernardi Delitiosi*, sentence, p. 211: *quia super machinatione in mortem prefati domini Benedicti, ...ipsum fore de ea culpabilem nequivimus invenire, eum super illa sententialiter absolvimus, justitia mediante.*

252. Lacger, p. 218.

253. Jean de Saint Victor, p. 644: *contra eum nihil probare potuerint.*

254. Godefroy Ménilglaise, p. 195 and sq.

255. *Parlement criminel*, X2a 15, f. 224 v and X2a 16, f. 35 v–36. The relative lightness of the sanction shows that the rigor of the law that prescribed that false witnesses be punished in the same way that the accused would have been if the accusation had been proved was seldom followed.

256. *Registres du trésor des chartes*, JJ 84, f. 145.

257. *Parlement criminel*, X2a 6, f. 368 v.

258. *Parlement criminel*, X2a 14, f. 214 v–217 v and X2a 18, f. 11 v–14.

259. Labande, pp. 137–144.

260. Jean de Roye, p. 275 in Michaud-Poujoulat's edition.

261. Recent research has shown the persistence of private arrangements to settle disputes in the late Middle Ages, despite the adage *omnis delinquens offendit rem publicam*; see T. Dean, Criminal justice in the mid-fifteenth-century Bologna, *Crime, Society and the Law...*, p. 32; C. Gauvard, De la difficulté d'appliquer les principes..., p. 96.

262. *Registres du trésor des Chartes*, JJ 106, f. 191 v–192.

263. Juvénal des Ursins, p. 364 in Buchon's edition: "asked and requested immediately that no investigation or punishment be carried out" (*pria et requit tres instamment que nulle enqueste ou punition en feust faicte*).

264. *Code théodosien*, IX, 38, 7.

265. *Lois d'Henri Ier*, p. 251: *Si quis veneno vel sortilegio vel invultuacione, seu maleficio aliquo faciat homicidum, sive illi paratum sit sive alii, nichil refert quin factum mortiferum et nulo modo redimendum sit.*

266. The reform edict of 1357 does not mention it explicitly.

267. C. Gauvard, La justice pénale du roi de France à la fin du Moyen Âge, *Le pénal dans tous ses états. Justice, États et société en Europe (xiie–xxe siècle)*, s.d. X. Rousseaux and R. Lévy, Bruxelles, 1997, pp. 81–112, p. 100.

268. *Registres du trésor des Chartes*, JJ 106, f. 191 v–192: the accused "is likely to suffer corporal punishment because of which he and his entire family will be dishonored" (*est en aventure de souffrir peine corporele dont eulx et leur lignages soit deshonnorez*).

269. *Registres du trésor des Chartes*, JJ 120, f. 85–85 v.

270. *Registres du trésor des Chartes*, JJ 162, f. 76 v. Note, however, that his name was retained in the records.

271. *Registres du trésor des Chartes*, JJ 234, f. 107 v–108.

272. *Lex romana Wisigothorum*, p. 435: *Consilium, non factum puniendum est.*

273. Bartole, *Commentaria in Digesti partes*, t. 2, p. 177 v: *statuta per Italiam puniunt factum et non animum.*

274. Placentin, *In codicis libris IX summa*, p. 435.

275. Gundersheimer, p. 111. Note that the *Statuto di Forli*, II, 46, pp. 240–241, punishes the intention as it does the act.

276. Des Godins de Souhesmes, pp. 134–135.

277. Grégoire de Tours, t. 1, p. 226 in Büchner's edition.

278. *Registres du trésor des Chartes*, JJ 196, f. 104–105.

279. C. Gauvard, La justice pénale du roi de France..., p. 100.

280. Without going back to the early Middle Ages, it suffices to read *La mort li roi Artu* (first third of the thirteenth century) to see Arthur's response to Guinevere when she protests her ignorance of the poison in the apple that had been given to a knight: "Lady..., however you present it, the act is evil and villainous" (*Dame..., comment que vos li donnissiez, l'ouvraige en est mauvese et vileinne*), p. 77.

281. Ferretus Vicentinus, col. 1013.

282. See E. Bozoky, Les miracles de châtiment du haut Moyen Âge, in *Violence et religion*, s.d. J.-M. Delmaire et P. Cazier, Lille, pul, 1998, pp. 151–167.

283. Grégoire de Tours, t. 1, p. 226 of the Büchner edition.

284. Grégoire le Grand, *Dialogues*, II, *Vita Benedicti*, 8, p. 160 and sq.

285. Grégoire de Tours, V, 36, t. 1, p. 300 in R. Latouche's tr.

286. *Le livre des trahisons*, p. 70.

287. Guillaume de Malmesbury, t. 1, pp. 211–212. The English chronicler does not connect the poisonings himself.

288. Grégoire le Grand, *Dialogues*, III, 5, t. 2, p. 274 and sq.

289. *Le livre des trahisons*, p. 30.

290. Grégoire de Tours, t. 1, p. 152 of the Büchner edition; *Cronica Najerense*, ed. A. Ubieto Arteta, Valence, 1966, pp. 85–87.

291. *Chronique de France et de Flandre*, f. 12.

292. *Grandes Chroniques de France*, t. 2, p. 84; Roger de Hoveden, t. 3, p. 162.

293. *Registres du trésor des Chartes*, JJ 81, f. 258 v, 1352; JJ 196, f. 56, 1469, JJ 207, f. 148, 1481.

294. De Gaulle, p. 90, deposition of the legate Simon reporting the words of the Bishop of Bayeux, who was close to Pierre de la Broce.

295. Froissart, t. 3, p. 243 in Buchon's edition.

296. *Renart le Contrefait*, t. 1, p. 294: "the common people carried out justice without calling either the provost or the baillif" (*faisoit le commun peuple justice sans appeller prevost ne baillif*). Bernard Gui emphasizes that the lepers were put to death outside the justice system (t. 1, p. 164 of the Baluze edition).

297. Jean le Bel, t. 2, p. 225: "everyone, large and small, was so angry with them that they were all burned and put to death in the border country, where the flagellants went, by the *seigneurs* and the judges of the area" (*chascun, grand et petit, fust si animé sur eulx qu'ilz furent tous ars et mis à mort es marches où les flagelleurs aloient par les seigneurs et les justices des lieux. . . .*) See the order of instructions against the Jews given August 10, 1348, by Louis de Savoie, Seigneur de Vaud, et Amédée, Comte de Genève, *in* A. Nordman, Documents relatifs à l'histoire des juifs à Genève, dans le Pays de Vaud et en Savoie, *REJ*, 1927, n°83, pp. 63–73, p. 71.

298. *Recueil des anciennes lois . . .*, t. 19, p. 398.

299. Bernardus Papiensis, *Summa decretalium*, V, 9, p. 219; two successive chapters (V, 32, then 33) treat, on the one hand, punishments, and on the other penances.

300. Bernardin de Sienne, *Sermons de Carême*, sermon XXXVI, p. 207: *Quis autem insanus est ut non credat esse peccatum preparare venenum ad homines occidendos?*

301. *Die Bussordnungen . . .*, c. 112, p. 173: *Si laicus occidit alium odii meditatione, si non vult arma relinquere, VII annos peniteat, sine carne et vino III; si par casum I annum; si pro ira, III; si in proelio cum rege occiderit hominem XL dies peniteat, si per poculum aut per artem aliquam VII annos peniteat aut plus.*

302. *Capitularia regum Francorum*, n°252, *Concilium triburiense*, chap. 50, t. 2, p. 241: *si quempiam veneno vel herbis aut diversi generis maleficiis perdiderit, velut pessimus homicida duplici mulctetur poenitentia.*

303. Alain de Lille, *Liber poenitentialis*, II, 37, t. 2, p. 66, according to Burchard de Worms (XIX, 5): *Confecisti aliquem mortiferam potionem et cum ea aliquem occidisti? Si fecisti, carinam unam cum septem sequentibus annis jejunare debes et nunquam sis sine aliqua poenitentia.*

304. Reginon de Prüm, *Libri duo de synodalibus causis*, II, 15, p. 220.

305. Id., II, 84, pp. 246–247: *Si mulier maritum suum causa fornicationis veneno interficit, aut quacumque arte perimere facit, quia dominum et seniorem suum occidit, X annis poeniteat.*

306. Barthélemy d'Exeter, *Poenitentiale*, p. 218: *seculum relinquat et in monasterio peniteat . . .*

307. Jacques Fournier, t. 2, pp. 134–145. See *Le livre des sentences de l'inquisiteur Bernard Gui*, p. 1289 and 1293, where appears the punishment of Guillaume Agasse announced during the sermons of July 4 and 5, 1322.

308. Alain de Lille, *Liber poenitentialis*, II, 37, t. 2, p. 66: *Si autem voluisti et non perfecisti homicidium, unum annum poeniteas.*

309. Suétone, *Vie des XII Césars*, Galba, 9, t. 3, p. 9.

310. *Digeste*, XLVIII, 19, p. 852. Mentioned by Bernardus Papiensis, *Summa decretalium*, V, 9, p. 219.

311. *Capitularia regum Francorum*, n°278, t. 2, p. 345: *regis ministerium est... maleficos et veneficos non sinere vivere.*

312. *Leges Burgundionum, Lex romana*, titre XXI, *De divortiis*, pp. 143–144.

313. Jordanès, *Histoire des Goths*, tr. O. Devillers, Paris, 1995, p. 72.

314. *Lex salica*, pp. 81–82.

315. *Lex Alammanorum*, IV, 21 and 22, p. 330.

316. J. Halsall, Violence and society in the early medieval west: An introductory survey, *Violence and Society in the Early Medieval West*, ed. G. Halssall, Woodbridge, 1998, p. 16.

317. T. Dean, Medieval justice in mid fifteenth-century Bologna, p. 32; a fine always constitutes part of the logic of pacification, even in the most serious crimes.

318. *Lois de Guillaume le Conquérant*, article 36: *Si quis alterum veneno occiderit, aut occidatur aut in exilium perpetuum agatur.*

319. Jean de Saint-Victor, p. 651.

320. *Documents nouveaux*, pp. 29–31, example of the humble Willemine la Barbière banished by the court of Aire in 1459.

321. Jean de Roye, t. 2, p. 30. J. Favier, *Louis XI*, Paris, Fayard, 2002, p. 290, mentions a John Boon, an agent of Edouard IV sent back by Louis XI in 1469.

322. A.-M. Courtray, p. 58 and 144. The question of the admissibility of the appeal arises with regard to Roman law that excludes it: cf. Balde, *Consilia*, n°221, p. 44 or Pierre de Fontaine, *Conseil à un ami*, XXII, 28, p. 308.

323. *Parlement criminel*, X2a 14, f. 176 v.

324. *Leges Wisigothorum*, VI, 2, 2, p. 259, Chindasvinde's law: *ingenuos sive servos veneficos, id est qui venena conficiunt, ista protinus vindicta sequatur, ut, si venenatam potionem alicui dederint, et qui biberit mortuus exinde fuerit, illi etiam continuo suppliciis subditi morte sunt turpissima puniendi. Si certe poculo veneni potatus evaserit, in ejus potestate tradendus est ille qui dedit, ut de eo facere quod voluerit.*

325. *Leges Langobardorum*, Rothari's edition, articles 139 to 142.

326. Id., p. 584: *Quicumque veneficio seu quolibet modo furtivae mortis aliquem peremerit aut inde consentiens fuerit, mortis sententiam incurrat omniumque suarum rerum mobilium seu immobilium facultatem amittat, ita tamen ut pretium decem librarum pro legitimo widrigildo propinquis perempti primum inde detur, reliqui rursus medietas eisdem propinquis veniat, altera autem medietas ad fiscum accedat.*

327. *Siete partidas*, Partie 7, titre 8, loi 7, t. 4, p. 495.

328. J. Chiffoleau, *Les justices du pape*, p. 238, points out the relationship between types of crimes and forms of execution, but he emphasizes the great variety of the latter.

329. *Gaydon*, v. 640. Note, however, that the real guilty party was finally hanged.

330. J.-M. Carbasse, *Introduction historique au droit pénal*, p. 275; N. Gonthier, *Le châtiment du crime au Moyen Âge*, p. 106.

331. Vigneulles, t. 3, p. 34: a woman who was both an adulteress and a murderer demands in vain that she be decapitated as was her lover "because of her great fear of fire" (*pour le grant doubte du feu qu'elle craindoit*).

332. Azon, *Lectura sive commentarius...*, p. 696: *ita maior poena debet imponi, quia comburetur.*

333. Adenet le Roi, *Li roumans de Berte aus grans piés*, ed. A. Scheler, Bruxelles, 1874, v. 2266. In a story in the *Decameron* (IV, 7) the companion of man who was allegedly poisoned demands that his female murderer be burned at the stake.
334. J. G. Bellamy, *Crime and public order . . .*, p. 186.
335. Jean de Saint-Victor, p. 651.
336. Géraud de Frachet, p. 39.
337. Albe, p. 109 et Ch.-V. Langlois, La fin d'Hugues Géraud, p. 543.
338. F.-O. Touati, *Maladie et société au Moyen Âge . . .*, p. 734.
339. *Registre criminel du Châtelet*, t. 1, p. 480.
340. Id., p. 322, 469, 474, 479; t. 2, p. 6.
341. See S. H. Cuttler, *The Law of Treason . . .*, op. cit.
342. *Chronique des règnes . . .*, t. 2, p. 301: treason is given as the reason for this form of execution.
343. *Chronique du Religieux de Saint-Denis*, t. 1, pp. 355–357 and 467.
344. Jean de Roye, t. 1, pp. 303–309. In addition to execution were added confiscation of belongings, the house to be razed and planted in its place a sign indicating the infamy of the convicted person.
345. Zantfliet, col. 417, et Dynter, t. 3, p. 441.
346. F. Mercier, *L'enfer du décor. La Vauderie d'Arras (1459–1491) ou l'émergence d'une nouvelle souveraineté autour des ducs Valois de Bourgogne*, Thèse de l'Université de Lyon II, s.d. J. Chiffoleau, 2001, p. 441 and sq. It is true that Chastellain describes the crime as divine and human treason (p. 260), but the form of the execution of the guilty party does not take this fact into account.
347. Du Clercq, p. 637.
348. Geoffroy de Salagny, p. 107 v.
349. Exemple *Parlement criminel*, X2a 18, f. 11 v–14.
350. Gundersheimer, p. 111.
351. *Parise la Duchesse*, p. 6.
352. K. J. Kesselring, A draft of the 1531 "Acte for Poysoning," p. 899: *that detestable offence nowe newely comytted requireth condigne punisshment . . .*
353. Monstrelet, t. 5, p. 470.
354. *Liber augustalis*, titre 72, p. 66.
355. *Chronicon turonense*, p. 470.
356. Matthieu Paris, t. 5, p. 702 and sq.: *tractus et in patibulo horribiliter suspensus*.
357. *Choix de pièces inédites relatives au règne de Charles VI*, n°106, t. 1, p. 245.
358. Vigneulles, t. 3, pp. 301–302.
359. J. Bellamy, *Crime and public order . . .*, p. 57.

6

Beyond Crime: Issues and Uses of Poison

In an article dedicated to Jean de Touraine, the heir of Charles VI who died in 1417, Y. Grandeau wrote that after this death nothing was left to the Duc de Bourgogne except "the sterile consolation of accusing the Armagnacs of having poisoned Jean de France."[1] Sterile with regard to the truth of the facts, the accusation was certainly not sterile, on the other hand, in the struggle that occurred among the factions to control the government of the kingdom. By throwing out libelous accusations, Jean the Fearless (*Sans Peur*) was acting as an expert in public discourse. Poison held a distinct place in the public mind. Easy to attribute to an individual or to a group, the crime of poisoning was one element in a political struggle or ideological "communication." In the work of Roman historians in the second century, the improved status of the Antonins at the expense of the Judeo-Claudians resulted from the denunciation of the propensity of this dynasty for *toxicatio*. The phenomenon seems all the more pronounced in the Middle Ages, particularly in the last part, because the loathing of criminal poisoning was strongest and its image more sensational in a "public opinion" in the process of being formed. That is why it seemed necessary to conclude this essay with a reflection on the diverse ways that stories and cases of poisoning were used.

POISONOUS AGGRESSION, HEROISM, AND SAINTHOOD

Before examining the uses of the accusation of poisoning at the expense of those who are accused comes the question of the "benefits" that certain victims were able to derive from the poisonous aggression that allegedly targeted them. We will consider athletes of both faith and sword while wondering if there is some glory to be gained in a confrontation with poison.

Poisoned Beverages and Certificates of Sainthood

Less edifying than the interminable torments inflicted on champions of the faith, *veneficium* is not any less an instrument of martyrdom that a twelfth-century author from Liège does not hesitate to raise to the level of fire and iron.[2] It is also an indication of sainthood. The poison that the pagans made the Christian faithful drink in order to test their God with their body served, on the contrary, to demonstrate, by the assimilation of the toxic substance with no consequences, the superiority of divine strength over the forces of evil represented by the poison. Saint John and Saint George resisted valiantly the cups of poison that the polytheists gave them. Saint Mathias was the victim of a poisonous trap prepared by the idolaters.[3] These saints conquered the poison they drank in the name of Christ who had promised them invulnerability.[4]

The toxic traps set for Benoît de Nursie tested not only his body, since it did not absorb the poison, but also his foresight,[5] which distinguished him from ordinary mortals.[6] The two episodes, symbols of his inaccessibility to sin, also show divine election that Samson, the future Bishop of Dol, also demonstrated when he triumphed over the *poculum mortis*.[7] This dimension continued to exist to the end of the Middle Ages, as the story of Saint Jacques de la Marche demonstrates.[8] The model of the founder of Mont-Cassin is, of course, Abélard, whose misadventures contributed to establish not sainthood, of course, but a form of grandeur. The persecution that he suffered at the hands of his monks permitted his person to rise to the level of Saint Benedict, who was evoked with total innocence to justify the abandonment of the establishment whose head he had become. Repeated poisonous attacks put their victim in the company of saints.[9]

An episode of the third crusade presents a case of a collective test of poison. On the road to Andrinople, the crusaders of Frederick Barbarossa were offered poisoned wine by the Greeks. Warned of the threat, the imperial *senechal* gave the order to not drink the wine. But a group of intrepid young men paid no attention and drank the wine with no ill effects, while a native of the region almost died. The author of the *Gesta Friderici* saw no other explanation than a miraculous invulnerability to poisoned drinks possessed by Christ's soldiers, and he linked the episode to the biblical story of the water that was unhealthy for the Egyptians but drinkable for the Jews.[10] Resistance to poison distinguished the knights in the holy war just as it characterized saints.

This resistance also demonstrated the infinite superiority of the Christian faith to the Muslim religion. Conceived about 900 as an exchange of arguments between a Christian and a Muslim, the *Risala* by the pseudo-al Kindi, translated at the request of Pierre le Vénérable in order to be more familiar with the adversary who was being fought,[11] relates the poisoning of Mohammed by a Jewish woman who wanted to avenge the extermination of her people by the Messenger of God. Considering his poison as a sort of testing poison that was to demonstrate either the imposture of the Prophet (if he succumbed) or his authenticity, the Jews succeeded in killing a guest but not the Master from Medina, who was warned by the poisoned mutton shoulder. The so-called prophet showed himself to be lacking in the virtues of the prophets, the apostles, and the saints.[12] Matthieu Paris ridiculed the salutary speech of the piece of meat and demonstrated the double miraculous inadequacy of the false prophet, powerless to prevent the death of a companion and incapable of neutralizing the poison that was destined for him[13] : a cruel test of poison that revealed the deception of Islam.

The hagiographic dossier of Saint Louis includes a toxic episode told by dionysian historiography and its derivatives. It does not concern an infidel trap but an attempted poisoning instigated by the Comtesse de la Marche in 1242. Certainly, the circumstances of the discovery of the harmful project were not linked to foresight. Besides, he was not the sole beneficiary of Providence since his brothers, also targeted for death, were also spared. Finally, neither Joinville, Guillaume de Saint-Pathus, nor other authors of the *vitae* mention the episode, thereby showing the necessity of discretion.[14] That does not prevent other authors who do mention it from emphasizing that God protected Saint Louis from being affected by the poison, and this particular protection is a part of the sainthood of the king who was in other respects merciful.[15]

A poisoning can be considered as a form of martyrdom in the case of sovereigns who, because they have not been carried onto the altars, have been close to it or at least have been considered worthy of being honored in this way. Criminal poisoning opens two paths by which the victim can reach the proximity of the saints. The first is a death that occurs innocently and piously. Like a sacrificial lamb walking to its death, Henry VIII experienced in 1313 a death of edifying saintliness.[16] His partisans did not fail to make clear that the death of the emperor occurred on Saint Bartholomew's Day, the first martyr to have his blood spilled,[17] and that death had carried into the other world a man of great faith,[18] who had refused all emetic treatment in order not to reject the Eucharist along with the infected substances in his body, preferring to die with Christ than to live without him.[19] The other path of sanctification, sometimes resembling the first, was the *passio corporis*[20] with its accompanying suffering and stigmata. It is not a question of seeing behind each description of the suffering of people who have been poisoned an effort to promote them to sainthood. It can be said, however, that mentioning the circumstances of their deaths could lead to their glorification. That was true for Louis VI, who was marked for life by the poison from his stepmother whose despicable act he pardoned, more evidence of his Christian virtue.[21] The misadventure of 1191 does not seem to play any part in the arguments of the partisans for the canonization of Philippe Auguste, who bore for his whole life the stigmata from an attempted poisoning.[22] The case of Charles V is more delicate. Did an attempted poisoning become one of the reasons to praise a monarch? Christine de Pizan clearly indicates that suffering marked the entire existence of the king, but she does not link the suffering to poison, for reasons that remain to be clarified: did she receive indirect information from her father on the true origin of the royal suffering? Is it modest silence on an episode that illustrates divisions in the kingdom?[23] On the other hand, she emphasizes the providential protection of the servant of God in the affaire of 1378.[24] Other authors state that from the middle of the 1350s or 1360 to 1380, the life of the king was a constant state of suffering and illness because of poisoning attempts by his enemies.[25] Such a path of suffering certainly did not lead the good king to Paradise, but the story of his slow poisoning contributed to the valorization of a sovereign who was, moreover, endowed, in the same way as the saints, with the ability to know in advance the moment of his death since the cessation of the flow from the fistula in place to evacuate the poison announced to him that he would die within the next two weeks (Froissart).[26] This "passion" of the poison is, however, not to be taken as an important factor in the promotion of Charles V, for it does not come from the prince's most enthusiastic admirers.

Without maintaining that poisoning could lead to sainthood by itself,[27] it can be stated that poison conferred a certain aura on some of its victims who were either killed by it or who managed to survive despite it. The cruel suffering that it caused, or the lack of vulnerability that neutralized it, the gift of detection that it revealed in some emerge in the hagiographic and historiographic imaginary.

Heroic Poison?

Just as poisoning seems to be able to be associated with candidates for sainthood or blessing, its contribution to the glorification of knights that it strikes down is uncertain. Putting its victim between grandeur and finiteness, it involves an insult that is close to infamy.

Alexander's place in medieval culture is immense. Important leaders knew his history and willingly identified with him, the model of bravery, an invincible and conquering warrior. Like that of another hero, Hercules,[28] his death emphasizes the invincibility of a warrior, circumvented by poison, the only way to overcome unsurpassable fighting virtues: "He could not die by the sword, but evil poison killed him" (*De fer ne pot morir, mis maus venin l'ocist*) observes the *Roman d'Alexandre* about 1200, which states that this sentence was put on the statue erected on the tomb of the king, who was represented in *pantocrator*.[29] Poison then played an important role in fashioning the image of a hero. From the twelfth century on, the figure of Alexander inspired authors who were reporting the deaths of certain warriors. The chroniclers who lingered over the death of Robert Guiscard, the model of audacity and of fighting spirit struck down in the middle of a campaign against the *basileus*, do not fail to point out that the Norman warrior was brought down because of the deceit of his wife, and not by the force of the sword against which he was invincible.[30] The parallel is more explicit in the case of Henri de Luxembourg. Like Alexander, Henry VII, *invictissimus imperator*, had to admit that he was conquered by poison.[31] Killed in the middle of the peaceful reconquest of northern Italy,[32] the sovereign described as "worthy, brave, chivalrous and very noble in his acts" (*preu, hardi, chevalereux et très noble en ses fais*) (*Grandes Chroniques de France*) was the equal in death of a hero of antiquity.[33] Written about 1315 by the canon from Metz Simon de Marville, the *Voeux de l'Epervier*, elevates the monarch, reputed to be the best tournament combatant of his time,[34] to the level of a hero of antiquity: "You have today put to death the best emperor/Who was after Alexander the most gallant" (*Avez heus mis a mort le meudre emperour/Que fut pués Alixandre le lairge donneour*) state the last verses of the poem.[35] The Alexandrine model stands out and surpasses the less certain one of another brave man reputed to be the victim of *venenatio*, Godefroy de Bouillon.[36]

The medieval image of Alexander is far from being only positive. The clerical perception of the warrior is that of a powerful man so blinded by his power that without a second thought he drank a deadly *poculum* presented by his enemies. His fate reminded contemporary princes of the vanity of terrestrial glory. As stated in the *Roman de Rou*, "Alexander was a powerful king / But his conquests were of little value to him / He was poisoned, and he died." (*Alexandre fu roy puissant / Mais cil conquist poi lui valut / Envenimez fu, si morut*).[37] Poison marks the end of all human power in contrast to divine omnipotence and eternity. Eustache Deschamps wondered: "Why did Alexander die by poison / He who was so powerful and so lucky / He who conquered the world at a tender age / And who began to conquer 15 years after his birth? . . ." (*Pour quoy fina par venin Alixandre / Qui si puissans fut et si fortunez, / Qui le monde soubmist en aige tendre, / Et commença XV ans puis qu'il fut nez / A conquérir? . . .*) And he answered that it was in order to illustrate the fact that what must happen will happen to the powerful who are subject to divine decrees.[38] The striking character of poison makes sense in that it destroys in a short time the efforts of many, many years.

The military force of Robert Guiscard was so vulnerable that his wife's betrayal was sufficient to wipe it out.[39] What Henri de Luxembourg had labored to built crumbled with a meteoric rapidity in a few days in August 1313: "In an hour everything was destroyed / What it had taken him five years to create / When he lost both kingdom and empire" (*en une heure a tout desfait / Ce qu'en V anz il avoit fait / Quand il perdi royaume et Empire*).[40] And the image of power ruined by *fortuna volubilis* remained lastingly associated with the death of Henry VII.[41] Poison received and given associates its victims with Alexander's fate, but in a negative way.

Let us go further. Is succumbing to poison undignified for a knight who is destined *ex officio* to die with his weapons in his hand? The cruelty of *veneficium* resides also in the fact that it steals from the one it kills, along with his life, his dignity as a warrior. To be defeated and killed without combat, and even more by the act of a weak being, is a death without honor. The reaction of medieval literature to ancient heroes who are poisoned betrays a desperate refusal to die from poison in such an unheroic death. As soon as he was poisoned, Alexander ran to drown himself in the Euphrates River. Did he want to escape the pain or the shame of dying on a pallet?[42] Chaucer tells that Hercules preferred to throw himself onto burning coals rather than be the victim of poison.[43]

Upon reflection, besides the compassion it expresses, doesn't the adverb *miserabiliter*, frequently used to describe death by poisoning,[44] include also the pitiful victim of the disgrace of the crime of poisoning? Surprised by poison, Robert Guiscard had deserved a better death.[45] The words engraved on the tomb of the knight poisoned by Queen Guinevere were, first of all, a derogatory inscription. But her act gave to the *miles* an end not in keeping with the chivalric ideal, a bad death that was the very opposite of Roland's.[46] A milder form of poison, the love potion dispossessed the knight of himself and subjected him to a woman, which did not increase his value.[47] A weapon used without combat, poison deprived the *miles* of his worth and caused him to die without glory.

The evoking of poison then can serve objectives of valorization and of promotion of the victims raised to the rank of saints or the worthy.[48] Nevertheless, this pattern can not be applied very well to princes over the centuries or to athletes of the faith, since death by poisoning appears to be ambivalent as to the benefit that its noble victims can get from it. The Alexandrine model is itself ambiguous. The allegation of poisoning conferred a clearer image on those who performed the crime. It proves to be more operational.

THE ACCUSATION OF POISONING, REGULATION, AND CATHARSIS

The political role of the accusation of witchcraft in the fourteenth and fifteenth centuries has for a long time been presented in its role as a social function, an outlet for neighborhood quarrels. The application of these interpretational grids to the accusation of *toxicatio* is appropriate because *maleficium* and *veneficium* are similar in both the form of the accusation and the motives behind it. The accusation permits the purging of society of those who, in the village as at court, are considered harmful to it. The continuation of the Roman idea according to which the intention is as culpable as the act opens interesting dimensions to the accusers, for it is more convenient to allege a simple *voluntas occidendi* than a crime that has been committed. Certainly, there is not a hidden plot behind each case designed to ruin an individual who is necessarily innocent. But it is interesting to analyze the many implications implicit in the accusation of *venenatio*, beyond the obvious attempt to exploit the law to the detriment of an enemy.[49]

A Political Regulator

A phenomenon often attested in the late Empire,[50] the accusation of poisoning proved to be a convenient way to eliminate troublesome rivals, arrogant upstarts, or undesirable queens. In literature, the theme of the princess accused because of spite or a desire for revenge serves especially to depict and to sympathize with persecuted innocence as well as to exalt the courage of the knights who became the champions of a desperate cause. In historical reality, the accusation of poisoning follows a more prosaic logic, linked to the politics of matrimony. Civil law like canon law authorized the separation of spouses when one of the two presented a threat to the life of the other.[51] The use of poison is an example of such an incident. Even in eras when the union of spouses was not yet strictly controlled by Church law, the brutal repudiation of a princess did not occur without arousing the hostility of ecclesiastical authority. Lothaire II's divorce was one such case. That is why invoking a pretext to send away a spouse who has become useless is not without reason. Conforming to the expected image of *venenosa conjux*, the accusation of poisoning was difficult to invalidate. Based only on the suspicion of preparing a poison, a Wisigoth princess was sent back to her father by her husband, the son of the King of the Vandals (about 440).[52] The accusation brought against the Frankish Gundeberga had, perhaps, also as a goal to reorient the foreign policy of her Lombard husband Charoald, in addition to the immediate origin of the affaire, the vengeance of a spurned suitor.[53]

During subsequent periods, the accusation of poisoning remained convenient to legitimate the repudiation of a wife or separation from her, but the accusation of witchcraft was just as popular. Among all the reasons that Louis VII had to divorce Aliénor d'Aquitaine, the threats that she presented against the life of the king (by enchantments or by poison?) are mentioned in the *Chronique de Rains*.[54] Philippe Auguste was content to invoke evil spells to obtain the departure of Ingeborg of Denmark.[55] But was poison really different from enchantments? The hypothesis of William of Newburgh according to which the King of France was disgusted by the breath of his new Scandinavian bride[56] recalls the story of the Poisonous Virgin whose origins some traditions trace to the northern countries not to India.[57]

When princesses played a political role, the purpose of accusing them of poisoning was to eliminate their credibility. The rumors that incriminated the Comte de Champagne reflected back on his alleged lover, the regent Blanche de Castille, whom the baronial milieux wanted to oust. According to Philippe Mousket, the accusation directed against Thibaut IV came from the uncle of Saint Louis, Philippe Hurepel, who also was a candidate for the regency.[58] Philippe Hurepel's death in turn put Thibaut IV's role in question along with the regent who was the focus of envy.[59] Manipulation of Mahaut's accusers, Jean and Isabelle de Férienne, is well known. They acted on the promises of persons whose names were voluntarily concealed in the act of October 1317. There is little doubt that Robert, the nephew and rival of the countess, was involved in the affair that improved his prospects of recovering the duchy of Arras allocated to his aunt in 1309. Disqualifying her as title-holder would contribute to her political downfall but not without putting at risk her son-in-law King Philippe V. Philippe's zeal in organizing a second inquest, when the widow and the family of the late king claimed to be satisfied with the results of the first, was motivated by the desire to clear up all the ambiguity surrounding the death of Louis X and all doubt about the legitimacy of his own accession.[60]

Accusations of crimes of poison brought against powerful men took on an increased gravity and thus an additional effectiveness since a traitor to his victim, the accused was, in addition, a traitor to his position. At the beginning of the reign of Edward III, rivalries ignited around the young king. His mother's lover, Mortimer, tried to counter the influence of Count Edmund of Kent, the monarch's uncle, by accusing him of holding a grudge against the royal personage (1330). The form that this attempt against the sovereign was to take is unclear since Jean le Bel speaks about a simple capture while Froissant talks about poison.[61] The fact remains that the accusation succeeded in its purpose since as soon as he heard the accusation, king commanded the decapitation of the accused. As the chronicler of Valenciennes says, the maneuver was successful because of the inexperience of the monarch whose impulsiveness and naïveté made him inclined to listen to slanderers.[62]

Somewhat earlier (1320), "the Comte de Nevers was accused of wanting to poison his father" (*l'en mis sus au comte de Nevers qui vouloit empoisonner son pere*).[63] Son and presumptive successor of Robert de Béthune, count of Flanders, Louis de Nevers did not have a fate as cruel as that of Edmund of Kent, but the attempt to ruin him was similar. His plot to kill his father that was suddenly divulged by a member of the plot takes its meaning from a double-crossing political plan. On the one hand, the role played by the brother of the accused shows that the issue that inspired the accusation was the succession in Flanders.[64] On the other hand, the informer, Ferry de Picquigny, the declared enemy of Mahaut d'Artois and of her son-in-law Philippe le Long, made the Flemish count very hostile against the latter, his heir,[65] who was captured then detained on land belonging to the Empire, thus out of reach of the King of France who demanded his freedom.[66] Once freed, Louis de Nevers perished from a poison that was more efficient than the poison of slander, but the legacy of Flanders finally returned to the son of the poisoner, who was poisoned in turn.[67]

The court in Savoie during the 1390s presents another example of the political use of the crime of poison.[68] The act attributed to Jean de Grandville involved more than just him. The alleged murderer of Amédée VII permitted the implication of people of high rank in Savoie and served very precise interests.[69] The exercise of power during the long minority of the young Amédée VIII (8 years old) was the true issue in this case. Those who wanted to remove candidates for the direction of the principality alleged their initiation of the crime. Two eminent figures were targeted, the mother, Comtesse Bonne de Bourbon and her protégé, *Seigneur* Othe de Grandson. In spite of the official recommendations for severity against his poisoner who was thought to have been manipulated,[70] the doctor benefited from support to escape his interrogators.[71] Othe de Grandson was thought to have acted together with the mother of the dead prince, the sister of Louis de Bourbon, whom Jean de Grandville had accompanied during the expedition of Mahdiya in 1390.[72] Two individuals had reason to throw suspicion on the princess: the Duc de Berry, father and protector of the widow, Bonne de Berry, as well as of her son; the Prince de Morée, a relative of Amédée VII, and a partisan of a *reformatio* of the regime. The first charged the second with knowing "the guilty parties and consenting to the poisons" (*les coulpables et consentans d'icelles poisons*).[73] Jean de Berry held in his prison the presumed murderer recaptured as he fled, but obviously he sought to get at Bonne de Bourbon. Bonne's fears concerning a confession that would compromise her having been extracted from the physician under torture are evident in a letter sent by Louis de Bourbon to his sister January 18, 1393. Jean de Grandville revealed that he wanted to flee to lands owned by the Bourbon family and that the mother of Amédée VII did not approve of the fact that her son, who was in his thirties, governed alone.[74] March 30, 1393, the accused made admissions that were still more embarrassing for the princess and for Grandson. He indicated that Grandson was embroiled in a controversy with the prince and wanted revenge. Also, he stated that Bonne had had prepared harmful substances to administer to her son and his wife.[75] Having returned to Bourbon territory, the principal accused retracted his statement on September 10, 1395. It is quite possible that the case of Bernard de la Roche, which broke the same year, was a sort of backfire lit against the Prince de Morée who was also suspected of wanting to poison the young Amédée VIII. The conditions under which the suspect confessed and its variations make one suspect manipulation. This second case shows, in any case, the important place of accusations of poisoning in the principality of Savoie during the last decade of the fourteenth century. These accusations were linked to the high political society of the kingdom of France since the Ducs de Bourbon and de Berry were involved as well as the Duc de Bourgogne, who was the father-in-law of Amédée VIII.[76]

In ecclesiastic society, our cases can be read in the same way only if those accused are considered victims of settlements of scores. The anticlerical historiography of the 1900s took this approach systematically.[77] Without following clues that were sometimes quite obvious, one can nevertheless observe that the accusations that were aimed at the Bishop of Cahors, Hugues Géraud, the protégé of Clement V, betray also the desire of John XXII to neutralize the "Gascon party" to which belonged the Bishop of Toulouse who was also implicated in the affaire, and to punish a prelate whose methods inconvenienced certain families of Cahors that were close to Jacques Duèze. The career of Hugues Géraud, who had already been prosecuted for abuses exercised in his episcopal functions, was already quite compromised at the moment that the cases of poisoning and bewitchment surfaced, but they were the final blow. For Jean de Winterthur, who was very "hostile" toward John XXII, the bishop was unjustly tortured after false accusations based on a bad dream had by the pope.[78] In the same way, (incorrect[79]) rumors of poison spread after the death of Alexander V were linked to the necessity of eliminating his inconvenient successor John XXIII when the Council of Constance met. The 29th article in the charges made against Bathasar Cossa at the time of the XIth session included, among other grievances, that of being *criminosus de veneficio*, an allusion to the "arranged" death of Alexander V.[80] At the end of the fifteenth century, the subtle Alexander VI knew very well that poison, which he used skillfully, could be traded advantageously against a simple accusation of using it to ruin an enemy. With the goal of serving the expansionist plans of his son Cesar, who did not succeed in taking Forli and Imola, the pope accused Catherine Sforza, who was holding them, by means of false accomplices whom he had opportunistically arrested,[81] of having attempted to kill him [the pope] by a poisoned letter (November 1499).[82] Then he kept her imprisoned in the château of Saint-Ange, without risking instituting proceedings against her that might embarrass him. Catherine Sforza remained firm in her denial of the pope's accusations and, in addition, threatened to make public the turpitudes of the Duc de Valentinois, who desired Catherine's land and was free to take it over as long as she was imprisoned. This *faire-savoir* worked as skillfully as the expertise of the pope since almost all the authors, with the exception of

Burchard,[83] judged the charge to be consistent with the personality of the princess, who was so adept at *experimenti* that she put them in writing in a book posterior to the affair (1508).

In the political sphere, the accusation of poisoning still conformed to a logic very characteristic of the last three centuries of the Middle Ages, in which the development of the States favored the promotion of servants of modest origin who aroused the hate of the "natural" elite groups, the barons, and nobles. Not always occupying positions that involved decision-making, a certain number of advisors present in noble circles exercised an influence that was considered excessive. Deaf to warnings, princes had to be faced with evidence (more or less fabricated) of the guilt of their protégés before agreeing to send them away, returning them to their humble origins. Such operations assuredly made use of the horror of a crime that was literally vile. To accuse these upstarts of using poison was to move the wheel of fortune in such a way that it made them tumble down a slope that they had climbed illegitimately.

In France, the case of la Broce began the process.[84] Many chroniclers observed that the fall of the "favorite" (an anachronistic but convenient term) of Philippe III occurred "more because of envy than because of any deed" (*plus par envie que par fet*).[85] The envy came from the barons who were irritated by the access to the king enjoyed by the Seigneur de Langeais, the former barber of Louis IX, and whom the king showered with kindness and honors and also with generous gifts. Through his functions as chamberlain, he controlled the distribution of large sums to important personages.[86] Reluctant to compensate the Duc de Brabant for his claimed expenses incurred on some expedition,[87] and instead crediting his funds to the Comte d'Artois who called him "his faithful friend" (*son amé et feal*),[88] Pierre de la Broce exasperated the aristocracy by his "foolish impertinence" (*fole outrecuidance*).[89] The advice of the barons was followed only if the chamberlain approved.[90] The motives behind the implication of Pierre de la Broce are obscure and the slandering of Marie de Brabant played a determining role in the fall sought in the first place by the queen's brother, who was worried that the princess's honor had been compromised. But certain authors imply that a transfer of guilt occurred from Marie de Brabant to Pierre de la Broce, concerning the death of Louis de France. The accusation of poisoning came to fill a heavy file of betrayals that led the "favorite" directly to the thieves' gallows. Fourteen barons singing at the top of their voices led him there, probably with the regrets of Philippe III.[91] At the head of the procession, the Duc de Brabant and the Comte d'Artois were pleased with the spectacle until the victim had stopped moving.[92] The infamy had been avenged, the hierarchy reestablished, and certain debts eliminated.... Considered by Dante as a complete fabrication,[93] the accusations brought against the chamberlain ruined him to the great surprise of the Parisians who "could not believe that a man who had risen so high could be brought so low" (*ne pooient croire en nulle maniere que home de si haut estat fust devalé en bas*).[94] Poison played a central part in this instructive disgrace.

The purge that occurred soon after the death of Philippe le Bel at the expense of the people whom he had promoted also made use of the accusation of poisoning, along with that of evil spells. Bewitchments were also used against a chamberlain of political importance far superior to Pierre de la Broce: Enguerran de Marigny, accused of wanting to cause the "death by poison" (*de male mort*) of Charles de Valois and Louis X.[95] Another advisor, who had become the guardian of the royal seal in 1313 and was too well considered at court, the grim jurist Pierre de Latilly was accused of having his predecessor poisoned on the Episcopal throne of Châlons, but he was cleared once the passion for purging was reduced, of which Charles de Valois was the main instigator.[96]

Much more than for the preceding accused, the implication of poisoning made against Jacques Coeur, in the middle of the fifteenth century, played a central part in the process of the decline of a man who had climbed very high.[97] A certain number of people had an economic interest in seeing the opulent merchant of Bourges eliminated. It was necessary to find a charge that started legal action even if it was soon abandoned. The offensive was launched at the end of July 1451 by the accusation that he had caused the death of Agnes Sorel, who had died eighteen months earlier.[98] The accusation was effective because it was very painful for the king, who was extremely angry with his "argentier."[99] Jeanne de Mortagne, who accused Jacques Coeur, went along willingly with the plot all the more because she was, like so many others, in debt to him. She was then banished from the king's dwelling because she made a false accusation.[100] But as false as it was, the accusation permitted the process to get under way, a process that was to ruin le Berruyer, giving his enemies the time to assemble other more serious charges. Although relatively favorable to Charles VII, Thomas Basin was surprised that the monarch, who kept the accused in his *familiaritas* and his *amicitia*, could have listened to those who were jealous of him. They knew how to touch him deeply. At the moment of making an assessment of the reign, the subtle Bishop of Lisieux put the case among the liabilities of a victorious king by demonstrating very clearly the mecanism.[101]

Instead of serving to put the pursuits in motion, the accusation was sometimes added to other charges to complete the ruin of the cause of the individual targeted to bring down. Enemy of Queen Anne de Bretagne in the eyes of whom he incarnated the evil Breton allied with France, the rival of the Cardinal of Amboise, the marshal of Gié was subjected to a trial in 1505, which not only revealed his betrayal but also revealed the proclivity of his lineage to betrayal. That is why witnesses were solicited to report, half a century after the facts, the poisonous crimes of his relatives, of his mother against her husbands and of her family against Gilles de Bretagne, whom a secret act countersigned by the chancellor of Duc François doomed to death.[102]

This kind of situation did not occur exclusively with French royalty. Mentioned by Dante as the consequence of the envy of courtesans,[103] the disgrace of the ***logothete*** Pierre de la Vigne, the son of a notary of Capua who had become a powerful man in the Sicily of Frederick II, rested, according to Matthieu Paris, on an accusation of poisoning perpetrated against his master, backed by the papacy, when he was returning from a mission in Rome.[104] In the particular atmosphere of the end of the reign of the excommunicated emperor, this fall illustrates without doubt the paranoia that had seized the emperor, but his implication (erroneous[105]) in a case of poisoning by the chronicler of Saint-Albans shows also the political role that was played in a already current accusation. In the fifteenth century, an author who is considering the brutal fall of the upstart advisors, associates Pierre de la Broce and Pierre de la Vigne.[106]

The case of Pierre Gerbais, which occurred in Savoie in the 1380s, seems at first glance not to depend on the same logic. The accusation was brought by the brother of Hugues de Grammont, a penniless *sire* from a family of the old nobility of Savoie, against the bourgeois de Belley, who had become general treasurer in 1354. It concerns a crime committed not against the holder of princely authority but against a noble who had made an alleged murderer his legatee after having been his constant debtor. But the case does not fit only in a context of settling of private accounts. Behind the Grammont family and the numerous witnesses that it brought together, the nobility of the sword of Savoie put the blame on a man of finance who had become indispensable to the successful functioning of principalities and who was pitiless toward penniless nobles who gave up fiefs and possessions to newcomers in order to maintain an elaborate lifestyle.[107] The allegation of poisoning coincides quite well with the profile of a covetous person, also convicted of diversion of public funds. In accordance with the social prejudices of the nobility, the allegation reflected the revenge of the traditionally elite groups against an upstart with disgusting manners; revenge that remained unaccomplished, for the accused was spared capital punishment because he had become so necessary to the development of the principality that he had to again enter the service of the count after his release (1384).

In the principality of Bourgogne, the story of Jean Coustain gives an even more eloquent illustration of the phenomenon, on the one hand, because the origins of the accused were much more humble than those of Gerbais and then his ascension more scandalous and his arrogance more insufferable; also, because the goal sought by the accusers was crowned with success; and finally because the victim targeted with poisoning was no one less than the heir of the principality. Whatever the grounds of the charges made against Jehan Coustain—the letters that have been found prove nothing, the impunity of their author makes them even highly suspect[108] —the meaning of the maneuver was clear: to separate Duc Philippe from his chamberlain in order to rid the political society of Bourgogne of an individual who had climbed "so high in credibility and in authority that everyone treated him with great respect" (*tant en credence et en autorité que toutes faces lui monstrent reverence*).[109] He disturbed the hierarchy and humiliated the nobles from whom he took land and his proximity to an aging and easily influenced prince was troublesome.[110] The purging of the court of Bourgogne began with the elimination of this harmful element to whom the use of a weapon appropriate to his condition was attributed without much imagination but not without effectiveness. It is advisable to point out that Philippe le Bon "sad about the outcome of the case and missing his lost *valet de chambre*" (*dolent du cas advenu et assez en regret de son valet de chambre perdu*),[111] was extremely difficult to convince of the perfidy of his servant. Every precaution was taken to assure the success of the operation: quick inquest and investigation, quiet execution, in the fortress of Ruppelmonde whose keys the Comte de Charolais kept personally; finally, safeguards were taken to prevent the "great duke of the West" "reluctant to extreme punishment" (*Tardif a extresme rigueur*) (Chastellain)[112] from revoking the authorization that he had given to punish the guilty man. By the elimination of Coustain, the impatient heir of the duchy did not only get rid of an enemy; he also affirmed his will to influence from then on affairs from which he had been too distant.

The accusation of poisoning committed or planned was therefore used to purge and regulate political society. It rid society of "stinking serfs" (*serfs de put aire*) that were fatal to Alexander[113] and in itself gave voice to dispute. In 1422, behind the *Seigneur* de Robays, a close advisor of Philippe le Bon, it is the ducal power itself that the people of Ghent targeted, a people who were chronically rebellious and attached to their dead Duchesse Michelle whom they believed was sacrificed to ducal interests. The rumbling did not become a riot but the alert was serious.[114]

The Accusation of Poisoning and Social Regulation

Beyond the courts and the palaces, the accusation of poisoning was a form of expression and a way of moderating the tensions that permeated society. To allege the use of poison against an enemy offered more that just a chance to settle domestic issues (especially) or neighborhood issues (much less often). As for witchcraft, the process also permitted the identification of the source of the misfortunes and then a way to get rid of it. In periods of difficulty, the incriminating explanation played a cathartic role of primary importance.

In 1481, Anthoine de la Brosse, a laborer from Agen blamed a chambermaid as the cause of the illness he suffered and he killed her in the passion of his anger.[115] His sincerity appeared to be genuine. That was not always the case. Jealousy of the prosperity of a neighbor or the desire to avenge an insult also led to accusations of *toxicatio*. It is quite probable that the numerous favors granted by the Bishop of Châlons to Guillume de Béthune, his barber, who managed to ease his suffering and who had cut him off from his entourage, had aroused such jealousy that the implication of the prelate's loyal servant became inevitable (1405).[116] Linked to the rejection of the remarriage of widowers,[117] the accusation was frequently brought against husbands in second marriages of having killed the first husband with poison.[118] In 1409, a servant and her husband accused a couple of having caused the death of the first husband of the implicated woman.[119] One can guess the concrete motive behind this accusation: the change of master had made the situation of the false accusers insecure and they then sought revenge. In an affaire of 1498, socioeconomic jealousy inspired the inhabitants of a village on the banks of Lake Geneva to rise up against François Marguet, a sexagenarian of note, accused along with others of having poisoned a neighbor with whom he had quarreled over wood. Thus, hidden rivalries in a neighborhood were combined and served as motivation for accusations of poisoning.[120]

The allegation of using poison served equally to settle accounts of a community with authorities who suppressed it. Bernard de Castanet, an authoritarian Bishop of Albi, who applied to the letter the Roman program of fighting against heresy and of the purity of the clergy, exercised a power that many found stifling. J. Théry has clearly demonstrated the close link that existed between this "Episcopal tyranny" and the accusations brought against the bishop by individuals linked to the heretical milieux, in hopes of making him leave. The people of Albi reached their goal, for their pastor, even though restored in his *fama*, had to leave his Episcopal post for that of Le Puy.[121] In lay society, the case of Jean de Jaux is exemplary in the middle of the fourteenth century. This Provost of Compiègne rendered iniquitous judicial decisions, used torture to kill victims, and tried to improve his modest salary by extortion and a fine marriage contracted with a widow whom he married very soon after the death of his wife. Eager to be liberated from such oppression, the people of Compiègne revealed these crimes to the bailiff of Senlis, who would probably not have been convinced by a single denunciation of ordinary abuse.[122] In the same way, in 1404, the ten persons who attacked the chamberlain of the *Seigneur* de La Flocelière, the squire Jean Guillereau, accused him and others of having tried to poison his wife. His adversaries described him as an extortioner, feared by his underlings. The deep resentment and seriousness of the accusation led to the arrest of the local petty tyrant.[123] At a still lower social level, a chronicle of Rouen points out that a Norman executioner was accused in 1397 of poisoning the wells with powder. The allegation served the will of the community by eliminating an impure element among them. He died a miserable death at the hands of a colleague.[124]

At a higher scale of communities affected by widespread disturbances such as famines and epidemics, the invocation of poison as the cause of misfortunes seldom worked,[125] especially at the end of the Middle Ages, with the accusation of groups who served as scapegoats and suffered avenging attacks to purge society. Sociologists and anthropologists have shown the cathartic logic of these allegations that responded equally, as for the misfortunes of individuals, to a need for an explanation.[126] The idea that an epidemic was *manu facta*[127] improved in no way its objective therapy but gave a sense to the incomprehensible and designated an enemy to pursue. In 1090, not far from Freising, the accusation of some poor women who were soon executed, despite the absence of any proof, responded to the anguish provoked by multiple difficulties (epidemics, epizootic disease, famine) and the vacancy of the Episcopal seat that prevented the solving of the *fas* and the *nefas*. The accusing words and the acts that followed relieved the fears inspired by the calamities.[128] A miracle of Our Lady of Rocamadour illustrates this mechanism at the end of the twelfth century. The inhabitants of Saint-Sever were dying one after the other. Wanting to avenge their mourning and exorcise the misfortune, they accused a poor woman of Rocamadour of being *venefica*. She was condemned to death by fire and saved by the Virgin of Rocamadour, who made the flames ineffective.[129]

The episode of 1321 took place in difficult circumstances that led to a search for outlets and solutions. The end of the troubled reign of Philippe le Bel, the unprecedented famines of the years 1315–1317, the outbursts of the second wave of the Shepherds' Crusade (*les Pastoureaux*) already looking for those responsible for the crisis,[130] made social relationships tense, and set the stage for accusations of the poisoning of the water. To the psychosocial and liturgical situation (the time of Easter stimulated anti-Jewish feelings)[131] were added concerns about the fiscal policy of Philippe le Long. The great movement of the persecution of lepers and their accomplices permitted an outlet for people gripped with anguish. Eager to accumulate resources, when a tax in a time of peace[132] loomed in front of them, urban communities exploited the accusation of poisoning in order to seize the sometimes rather great wealth of the leprosariums.[133] The local elite had, in addition, every reason to make the lepers confess the participation of the Jews in the plot. They conjectured that Philippe V would expel the Jews after confiscating their belongings, or at least impose a fine sufficiently high so that he could abandon his disastrous plans for a new tax.[134] D. Nirenberg was probably correct in seeing in the letters that reveal the judeo-pagan plot conveyed on the order of the bailiff of Mâcon a forgery by the municipal authorities of Mâcon motivated by greed.[135] Let us add, but it is only a conjecture, that the implication of the "sultans" in the judeo-leper plot could justify the relaunching of the crusade still planned and continuously put off, but an excellent pretext for raising funds.[136] In any case, it is certain that the accusation of poisoning served in France as an outlet in a tense situation, according to the logic of violence that was both "systemic" and regulating as demonstrated by D. Niremberg. C. Ginzburg is entirely right when he sees in the situation something entirely different from an "obscure collective convulsion."[137] The crime that was held against the lepers was remarkably coherent with the nature of the group being accused, who were associated with poison in several ways. The well-thought-out furor of 1321 had played its part: to bring to those excluded from society the bloody weight of a fiscal draining that no one wanted.

In 1348, the mechanism was quite similar—the memories of 1321 were still quite present in all minds—if it is only that the accusation targeted essentially the Jews who were held responsible for the demographic crisis that was developing.[138] The unexplained numbers of deaths raised the suspicion of poisoning.[139] A reaction both cultural and spontaneous,[140] the massacres in the Jewish communities served as a catharsis at the same time as, perhaps, social revenge: a chronicler from Strasbourg suggested that the poison that killed the Jews was their wealth.[141] According to the very precise study by F. Graus, the accusation resurfaced because of the epidemics, in particular in the Empire (Halle, 1362; Colmar, 1401; Cologne, 1424[142]) more than in Italy (because of the medical culture?), and without a direct relationship to the size of the communities in these places.[143] It was no longer a question of a calculating exploitation but of a compensatory incrimination of the lack of understanding, of fear and of vulnerability in which the disease left people.[144]

Whether they affect only political society or society as a whole, tensions were thus manifested by the accusation of poisoning. This phenomenon does not belong to any period of the Middle Ages in particular, but it proved especially obvious in the thirteenth, fourteenth, and fifteenth centuries when the times of conflict became more numerous both for the heads of State and in the social fabric, and when the interrogations on the causes of death became more numerous, opening the way for accusers of all sorts to appear, some motivated by jealousy, malevolence, or calculation, others by the need to find an explanation for the misfortunes of the times. Beyond individual rivalries, the allegation of poisoning participated by setting them in motion, the mechanisms of regulation and stabilization of a society confronted with imbalances as much hierarchic as demographic: a bitter potion to purge a social body that felt soiled.

POISON, PROPAGANDA, AND IDENTITY

Toxicatio inspired a discourse that aimed not only to ruin physically or materially an enemy but also to discredit him ideologically. From a planted rumor to orchestrated propaganda, the accusation of poisoning functioned in several ways. It participated not only in the defamation of political order, but also in a process of identity that designated the other as a vile poisoner and oneself (the king, his people, the nation) as totally innocent of such a heinous crime.

The Use of Poison: A Theme of Propaganda

As pathetic as were the means of diffusion of ideas and as uncertain as were the conditions of forming a "public opinion," powers constructed their legitimacy by an ideologic activity in rapid development during the last centuries of the Middle Ages. It would be ridiculous to say that poison occupied a central place in this process, but it did play a certain role, since the discrediting of the enemy constituted one of the cornerstones of self-legitimization.

Before the eleventh century, for reasons that were linked at the same time to political structures and to types of extant documents, no use of the accusation of poisoning as propaganda has been found. The allegations of poisoning following the deaths of Eudes in 898, of Lothaire in 986, and of Louis V the following year do not seem to be an attempt to disqualify one or another dynasty in competition for occupying the Frankish throne in the West. It does not seem that the black legend of the Capetian line, developed during the eleventh and twelfth centuries, involved the accusation of crimes of poisoning committed against the last two Carolingians. On the contrary, allegations related to the deaths of the last two monarchs descended from Charlemagne against their wife and mother respectively sought to heighten, in contrast, the purity of the mores of the Robertonian spouses.[145]

The first episode that illustrates the articulation between the accusation of poisoning and political "communication" is related by Orderic Vital. In 1075, two earls, Roger of Hereford and his brother-in-law Ralph of Norfolk—one of the rare natives to still retain an earldom—joined by another native, Walteof, attempted to profit from a storm that cut England off from the continent, in order to stir up opposition against the new master of the country, William, who was then in Normandie.[146] In a speech destined to justify their undertaking and to galvanize their partisans, they claimed that in addition to being a bastard, the Duc de Normandie was guilty of hideous crimes, among them the poisoning twelve years earlier of the Comte du Mans, the nephew of Edward the Confessor, and of his wife, who were then hostages held by the Conqueror in Falaise before having them killed, without any consideration of chivalric ethics. He was also accused of having killed Conan, the Comte de Bretagne, with poison.[147] The uprising was short-lived, but the rhetoric of the insurgents showed the ideologic function that can be attached to the horrible grievance of *toxicatio*, with a possible xenophobic connotation that will be discussed below.

Among the minor themes of the quarrel between the papacy and the Empire, the use of poison arises several times in the propagandist argumentation of both sides. The intention was to present the enemy with the hideous features of a tyrant thirsty for power and to destroy in that way his legitimacy in order to justify, if need be, deposing or excommunication, and to win the support of other powers. The struggle between Gregory VII and Henry IV began the tradition. The argument of poison evidently did not hold the first place in a conflict with such great stakes.[148] But with other grievances put to good use—the pope was also accused of being a heretic, a magician, idolator, and soothsayer[149] —he had served against Hildebrand and his supporters. From 1080, the synod of Brixen, a veritable antigregorian forum, denounced the poisonous activity of the pontiff by attributing to him the death of at least four of his predecessors, according to the last confession of his agent.[150] Cardinal Benno, a partial author of a *Vita Hildebrandis*, who was from Lorraine and close to Henry IV, described Gregory as a serial poisoner. In fourteen years (1047–1061), with the help of his damned soul Brazutus, Hildebrand allegedly killed six pontiffs with poison, without counting a seventh, who was put to death violently.[151] The charges were serious, almost a caricature of a pope and were meant to demonstrate, in order to ruin the memory of Gregory VII (for the text is probably posterior to 1085) and disqualify his partisans and supporters, that such an individual had no place on Peter's throne and that his doctrines were harmful to the order of the world.

The very serious tensions between the Staufens and the popes of the thirteenth century were the occasion for both sides to unfurl propaganda, in particular in the form of letters addressed to the authorities in many countries in the West. Although, once again, many other arguments of heavier weight were exchanged,[152] the accusation of poisoning held an important place in the slanderous arsenal of the two adversaries. The accusations become integrated in the polemic as if the accusation of using poison almost naturally portrayed the enemy in the most evil light. On the side of the papacy, the attempt to discredit the emperor and then his heirs through the accusation of poisoning did not lack reason. On several accounts, Frederick II and those who sought his succession presented a perfect profile of a poisoner: tyrannical, they were assumed to have teamed up, moreover, with the Infidels whose contact (in Sicily and overseas) contaminated bad Christians with their poisonous customs; educated in the occult sciences, they were in a position to use the services of the dangerous keepers of the secrets of nature.[153] The first recorded accusation concerns the death of the *landgrave* [the title of certain German princes] of Thüringen, Louis IV, in 1227 at Brindisi, while he was awaiting the departure of the Staufen for the Holy Land. Suffering from fever, the *landgrave* apparently died from the epidemic cited by the emperor for delaying his departure, to the great horror of the papacy.[154] The Pope pretended to doubt the validity of the pretext as the natural causes of the death of the *landgrave*. It is probable that from the day after this episode the pope spread the rumor that the Thuringian had died from poison. Kantorowicz indicates that the emperor had a response to the papal accusations read in public, during the absence of the pope, who had fled.[155] Twelve years later, the sovereign pontiff insinuated in an encyclical letter in which the enormous mistakes of the former pupil of Innocent III were listed, that the death of the Germanic prince was caused by poison. Frederick was presented as the murderer of a crusader.[156] At the time of the Council of Lyon in 1245 that was expected to make a pronouncement on the deposition of the emperor, a partisan of the papacy addressed a letter condemning, in terms altogether innocent, the "serpentine" nature of the sovereign who bit, just like the asp or the grass snake, the side of his nurturing mother, the Church. This missive denounced more concretely the fate that he had inflicted on his successive wives, who had been deprived of life by the harmful action of some cook, a way of referring to poisoning.[157] Continuing the toxic metaphor to apply it to his own case, this self-serving man evidently challenged what he called the "poisonous insinuations" of the Pope.[158] But the rumored poison did its work and Matthieu Paris considered that all these accusations had no other purpose than to incite antiimperial hate.[159]

The descendants of the Staufen whom the papacy wished to dispossess of the kingdom of Sicily, were similarly targeted by pontifical propaganda. Against Conrad, the rumor was spread that he had ordered the death by poisoning of his nephew Frederick (son of Henry "VII" who also was brought down by an accusation of poisoning[160]) and his young brother Henry (born from the union of his father with Isabel of England), killed by the intermediary of Jean le Maure.[161] The polemic became so great on this subject that the heir of Frederick II was obliged to send a representative to Rome in February of the year 1255 in order to formally deny the allegations.[162] On this occasion, he demonstrated the seriousness of this kind of accusation that could have been treated simply with scorn if the common mind had not taken it seriously.[163] Matthieu Paris believes that these Roman lies played a role in the death of the Staufen, who was afflicted psychologically before succumbing to a quite concrete poison that finished the job that the poisonous words had begun.[164] Very unfavorable to Innocent IV, the English chronicler explains that if Rome accused its enemy of having had the young son of Isabel of England poisoned, the reason was to bring to its side, fiscally and militarily, the Plantagenets in a crusade against Conrad.[165] Nine years later, Urban IV warned Charles d'Anjou that Manfred, the bastard of Frederick II and partisan of his cause, was manipulating incessantly to have his neighbor the Pope killed by the assassins whom he had also sent to the Comte de Provence, armed with innumerable kinds of poison. The continuation of the letter is a pressing invitation to come to Italy to overthrow the tyrant. It is not possible to find a better political and ideological exploitation of the accusation of poisoning.[166]

The opposing camp did not act any differently. If one believes the sources that are favorable to him, Frederick II did not experience fewer than six attempts to poison him. At the end of his reign, the excommunicated emperor alerted the West about the papal traps. The *fama* of the papacy suffered serious damage, if one believes Matthieu Paris.[167] In a letter from March 1249 addressed to all the Christian princes, the Staufen attacked the Holy See in hyperbolic tones meant to emphasize the enormity of the crime. "Listen, all people through the centuries, to the enormous wickedness that has remained unknown during the past centuries" (*Audite gentes degentes per secula ingentem nequiciam a seculis inauditam*). Thus begins the document that continues by saying that such an atrocity cannot remain hidden. The formulas were carefully chosen to strike the reader: false father, the Pope has dispensed *veneficium* instead of the *beneficium* expected from a good pastor.[168] The papal action is attributed to the desire for power whose final stage is the elimination of the imperial majesty that has been outrageously damaged. If the correlation is not made explicitly between this form of tyranny and the use of poison—the pontifical traps that are denounced were not only those associated with poison—the accusation of poisoning participated in a large way in the propaganda against the Roman pretensions to monopolize both the political and religious realms. In 1252, suffering from an illness, Conrad had the rumor spread that the cause was poison from the Pope who was continuing the persecutions that victimized his father. Uncertain about the reality of these allegations that he hoped were false—another way of saying that he feared that they were well-founded—Matthieu Paris notes once again the damage that the Pope suffered following these accusations.[169]

The accusations that followed the death of the emperor Henry VII in 1313 constitute, in a way, simply a continuation of the polemics of the thirteenth century. Certainly, the papacy was not directly implicated in the affair and the victim did not have as terrible a relationship with the Pope as Frederick II did with Innocent IV. Clement V had even hoped and prayed for the descent from Luxembourg into Italy. But the Dominican Order of Preachers (*Prêcheurs*), to which is collectively attributed the crime that one of its members had committed,[170] was considered the militia of the papacy, which had become worried about the successes of the

Empire. And the quarrel that arose between the new emperor, Louis of Bavaria, and Avignon gave the affair a dimension that recalled the quarrels of the preceding century. The accusation served the anti-Roman positioning of the Germanic sovereign linked to the spiritual group among the Order of Friars Minor (Franciscans), itself targeted somewhat later through Bernard Délicieux by an accusation of poisoning.[171] The popular condemnation of the brothers of Bernardin was, if not upheld, at least not hindered by the emperor in the hope of strengthening the Germanic population against the representatives of the Holy See, itself perhaps the origin of another accusation made in 1340 against Louis, the presumed poisoner of Henry of Bavaria, then of his widow, a member of the house of Luxembourg.[172]

Behind the Dominican Order, it was indeed the papacy and its theocratic pretensions that are targeted. Their radical challenge by the theories of the Church councils during the fifteenth century did not forget to recall the image of the pontiff as poisoner applied to Gregory VII: "several popes have truly covered their poison with honey" (*pluisieurs papes vraiement/Soubx miel ont couvert leur venin*) says Franc Vouloir, the spokesman for the man from Bâle, Martin le Franc.[173] The turpitudes of the Borgia also fed a propaganda that featured their poisonous practices. Lampoons based on stereotypes circulated in Rome in 1502 against Alexander VI and his son.[174] The place of accusations of poisoning in the Protestants' anti-Roman literature deserves to be researched. Luther condemned the evil act of the Dominican brother in 1313 behind which he certainly saw the hand of the Pope.[175] The publication of Cardinal Benno's text in Frankfort, in 1581, is probably not surprising in the middle of the reformed printers.

In the last decade of the fourteenth and the first decades of the fifteenth centuries, when new developments[176] occurred in the affair of 1313, the resurgence of hate against the Dominican Order of Preachers was no longer linked to the defunct quarrel between the Pope and the Emperor, but the doctrinal and social rejection targeted by an order that his role in the Inquisition and his murky involvement rendered unpopular.[177] The accusations of 1390 that the Religious of Saint-Denis considered with more circumspection than indignation[178] fit well into this context. Between the poisoning of the fountains and the poison of heterodoxy (at least in the eyes of the partisans of the Virgin's immaculate conception), the border is vague. It is, therefore, not impossible that this strange episode reflects also the hostility to an order further distanced from the general population than the Franciscans. In the Empire of the years 1400–1430, the enemies of the OFP (Order of Friars Preachers: Dominicans) used the accusation of poisoning as a weapon of the first order. Jacques d'Esch mentions a "proof" of his guilt that appeared probably in Germanic territory after 1367.[179] It is a question of the marks of infamy that the brothers bear as the humiliating mark of the impious crime of one among them. The chronicler indeed indicates that after the death of Henry VII, "it was ordained by the Holy Father, by the cardinals, bishops and legates, princes and lords that henceforth preachers would never celebrate nor use the body of Our Lord with the right hand only with the left hand, and that they would never more carry their capes to their feet but just to their knees, so that they would remember forever the evil stated above that the said preacher had done by poisoning the said emperor" (*fut ordonneit par le saint peire, par les cardenalz, evesques et liegalz, princez et signeurs que de ci en avant jamaix prescheurs ne celebroit ne ne useroit le corps Nostre Sgr. de la droite main for que de la clanche main, et que jamais ne pourteroient plux leur chappe jusqugs aux piedz for que jusques aux genoilz, adfinc d'ons heust memore a tous jours maix de la mauvistiet dessus dite que le dit prescheur avoit fait d'enherber le dit emperour*).[180] The slander was terrible because it was founded on the Dominican liturgy of the eucharist.[181] Certain members of the Order of Friars Minor [Franciscans] (*Mineurs*), quite aware of the advantage to be gained from the accusation, were at the forefront of the movement. About 1420, the Dominican from Lubeck Hermann Korner condemned the *sceleratissimi religiosi et perfidissimi* of the OFM (Order of Friars Minor: Franciscans), who unrelentingly tarnished his community with their accusations, more than a century after the fact, of a horrible crime.[182] The collective incrimination and its surprising perpetuation reveal the vision that a certain number of individuals, who were jealous of its success[183] or exasperated by its action against heresy, had of the Order of Friars Preachers (OFP: Dominicans). The brothers' hypocrisy, which has often been denounced, is in perfect harmony with a type of crime in which the perpetrator speaks in one way and acts in another. However, honesty requires us to say that one does not find connections expressed explicitly anywhere, including in the writings of the worst enemies of the mendicant friars, such as Rutebeuf. Is it necessary to go further and see in the rejection of the OFP (Order of Friars Preachers: Dominicans), after that of the Templars, a form of hostility against international institutions of the Church by young nations? This hypothesis collides with the fact that, in the case of Henry VII, it was a universal monarch, supported by certain Italians that the order was supposed to attack. In any case, it is not unthinkable that a "national" identity was nourished, in the Empire or in the France of the 1390s[184] by the hostility toward the Dominicans by means of a grievance of a poisoning from which the brothers of Saint Dominic had great difficulty freeing themselves despite all their efforts.[185]

The factions formed in France in favor of the dynastic disputes then resulting from the madness of Charles VI produced an intense propaganda. Poison played a role. The struggle between the Valois of France and the Capetian of Navarre Charles the Bad (*le Mauvais*) took on a certain ideologic dimension. Faced with Navarre, the Dauphin then King Charles knew how to mobilize the energies, including intellectual ones, to impose his legitimacy. The arrest of the poisoners that his cousin sent to him in 1378 gave the monarch the opportunity to condemn an enemy who was militarily weak and vile enough to have recourse to such an odious weapon.[186] As stated in the foreword of the text of the confession of Jacques de Rue, read in Parlement June 15 and June 16, 1378 before the whole political society and reproduced at length in the almost official chronicle of the reign, *Chronique des rois Jean II et Charles V*,[187] the sovereign desired that such a crime be known by all his subjects in order to expose his own rights and the iniquities of the King of Navarre.[188] The publicness of the torture of the agents served also to display the ignominy of the instigator. The events of 1385 do not seem to have resulted in such exploitation, even if the execution of the accused and the thanksgiving of the victims who were miraculously spared can appear to be a form of propaganda against Charles the Bad (*le Mauvais*).[189] It is sure in any case that Charles the Bad (*le Mauvais*) was not indifferent to the damage that his *fama* could suffer from this situation, for in 1374 he asked for a pontifical letter that would officially absolve him from another crime of poison, fatal, said his enemies, against the Cardinal of Boulogne the preceding year.[190]

The struggles between the Armagnacs and the Burgundians included, in their turn, the argument of the crime of poisoning. The disorder of the time makes the rumor of poisoning all the more powerful because the word of authority failed to authenticate the information.[191] With a certain coherence, the accusations came mostly from the Burgundian faction, draped in its ideal of the defense of freedom, toward the Armagnac faction considered adept with tyrannical power exercised notably by means of poison. The use of the accusation of poisoning went back to Charles VI's first attacks of madness. The chroniclers point out, in fact, that the rumor circulated in the streets of Paris that the king's condition was caused by *veneficia* (in every sense of the word) by his sister-in-law Valentine Visconti.[192] It is not possible to determine, at this time, if Philipple le Hardi sought to manipulate public opinion by creating what Froissart called "rumor and general scandal" (*fame et et esclandre generale*.)[193] The Augustinian brothers who tried to cure the king took refuge behind the criminal origin of his illness in order to excuse their failure.[194] Were their hostile insinuations against the Orléans dictated by the Duc de Bourgogne? It is difficult to prove, even more so because the Religious of Saint-Denis indicates clearly that "witches" often visited the duke.[195] The quick punishment reserved for them perhaps demonstrated the desire of Louis d'Orléans to respond to the attacks that came from above and that shocked a certain number of silent people, such as Honorat Bovet, into taking up the defense of Valentine Visconti.[196]

The famous defense of tyranicide made by Jean Petit to justify the assassination of the Duc d'Orléans because of the crimes that he had committed in a way formulated a propaganda that had been until that time more diffuse than frontal. Accompanied certainly by the accusation of other crimes, already committed or planned, with or without violence, the accusation of poisoning occupies an important place in the arsenal of arguments of Petit (as a minor premise of his syllogism) and the second version of the text (1409) adds even more material to this subject. Coville had indeed picked up the desire of John the Fearless (*sans Peur*) to give the greatest publicity to the words of his spokesman: his text was carefully copied and recopied even after its solemn condemnation in 1413. Copies were still circulating several years after the events.[197] The text illustrated the thesis of the tyranical power of the Armagnacs denounced with virulence during the years of power (1413–1418) of this faction of "plunderers, idlers, tyrants, traitors, poisoners, and murderers."[198] At the start of the allegations in 1408, Duc Jean the Fearless (*sans Peur*) accused the Armagnacs of having killed with poison the Dauphins Louis de Guyenne and Jean de Touraine, his protégés.[199] As early as December 1415 the rumor spread of the poisoning of Louis de Guyenne;[200] then, the duke orchestrated a libelous campaign to inform the population about the vilainous act of his enemies. April 26, 1417, a few weeks after the death of Jean de Touraine, letters of accusation were sent to the towns and posted at the churches,[201] notably those in Rouen where they caused discord.[202] The letters were solemnly refuted and destroyed in Parlement.[203] Less useful after the expulsion of the Armagnacs from power, the propaganda nevertheless had consequences and inspired counterattacks. Literature transmitted these events through works such as the *Pastoralet* (about 1422–1425)[204] or the *Book of the Betrayals of France* (*Livre des trahisons de France*), composed sixty years after the assassination of Louis d'Orléans.

These literary works reflected the newly current tensions between the "great duke of the West" and the French monarchy. The argument of poisoning was taken up again in order to justify the insubordination of the principality to the king. In 1461, the future *Téméraire* (Foolhardy) made it known that he refused to participate in the coronation of Louis XI for fear of poison.[205] In 1462, the Coustain affair gave an opportunity to the same Comte de Charolais to condemn the traps of his royal cousin whom he saw, along with the Sire de Croÿ, behind the attempt of the ducal chamberlain. From this moment, wrote Adrien de But, somewhat simplifying the affaire, resurfaced the discord between France and Bourgogne.[206] After the accession of Charles the Foolhardy (*le Téméraire*) the Burgundian enmity toward Louis XI manifested itself with propaganda campaigns as intense as the military campaigns that they justified. In 1470, the greatest publicity was given to the attempt attributed to the bastard Baudouin de Bourgogne to poison his half-brother. Certainly, the first accusation, put forth by the *fama publica atque vulgarissima*, remained vague on the exact methods used by the king to kill his enemy: *veneno, vel gladio seu telo*, wrote

Thomas Basin who relates with complacency the criminal nature of the new Domitian (a particularly cruel and ruthless Roman emperor 81–96), a name that in his eyes characterized the monarch.[207] Whatever it was, the duke sent on December 13, 1470 from Hesdin letters to the most important cities of the principality of Liège (*bonnes villes*) to inform them of the dark schemes of the king of France and to ask them to thank Heaven for having permitted the duke to be spared.[208] The Bishop of Liège actually had a mass said whose sermon devoted to the affair included the reading of the duke's letter.[209] In response, the Seigneur de Chasse, implicated in the so-called plot woven against the duke, rejected the "disloyal calumny" (*desloyale calomniation*) and, probably inspired by Louis XI, instructed a veritable indictment against the prince who was accused of contaminating the air with his morals: to a poisoner, a poisoner and a half.[210]

May 24, 1472, young Charles de Guyenne, whom the princes hostile to the sovereign planned to manipulate against his brother, died in conditions that implied the use of poison. The following July 16, "extremely upset and encouraged by others sad about the said death, [the duke] wrote letters to several towns charging the king" (*fort desesperé et enhorté par aucuns dolens de ladicte mort*, [le duc] *escrivit lettres a plusieurs villes a la charge du roy*).[211] While the *Téméraire* was camping before Beauvais, a manifest was produced by the chancellery of Bourgogne that spread the news that the brother of Louis XI had died "as a result of poison, evil spells, enchantments and diabolic incantations" from " the most pitiful death that can be remembered in this kingdom or elsewhere" (*par poisons, malefices, sortilèges et incantations diaboliques*) from (*la plus piteable mort que jamais ait esté memorée en cedit royaume ne ailleurs*). This nothing less than spontaneous reaction became part of a strategy consistent with justifying the opening of hostilities while the Duc de Bourgogne had already been in Picardie for three weeks: it was necessary to seek vengeance for the crime as honor and nobility required.[212] In September, another manifest of the same ilk came to legitimize the continuation of the war being waged against the king.[213] In the long term, in the eyes of the implacable censor of Louis XI, Thomas Basin, the accusation was to make the king as appalling to posterity as Cain. His exile from Utrecht, in Burgundian territory, shows by this consideration that the reach of the accusation of *veneficium* went beyond the political scene to enter into a logic of *damnatio memoriae* on a larger scale.[214] As the interpolator of Jean de Roye said, "the news of the poisoning of the said Duc de Guyenne was known by the majority of the Christian kingdoms" (*il fut sceu par la pluspart des royaulmes chrestiens la fumée de l'empoisonnement dudit duc de Guienne*).[215]

In response to the insistent and ringing accusations, Louis XI not only wanted to make known that he gave complete support to the search for the truth about the death of his brother against whom he curiously retained only the crime of evil spells.[216] He did not fail to use the same weapons as his enemy to whom was several times alleged the insidious and sacrilegious desire to attack the royal majesty with poison. The king gave the greatest dissemination to these affairs that were if not fabricated, at the very least skillfully exploited to overwhelm his Burgundian cousin. The arrest, in 1473, in the royal kitchens, of a man accused of having tried to poison Louis XI as the agent of Charles the Foolhardy (*le Téméraire*), was followed by a production destined to make known to everyone the latter's treachery. Having left Touraine where he learned about the attempt on his life, the king set out dragging behind him Jehan Hardy in irons, as far as the outskirts of Beauvais, a town well known as a symbol of Franco-Burgundian enmity. The guilty man was taken into Paris on January 20, 1474 during a sort of solemn entry during which the criminal placed on a high cart was protected from lynching. This ritual of mockery, the trial, and the punishment were meant "to publicize the enormity of the case" (*faire savoir l'énormité du cas*) for which the wronged monarch was obligated to seek vengeance publicly calling the entire kingdom as witness to a vassal's treason.[217]

The affair of 1476 (the attempted poisoning of the Dauphin Charles) does not seem to have produced the same kind of scenario. On the other hand, the betrayal of the new Judas, Jean de Chalon, charged with seizing Bourgogne in the name of the king before he became the ally the daughter of the *Téméraire* after Louis XI had given him the Order of Saint-Michel, was treated in the same way. A royal letter written from Cambrai on June 6, 1478 indicates the will of the sovereign: "the prince of Thirty Pieces of Silver wanted to have us poisoned, but God, Our Lady, and Saint Martin preserved and protected us, as you will see by the copy of the information that we are sending you, in order that you have it read in open court before everyone, so that everyone may know about this great treason and the evil character of the said prince" (*le prince de Trente Deniers nous a voulu faire empoisonner, mais Dieu, Nostre Dame et Monseigneur Saint Martin nous en ont preservé et gardé, comme vous verrez par le double des informations que vous envoyons, afin que vous le fassiez lire la salle ouverte devant tout le monde, et que chacun connoisse la grande trahison et mauvaiseté dudit prince*). Another letter received June 18 by the town councilors of Lyon contained "information . . . concerning the poisoning" (*information . . . touchant l'emprinsonnement* [sic]). It was published the following morning and "read before all the people gathered there in large numbers" (*devant tout le peuple illect amassé en grant nombre*).[218] The goal of this public reading was in the first place to promise a reward to whoever could deliver one of the accomplices of the Prince of Orange. But the reading had also the purpose of informing the good subjects of the King of France, who lived in Lyon, about the horrible crime that occurred when the monarch was involved in a campaign against the followers of the late Charles de Bourgogne whose partisans resorted to such underhanded methods. A dialectic of the accusation of poisoning thus punctuated the conflicting relations between the Valois de France and the Valois de Bourgogne during the years 1460–1480. More broadly, poison indeed played a role in the French civil wars, as an ideologic weapon, from the end of the fourteenth to the end of the fifteenth century.

To a lesser extent, poisoning also had a role in English quarrels. If the propaganda hostile to Richard II of England made little use of it,[219] at least to our knowledge, the Lancastrian royalty, on the other hand, did not neglect to use threats of poisoning allegedly directed against it in order to establish its legitimacy by inciting a feeling of belonging to it and a feeling of rejection toward its adversaries. The case of Stamford, Henry IV's confessor, who was accused by the aristocracy of poisoning the monarch, could have been instrumental in these decisions.[220]

Thus, there did exist a poison of propaganda, poison that was used against an enemy to undermine its ideological base and to take away from it possible partisans. Its use depended on situations provided by death or illness. Such propaganda spread an abstract toxin that poisoned public opinion and thus affected to a greater or lesser degree the reputation of the adversary. The deployment of counterpropaganda tended to prove the nuisance power of this kind of accusation. But it also participated in topics denouncing the enormity of the enemy's crimes in order to respond to his own accusations or to warn about them.

The Crystallization of an Identity Crisis

The discourse on the uses of poisonous substances outlines, at the same time as the contours of evil, those of good. The accusation of poisoning has as a corollary an idealized "toxic virginity" that contributed to the shaping of the identity of different scales of reference.

Gui de Chauliac affirms this statement in a peremptory fashion: in the West, "it is not customary for two parties to administer a mortal substance to each other."[221] A few decades earlier, Pietro d'Abano considered the crime of poisoning as originating in the East and the South.[222] This medical extradition of *veneficium* from its origins or its practice has as a corollary a discourse that tends to imply that criminal poisoning is essentially foreign to the countries of northwestern Europe, for ethical reasons that both the Islamic enemy and the false Greek ally lack because of the "general propensity of all the nations of the East" (*generale proprieté de touttes les nations d'Orient*), which is to betray.[223] In each *envoi* of his *Ballade des empoisonneurs: En Orient servent tel beuvrage*, Eustache Deschamps thinks of "those of the West" (*ceux d'Occident*), who are called to the greatest vigilance.[224] This opposition does not date from the medieval period. Rome was already defining itself at the moment that she felt her identity threatened by her own conquests, in comparison with this decadent and treacherous Orient, skilled with toxic weapons that the Romans scornfully rejected. Assuredly, the Western expansion at the expense of the Muslim and Byzantine powers nourished a reflection on the identity of the Latins in relation to their enemies or rivals (one needs only to read the letters of Jacques de Vitry). In part, abstention from the crime of poisoning in contrast with its usage in the Orient entered into the construction of the occidental identity that increased the value of the loyal and frontal combat.

Inside the nations in the process of forming in the West, the identity function of poison passed, in the same way, by an accusation of its usage against neighbors that is linked to its rejection as such. Among the "stereotypes of the national psychology,"[225] the propensity of a given foreign people or a given foreign region to resort to poison among themselves or against neighbors demonstrated the courage and the virtue of the inhabitants of the kingdom. Germanic identity also fed on the toxic setbacks met by the emperors at the time of their descent into Italy. Proud knights innocent of disloyal acts, the Germans fell into the toxic ambushes set in "Latin territory" as a chronicler said about Henry VII.[226] Castillian mythography affected very significantly the origins from over the mountains of the bad countess who tried to hand over her country to the potentate of Cordova. In a first version of the episode, written about 1160, her name was Ava, and her origins were local. But a second version dating from the middle of the thirteenth century in which her Castillian identity is confirmed, renames her Sancha and has her coming originally from the other side of the Pyrenees: in this version she was the daughter of a French count.[227] In comparison to its poisonous neighbors to the south and north, Castille was an island of purity.

The kingdom of the lily, reputed to be free of heresy, similarly rejected the stain of *veneficium* all the more because it was linked with evil spells. Beyond the political operation, the trial of Guichard de Troyes entered into the ideology of purification led by his most Christian majesty (*Très-Chrétien*) with a broad sense of "communication": on October 6, 1308 clerics and ordinary people met in the gardens of the palace to hear the crimes charged against the bishop.[228] The proclivity to believe itself the depositary *par excellence* of chivalric values led the most Christian (*Très Chrétien*) kingdom to deny the same claim by others. One of the ways of doing this was to point out the inclination of certain neighbors to resort to the weapon of poison. This inclination implies an offensive collusion with the Infidels (see Richard of England or Galeas Visconti), thus a betrayal of Christianity defended only by the King of France. It also reflects another basis for identity, a profound difference in political regime. To the perfect monarchical system of the French is contrasted the tyrannical regime of the lords of Milan that implies intrigue and murder to establish a questionable power by an unstable individual.

The fulfilling and false idea (see the history of Eadburh) although explainable—princely murders abound indeed in England during the tenth and eleventh centuries without the least trace of poison[229] — according to which poisoning would be foreign to the Island dwellers permeates national feeling from the eleventh century to the modern era. This idea probably provides the background of the accusations brought in 1075 against the continental William the Bastard whose toxic devices were unheard of among the Anglo-Saxons.[230] The great number of poisonings reported by Orderic Vital in Norman circles reflects the surprise of the *Angligena* faced with the deplorable mores of those from the continent.[231] Pride in their toxic virginity can be found explicitly in the writings of John of Salisbury when he affirms in the middle of the twelfth century that his country has always had a horror of poison and has never used it against its princes.[232] When poisoning is practiced in English political society, the users are necessarily foreigners, those cursed continentals. The episode of 1258 serves as an example. An authoritative heir of a power formerly centered in the west of France, himself tempted to use poison,[233] Henry III Plantagenet surrounded himself with advisors from Poitou, his half-brothers from Lusignan, considered by the English barons, even those of recent date, as exercising a bad influence on the king by drawing him away from the principles of the *Magna Carta*. It is hardly surprising that these men from Poitou, recipients of many royal favors, were accused of wanting to have the great English nobles punished at a time when famines, bad weather, and epidemics ravaged a kingdom confronted, in addition, with serious financial problems.[234] The sovereign, in accordance with the Provisions of Oxford in June 1258, had to exile his relations from Poitou along with other "foreigners." But it is most likely that these foreigners continued to do damage from the continent with the aid of the servants of the aristocratic households charged with poisoning the heads of these households. The account by the author of the *Chronica majora*, convinced of this theory despite the uncertainty of many of his compatriots,[235] is marked with a very interesting xenophobia, at the time when the insularity of the Plantagenet regime following the Capetian conquests was accelerating the feeling of belonging to the *communitas Angliae*.[236] Poison from the outside was attacking the baronial group, the natural elite of the kingdom whose inhabitants, opposed to all tyranny, were necessarily opposed to the use of poison. Faithful to this fictitious image of identification, Henry VIII considered in 1531 criminal poisoning as *nowe newely comytted*.[237] This imaginary particularity constitutes part of national pride: *Anglia abhorret a veneno*.

Certainly minor with regard to other positive themes such as that of glorious origins or of unsullied faith, the theme of the poison of the enemy is not used any less for terms of identity: To overcome and discredit the enemy in order to better glorify a party or a people. In the spirit of

Pierre Gringore in 1506, the "French People" set themselves apart from the "Italian People" notably on the question of the use of poison. But the risk was great when the French were "italianized,"[238] that is won over to the mores of the inhabitants of the peninsula, somewhat like, one is tempted to add, this group who had adopted the mores of the Infidels.

The allegation of physical poisoning was useful for the poisoning of minds in order to possess them. This image already existed in the Middle Ages. In a letter to the papacy dated August 1278, Queen Marie de Brabant complains that Pierre de la Brosse had flooded the streets with his poison.[239] This behavior extends well beyond the Middle Ages. The *Discours merveilleux* composed in 1575 and most likely of protestant inspiration accuses Catherine of Medicis of numerous poisonings or attempted poisonings, from the Dauphin in 1536, whose death at the time had been attributed to the servants of Charles Quint,[240] up to Jeanne d'Albret, to the brothers Châtillon and to the entire army of Condé.[241] A lampoon of 1582 accuses the King of Spain of wanting to poison the Duc d'Anjou, Henry III's brother, who had been chosen by the Netherlands during a rebellion.[242] The affair of West Indian poisons in the eighteenth century served the propaganda against the Company of Jesus whose members, defenders of the Blacks who had been unjustly accused, were thought to be the instigators of a plot that would have given them supreme control over the colony.[243] And the accusation continues to be part of the arsenal of propaganda in the contemporary era, with denunciation of the use of gas in combat or, on the contrary, the virtuous announcement of the refusal to use it.[244]

With no doubt whatsoever, the accusation or the allegation of poisoning functions in social, political, and ideological arenas. Sometimes, poison endows its victim with a certain glory. The nature of the crime, which is difficult not only to prove but also to disprove, makes it easy to charge individuals destined to fall, if not definitely, at least probably. It is consequently a way of reestablishing a socio-political balance that has been threatened. The horror that *venenatio* inspires also permits the discrediting of the enemy in the eyes of public opinion and unites the community behind its leader against the *gentes* with detestable characteristics with regards to which identities are composed. Relegated to the fringes, the poisoner with one action emphasizes the values that form the foundation of the *communitas*, in the words of the English barons who rebelled in 1258.

NOTES

1. Y. Grandeau, Le dauphin Jean de Touraine, p. 721.

2. *Vita Frederici*, p. 502. Having been given dreadful substances to drink several times, he succumbed to the poison, but his corpse rejected it through the

mouth, the eyes, and the ears, symbolizing the impossibility of evil remaining in the bishop (p. 506).

3. Jacques de Voragine, *Legenda aurea*, chap. 9, 45, and 58.

4. Marc, XVI, 18: *Et si mortiferum quid dederint, non eis nocebit.*

5. Grégoire le Grand, *Dialogues*, II, *Vita Benedicti*, 8, t. 1, p. 160 and sq.: *eum non latuit quae pestis in pane lateret*, and t. 1, p. 140.

6. Cf. Benoît de Sainte-More who said, on the other hand, speaking of Richard III de Normandie and of his household: "They died from poison; / But man cannot be divine (*Eissi furent mort par venin; / Mais ne pout l'om estre devin*) (v. 29998).

7. *La vie ancienne de saint Samson de Dol*, I, 16 to19 and I, 55.

8. *Bibliotheca Sanctorum*, VI, col. 388–401, according to the *Vita* written about 1500 by this Franciscan preacher (1394–1476) who overcame poison during a mission in the Balkans during the 1430s.

9. Abélard, pp. 106–107. On the episode related from the perspective of Abélard's life, see J. Verger, *L'amour castré. L'histoire d'Héloïse et d'Abélard*, Paris, Hermann, 1996, p. 103; M. T. Clanchy, *Abélard*, Paris, Flammarion, 2000, p. 302 and sq., as well as M. M. McLaughlin, Abélard as Autobiographer, *Speculum*, 1967, n 42, pp. 463–488.

10. *Historia de expeditione Friderici*, pp. 54–55: *Nunc etiam non minori miraculo vinum Grecorum veneno infectum et nostris ad exitium procuratum Grecis fuit exitiale, nostris vero poculum salutis . . . Dei clementia illud nobis mutatum in antidotum salutis.*

11. See N. Daniel, *Islam et Occident*, p. 24.

12. Id., pp. 144–145.

13. Matthieu Paris, t. 3, p. 351: *qui si verus propheta fuisset, potuit pro suo socio orasse ut viveret; vel salutem sibi et socio illi a cibo venenato praecavisse, sicut olim Elyas et Elyseus leguntur fecisse, dicentes "Mors est in olla"* (2, *Rois* IV, 38–40). See also Vincent de Beauvais, *Speculum historiale*, Douai, 1624, XXIII, 46, p. 914.

14. J. Le Goff, *Saint Louis*, Paris, Gallimard, 1996, p. 835 and sq., does not include the event of 1242 in the elements that lead to the sainthood of the king. The study of L. Carolus-Barré and H. Platelle on the canonisation process (Rome, 1994) is also silent.

15. Nangis, *Gesta Ludovici*, p. 334, French translation: "Our Lord who always protects His own, protect us from what this lady has planned" (*nostre Sires qui garde toujourz les siens, destourna ce que la dame avoit pourpensé*). R. Folz, *Les saints rois au Moyen Âge, vi^e–xiiie siècle*, Bruxelles, 1984, does not give any other examples.

16. Dynter, t. 2, p. 492: *Mortem subiens velut agnus*. Note the expression *ovis mansuetissima* (*Imperator Heinricus*, p. 129).

17. *Gesta Trevirorum integra*, p. 230.

18. *Imperator Heinricus*, p. 128: *virum pacis, justum, pium, sanctum et mansuetum.*

19. See for example *Annales de Lübeck*, éd. *MGH SS*, XVI, Hanover, 1859, p. 423; same content as the account of Gilles li Muisit and of the *Vœux de l'épervier*.

20. Thietmar de Mersebourg, p. 319, concerning a bishop who died after ten years of suffering caused by poison.

21. Orderic Vital, t. 4, pp. 106–107. Note, however, that it is not the king's cleric, Suger, but the "Norman" Orderic Vital who reports the fact.

22. See J. Baldwin, *Philippe Auguste et son gouvernement*, Paris, Fayard, 1991, p. 491 and sq.

23. Christine de Pizan, *Livre des fais et bonnes mœurs*, II, X, pp. 125–126. F. Autrand, *Charles V*, Paris, Fayard, 1994, p. 848: the author suggests that the very precise but anonymous account of his last moments would have served to contradict any suspicions of poison.

24. Christine de Pizan, *Livre des fais et bonnes mœurs*, II, 52, p. 138 of Solente's edition.

25. Zantfliet, col. 317.

26. Froissart, t. 2, p. 110 of Buchon's edition.

27. William of York was canonized in 1226, but the circumstances surrounding his death counted very little in this decision in comparison with the miracles that occurred on his tomb. (*Fasti Ecclesiae Anglicanae, 1066–1300*, VI, York, ed. J. Le Neve, D. E. Greenway, Londres, 1999, p. 3).

28. Eustache Deschamps, *Mirouer de mariage*, XXIX, v. 2660 and sq., t. 9 des *Œuvres complètes*, p. 89: "Deianira, the traitor / Who gave him such strong poison / And thus overcame Hercules / Who defeated so many monsters / That he was not defeated by any of them / He was conquered by his wife" (*...Dyanira la felonne, / Qui tel ardant venin lui donne / Et ainsis Herculès dompta / Qui tant de monstres surmonta / Que par nul ne fut surmontez / Cil qui fut par sa femme domptez*).

29. *Roman d'Alexandre*, v. 1551, p. 840.

30. Guillaume de Malmesbury, t. 2, p. 322: *invicibilis hostili ferro, et domestico obnoxius veneno*; Orderic Vital, t. 3, p. 187: *non militari robore prostratus sed livore femineo correptus, non armis sed veneno laesus.*

31. Jean de Winterthur, p. 65, and Dynter, p. 492 (verses inserted)

32. Cf. the words of Dante, *Divine Comédie*, tr. H. Longnon, Paris, 1962, Paradis, XXX, p. 547.

33. See Ch. Raynaud, Fin des temps et politique: la mort d'Alexandre au xve siècle, *Fin des temps et temps de la fin dans l'univers médiéval, Sénéfiance*, 1993, n°33, pp. 359–396, on the passionate dimension of Alexander's death in certain iconographic representations.

34. See M. E. Franke, *Kaiser Heinrich VII. im Spiegel der Historiographie*, Cologne-Vienne, 1992, p. 290. Mathias von Neuenburg, p. 93, then 354.

35. Jacques d'Esch, *Die Metzer Chronik über die Kaiser und Könige aus dem Luxemburger Hause*, ed. G. Wolfram, Metz, 1906, p. 55 and sq., v. 559–560; R. Blumenfeld-Kosinski, Historiography and Matière antique: The emperor Henry VII as new Alexander in the fourteenth-century, *Vœux de l'Épervier*, *Medievalia et Humanistica*, 1986, n 14, pp. 17–35.

36. *Godefroid de Bouillon*, p. 290 and sq. See p. 300 the praise of a bold prince, warned in advance of his death, like Alexander, and the perfect manager of his last moments.

37. Du Cange, *Glossarium*, article *venenare*.

38. Eustache Deschamps, *Œuvres complètes*, bal. 1155, t. 6, p. 88.

39. Orderic Vital, t. 4, p. 374: *mortalium robur fragile est.*

40. Geoffroi de Paris, p. 140.

41. *Gesta Trevirorum integra*, p. 230: *prospera in contrarium mutantur*; Chastellain, t. 1, p. 26.

42. *Roman d'Alexandre*, IV, 10, p. 754. Ch. Raynaud, Fin des temps et politique..., p. 361, considers only the first hypothesis.

43. Chaucer, *Contes de Canterbury, Monk's Tale*, v. 3324: *for with no venim deyned him to dye.*

44. Exemple *Parlement criminel*, X2a 4, f. 143. See also the case of Godefroy de Bouillon whom the *Roman* depicts at length verse 1320 the "great piety" (*grans pités*) of his agony (p. 290 et sq.).

45. Guillaume de Malmesbury, t. 2, p. 322: *meliorem exitum, si Deus voluisset, emeritus.*

46. *La mort le roi Artu*, p. 78.

47. Cf. C. Cahné, *Le philtre et le venin dans* Tristan et Iseut, Paris, 1975.

48. The (rich) tradition of chi'ite martyrology shares this vision: Tabari, *Chronique*, ed.-tr. H. Zotenberg, Paris, 4 vol., reed. 1984, V, 2, t. 4, p. 8, the murder of Hassan, brother of Hussein and son of Ali, by Mo'awiya, by means of a poisoned napkin, and V, 111, p. 518, the poisoning of Alide Ali ar Ridha, who was the victim, according to the chi'ites, of grapes that were contaminated on the order of the calife abbasside al Mamoun in 818.

49. J. Chiffoleau, Sur la pratique et la conjoncture..., p. 372: the term refers to the cynicism of the accusers, without taking into account the sometimes sincere belief in the idea that evil threatened Christianity.

50. Cf. Ammien Marcellin, *Histoires*, XXVIII, 1, t. 2, p. 60 to 71 and sq. of Seyfarth's edition: about 365, the vice-prefect of Rome Maximinus eliminated various senators on the pretext of accusations of poisoning.

51. *Code théodosien*, III, 16, *De repudiis*, 1; Alain de Lille, *Liber poenitentialis*, II, 118, p. 106.

52. Jordanès, p. 72.

53. Frédégaire, p. 145.

54. *Chronique de Rains*, ed. P. Paris, Paris, 1837, p. 7.

55. See J. Baldwin, *Philippe Auguste et son gouvernement*, p. 117 and sq.

56. Gullaume de Newburgh, t. 2, p. 78.

57. R. Caillois, *Le mythe et l'homme*, p. 66.

58. Philippe Mousket, t. 2, p. 576.

59. Id., t. 2, p. 582: ".. all the barons and the entire region blamed his death on the Count of Champagne because he hated him so much" (*...sour le conte de Canpagne / Maitent sa mort tout li baron / Et tous li païs environ / Pour çou qu'il l'ot haï ançois*). See J. Le Goff, *Saint Louis*, pp. 104–105 on the lies spread by the minstrels against the queen mother, but which did not include the accusation of poisoning.

60. Godefroy Ménilglaise, p. 214.

61. Froissart, t. 1, p. 87 in the ed. *SHF*: "And the jealousy rose to such a pitch that the Lord of Mortimer asked and exhorted the young king so much...that the Count of Kent wanted to poison him...in order to take over his kingdom" (*Et monta puis li envie si haut que li sires de Mortimer enfourma et enhorta tant le jone roy...que li dis contes de Kent le voloit empuisonner...pour avoir son royaume*).

62. *Ibid.* Voir W. M. Ormrod, *The reign of Edward III. Crown and political society in England, 1327–1377*, Oxford, 1993, p. 5. Edmund was also accused of preparing Edward II's return to the throne, since he was thought to be living hidden away somewhere.

63. *Grandes Chroniques de France*, t. 8, p. 354.

64. See l'*Istore et croniques de Flandre*, in *RHGF*, XXII, pp. 412–413; This work does not speak of poison but it indicates that desiring to seize the succession to the throne in Flanders, the brother of Louis de Nevers allegedly directed the writing of a lie in the name of his father to order Louis' decapitation.

65. J. Favier, *Philippe le Bel*, p. 506.

66. Jean de Saint-Victor, p. 673. Philippe V's demande confirmed Robert de Béthune in his idea of collusion with the King of France; Nangis, continuation, t. 2, p. 30.

67. Jean de Saint-Victor, pp. 676–677. Some thought instead that the death was due to an illness contracted in captivity.

68. G. Castelnuovo, *Ufficiali et gentiluomini. La società politica sabauda nel tardo medioevo*, Milan, 1994, pp. 65–69, attributes the death of the count to tetanus and shows the struggles for influence during the Regency. See also B. Galland, *Les papes d'Avignon et la maison de Savoie, 1309–1409*, Rome, 1998, pp. 339–341.

69. Carbonelli, PJ XXX, declaration of Brother Guillaume Franczon, OFM, confessor of Amédée VII, April 20, 1394.

70. Id., p. 240.

71. Id., p. 234 and p. 265.

72. Id., p. 275.

73. Id., PJ Xb, letter from Jean de Berry to the nobles and communes of Savoie to inform them of the mission entrusted to the Prince de Morée.

74. Id., p. 280.

75. Id., PJ XVII.

76. B. Galland, *Les papes d'Avignon et la maison de Savoie*, p. 340, indicates that receiving the Regency in May 1393, Bonne de Bourbon had to step aside in November, in favor of the Ducs de Berry and de Bourgogne.

77. This was the perspective of Ch.-V. Langlois in his controversy in 1906–1907 with the canon Albe and the future Mgr. Mollat (A bishop tortured to death in the time of John XXII, *Revue pratique d'apologétique*, 1907, pp. 753–767).

78. Jean de Winterthur, p. 98: *propter unum sompnium displicibile habitum*.

79. The text by his embalmer Pietro d'Argelata, *Chirurgiae libri sex*, the Bologne edition, 1520, livre V, traité 12, chap. 3, p. 102 v, lacks any allusion to poison.

80. *Sacrosancta concilia*, ed. Labbé and Cossart, t. XII, Paris, 1672, col. 88, 77 et 84: *legatus Bolonie existens, ad papatum illicitis mediis anhelans, in mortem bone memorie domini Alexandri papae extitit machinatus ut tam ipse quam medicus suus magister Daniel de Sancta Sophia . . . veneno extinguerentur*.

81. Pasolini, n°1097, p. 407, letter from an ambassador from Estonia in Rome to his master, November 22, 1499. See t. 2, p. 260 and sq., some details on the partisans and the results of the affair.

82. Pasolini, n°1096, p. 406: letter from the pope to Florence on November 21 to inform the city authorities that there had been an unsuccessful attempt to poison him.

83. Burchard, t. 2, p. 579: he also speaks of poison but does not directly implicate Catherine Sforza.

84. On the general context, see Ch.-L. Langlois, *Le règne de Philippe III le Hardi*, Paris, 1887, I, 2. The recent biography of the king published by G. Sivéry with Fayard does not supply any further information.

85. *Chronique de Saint-Magloire*, éd. *RHGF*, XXII, Paris, 1865, p. 84: "In the year 1278, all the barons were in agreement, / to seize Pierre de la Broce. / To my knowledge, he was defeated / More because of jealousy than for any action. (*L'an 1278, s'accorderent li barons tuit / A Pierre de la Broce prendre. /... Mien enscient qu'il fu desfet / Plus par envie que par fet*).

86. *Complainte de Pierre de la Brosse*, str. 4, v. 1: "I had the key of France" (*la clef de France avoie*). It is a question of the key to the treasury.

87. *Ancienne chronique de Flandre*, ed. *RHGF*, XXII, Paris, 1865, p. 348.

88. F. Schneegans, Trois poèmes de la fin du xiiie siècle sur Pierre de la Brosse, *Romania*, 1932, n°58, pp. 520–550, p. 522.

89. *Complainte de Pierre de la Brosse*, str. 18, v. 4.

90. *Estoire de Eracles*, continuation, excerpt published in the *Jeu et complainte de Pierre de la Brosse*, p. 14.

91. *Chronique anonyme finissant en 1308*, extraits, ed. *RHGF*, XXI, Paris, 1855, p. 138: "In the year 1278, the barons of France had Pierre de la Broce hanged contrary to the wishes of the king" (*L'an 1278 firent les barons de France contre la voulounté du roi pendre messire Pierre de la Broce*); *Grandes Chroniques de France*, t. 8, p. 61; *Ancienne Chronique de Flandre*, p. 348.

92. Primat, pp. 99–100.

93. Dante, *Divine comédie*, Purgatoire, VI, 19–24. The poet condemns Marie de Brabant.

94. *Grandes Chroniques de France*, t. 8, p. 61.

95. Id., t. 8, pp. 304–316.

96. Nangis, continuation, t. 1, p. 421, and Geoffroi de Paris, *Chronique rimée*, p. 161. See J. Favier, *Philippe le Bel*, pp. 26–27 on the career of this jurist.

97. M. Mollat, *Jacques Cœur ou l'esprit d'entreprise*, chap. XI, p. 280 and sq. on the downfall as well as chap. XIII, p. 350 on the Minister of Finance's image as an upstart.

98. P. Clément, t. 2, p. 140 and sq.

99. Escouchy, t. 2, p. 284: "to further anger Charles VII against the said Coeur... he was told that Jacques Coeur had poisoned or had had poisoned the said young woman, from which poisoning she went from life to death" (*pour le* [Charles VII] *plus enflamber contre ledit Cœur... lui fut dit que Jacques Cœur avoit empoisonné ou fait empoisonner ladicte Demoiselle, duquel empoisonnement elle alla de vie a trepas*).

100. Id., p. 289.

101. Basin, *Historia Karoli*, pp. 283–287: charges *confecta ab aemulis potius quam vera*.

102. Maulde, p. 394 and sq., memoire on the crimes committed by Rohan's family, May 28, 1505.

103. Dante, *Divine Comédie*, Enfer, XIII.

104. Matthieu Paris, t. 5, pp. 68–69.

105. The author confuses the imperial chief doctor's attempt to poison his master and the disgrace of the ***logothete*** with motivations linked to treason (E. Kantorowicz, *L'empereur Frédéric II*, p. 601).

106. Dynter, t. 2, p. 185.

107. See G. Castelnuovo, Physionomie administrative et statut social des officiers savoyards au Bas Moyen Âge: entre le prince, la ville et la seigneurie (xive–xve siècle), *Les serviteurs de l'État au Moyen Âge*, Actes du XXIXe Congrès de la shmesp (Pau, 1998), Paris, Publications de la Sorbonne, 1999, pp. 181–192, p. 189. Dans *Ufficiali e gentiluomini...*, pp. 84–85, he gives examples of men of finance, who were hated by the nobility and disgraced. Jean Lagaret fell from power in this way in 1416 because of magic and alchemy.

108. Du Clercq, p. 203 in Buchon's edition: Master Gilles Courbet, who was close to Coustain and *subtil en subtilité réprouvée*, fled to Paris and then returned quietly to end his days as a canon in Arras.

109. Chastellain, t. 4, p. 265.

110. Id., pp. 267–268. J. Bartier, *Légistes et gens de finance au xve siècle. Les conseillers des ducs de Bourgogne Philippe le Bon et Charles le Téméraire*, Bruxelles, 1955, believes that the Coustain family was among the most active reclaimers of land in the duchy of Bourgogne.

111. Chastellain, t. 4, p. 266; Adrien de But, p. 435.

112. Chastellain, t. 4, p. 260.

113. *Le roman d'Alexandre*, p. 752.

114. R. Vaughan, *Philipp the Good. The Apogee of Burgundy*, Londres, 1970, p. 8. Letters presented in Parlement cleared Robays in 1423 (Fauquembergue, t. 2, p. 101).

115. *Registres du trésor des Chartes*, JJ 207, f. 148.

116. *Parlement criminel*, X2a 14, f. 257 v.

117. See the thoughts of C. Gauvard, "*De grace especial*," pp. 590–591; this hostility toward those who remarried is based also on "economic" jealousy: remarriage reduced the numbers of marriageable people.

118. *Parlement criminel*, X2a 15, f. 217 v, 1408.

119. *Parlement criminel*, X2a 15, f. 224 v and X2a 16, f. 35 v–36.

120. Pfister, p. 190.

121. Théry, p. 44.

122. *Parlement criminel*, X2a 6, f. 178–181.

123. *Parlement criminel*, X2a 14, f. 153–155 v.

124. Chronique rouennaise adjointe à la chronique de Pierre Cochon, p. 325. F. Graus, *Pest-Geissler-Judenmorde*, p. 308, reports the similar case (1395) of an executioner in Zurich, who was accused of having provoked an epidemic among animals by spreading poison on the pastures.

125. The dysentery epidemic (about 575), mentioned by Grégoire de Tours (t. 1, p. 295 of the Latouche edition) as caused by poisoning, is not attributed to any individual.

126. On this subject, see the studies contained in the collective work directed by M. Augé, C. Herzlich, *Le sens du mal. Anthropologie, histoire, sociologie de la maladie*, Paris, Éd. des Archives contemporaines, 1983. R. Girard devotes the first chapter of his scapegoat "*bouc-émissaire*," to the accusations of 1348 and observes that "it is necessary to see in the poisoning of the springs of potable water a variant of the accusatory stereotype" (p. 20).

127. It is found in *De ira* de Sénèque; see P. Preto, *Epidemia, paura e politica...*, p. 5.

128. Cohn, p. 191.

129. *Miracles de Notre-Dame de Rocamadour au xiie siècle*, p. 276.

130. *Chronique rouennaise allant de 1282 à 1343*, ed. *RHGF*, XXXIII, Paris, 1875, p. 349 or *Chronique parisienne anonyme*, p. 47: movement joined by people eager to wipe out their debts by killing their Jewish creditors; Nangis, t. 2, pp. 31–36.

131. Remark by F. Bériac, La persécution des Lépreux . . . , p. 208.

132. *Grandes Chroniques de France*, t. 8, p. 361.

133. *Si sont plainnes lor abeïs* dit Geoffroi de Paris (F.-O. Touati, *Maladie et société au Moyen Âge . . .* , cited p. 728). On a local level, see G. Lavergne, La persécution et la spoliation des lépreux à Périgueux en 1321, *Mélanges Clovis Brunel*, t. 2, Paris, 1955, pp. 107–113; P. Borradori, *Mourir au monde. Les lépreux dans le pays de Vaud (xiiie–xviie siècle)*, Lausanne, *Cahiers lausannois d'histoire médiévale*, 1992, n°7, p. 84 and sq.

134. A letter written in the autumn of 1321 punishes the Jews for usury, excess, and disobedience and imposes a fine of 150,000 livres that saves them from expulsion: E. A. R. Brown, Philip V, Charles IV and the Jews of France: The alleged expulsion of 1322, *Speculum*, 1991, n°66, pp. 294–329; W. C. Jordan, *The French Monarchy and the Jews: from Philip Augustus to the Last Capetians*, Philadelphia, 1989, p. 245 and sq.

135. D. Nirenberg, *Communities of Violence*, p. 64.

136. See C. Taylor, French assemblies and subsidy in 1321, *Speculum*, 1968, n°43, pp. 217–244; G. Ginzburg, *Le sabbat des sorcières*, p. 58.

137. Id., p. 65.

138. See M. Ginzburger, L'empoisonnement des puits et la peste noire, *REJ*, 1927, pp. 34–36; V. Pasche, Les épidémies de peste en Suisse romande. Vers de nouveaux comportements?, *The Regulation of Evil*, pp. 125–137, on the existence of the persecutions prior to the beginning of the plague. Guillaume de Machaut and Gilles li Muisit (*Annales*, p. 222) place the outbreak of the epidemic following the crime of the Jews.

139. Guillaume de Machaut, *Jugement du roi de Navarre*, in *Œuvres*, v. 225–226, p. 70 in ed. Tarbé. *Est alia causa quam naturalis*, writes Alphonse of Cordoba in a treatise on the plague (*Pestschriften*, t. 3, p. 224).

140. F. Graus, Pest-Geissler-Judenmorde, p. 161 and sq. and p. 299.

141. Cité par J.-N. Biraben, *Les hommes et la peste*, p. 65.

142. Trachtenberg, p. 107.

143. J.-N. Biraben, *Les hommes et la peste*, p. 64. Giovanni Villani, who speaks at length about the plague, mentions nowhere any accusations brought against the Jews. In places that have no Jewish community, such as the Island of Gotland, accusations nevertheless are directed toward those who are absent. On the example of Aragon, D. Nirenberg, p. 234. It is to the spiritual poison spread by the Jews that is attributed the epidemic of the plague.

144. See J. Delumeau, *La peur en Occident (xive–xviiie siècle)*, Paris, 1978, pp. 174–175.

145. L. Theis, *L'avènement d'Hugues Capet*, Paris, Gallimard, 1984, p. 203.

146. Context clarified by D. C. Douglas, *William the Conqueror*, p. 231 and sq.

147. Orderic Vital, t. 2, p. 101 and p. 259. On the context of this affair, M. de Boüard, *Guillaume le Conquérant*, Paris, Fayard, 1995, p. 392 and sq.

148. The *Libelli de lite imperatorum et pontificum* published by E. Dümmler, *MGH*, Hanover, 1891–1897, do not appear to contain accusations of poisoning other than those that are found in Benno's work, also edited in this collection under the title *Gesta romanae ecclesiae contra Hildebrandum*, t. 2, p. 379.

149. F. Cardini, *Magia, stregoneria, superstizioni...*, p. 29.

150. *Constitutiones et acta publica imperatorum et regum*, ed. L. Weiland, *MGH, Legum sectio IV*, t. 1, Hanover, 1893, p. 119.

151. Benno, pp. 51–52.

152. See *Politische Propaganda Kaiser Friedrichs II. und seiner Gegner*, ed. H. M. Schaller, Munich, 1965; collection of twenty-four letters and documents addressed by Frederick II or his enemies to other princes or authorities.

153. See *Le scienze alla corte di Federico II, Micrologus*, 1994, n 2.

154. *Cronica Reinhardsbrunnensis*, ed. O. Holder-Egger, *MHG SS*, XXX-1, Hanover, 1896, p. 611.

155. E. Kantorowicz, *L'empereur Frédéric II*, p. 164. We were not able to find the source of the material found in Frederick II's biography. The act of October 10, 1227 that excommunicates Frederick does mention the death of the *landgrave* but does not give the causes. (*Epistole seculi XIII e regestis pontificum Romanorum, MGH*, ed. C. Rodenberg, t. 1, Berlin, 1883, p. 283).

156. *Epistole seculi XIII. a regestis pontificum*, t. 1, p. 647; the pontifical rhetoric pretends not to want to believe what the rest of the world proclaims, the unanimous thus indisputable *fama*: *utinam non veneni periculo sicut mundus clamat.*

157. *Politische Propaganda Kaiser Friedrichs II*, n 15, p. 54: *ipsas vero non eripuit a vivendi termino mors naturalis, sed mors per coquum procurata, ut opinio vulgata declarat.*

158. Matthieu Paris, t. 4, p. 540, letter of July 31, 1246 to the lords of England.

159. Id., t. 4, p. 607.

160. Id., t. 3, p. 323.

161. Id., t. 5, p. 412 et 448, t. 6, p. 302; Nicolas Jamsilla, *Gesta Friderici imperatoris eiusque filiorum Conradi et Manfredi regum*, ed. Muratori, *RIS*, VIII, Milan, 1726, col. 506.

162. Matthieu Paris, t. 5, p. 432.

163. Id., t. 6, p. 302.

164. Id., t. 5, pp. 159–160; Ptolémée de Lucques, *Historia ecclesiastica*, ed. Muratori, *RIS*, XI, Milan, 1726, col. 1146; Martin de Troppau, *Chronicon Pontificum et Imperatorum*, ed. L. Weiland, *MGH SS*, XXII, Hanover, 1872, p. 472.

165. Matthieu Paris, t. 5, p. 459 and p. 448.

166. *Novus thesaurus*, t. 2, p. 86. Letter dated July 28, 1264.

167. Matthieu Paris, t. 5, pp. 68–69.

168. *Constitutiones regni Siciliae*, t. 6-2, pp. 708–709: *Libentius utique (scit Deus) que nostra serenitas loquitur tacuissemus, nisi quod tam atrox hujus sermonis materia que nequivit non esse notaria, si profundo nostro in pectore meditamur, sub sigillo silentii non debuit contineri... ut mundus agnoscit...* [the pope] *temptavit (proh pudor) occultis insidiis perdere vitam nostram et cum medico nostro qui Parme pridem in carcere tenebatur per legatum suum qui ad tractatum hujusmodi medius intervenit, fuit inhumaniter et nepharie machinatus quod post ejus ad nos regressum nostro venenum haustui propinaret sub specie potionis... Ecce quomodo nos amabat iste karissimus pater noster, ecce*

laudabilis et diligentia pastoralis!... Ô quantus exhuberta in nostris visceribus ex hujusmodi dolo dolor! Ô quanta turbatio dum veneficium ab illis astruitur a quibus beneficium deberetur!

169. Matthieu Paris, t. 5, p. 301.

170. *Chronica Ordinis*, ed. B. M. Reichert, Rome, 1904 (*Monumenta ordinis fratrum praedicatorum historica*, VII-1), p. 21: his enemies accuse Bernardin *ut ipsum ordinem diffamarent*.

171. A. Friedlander, Bernard Délicieux, le marteau des hérétiques, *Heresis*, 2001, n°34, pp. 9–34, who emphasizes that, through the trial brought against Délicieux, John XXII intended to add to the file of the Spirituels.

172. Mathias von Neuenburg, p. 160. See H. Thomas, *Ludwig der Baier*, Graz, Vienne, Cologne, 1993, p. 328.

173. Martin le Franc, *Le champion des dames*, t. 4, v. 18867–18868.

174. Burchard, *Liber notarum*, ed. Celani, *RIS*, XXXII-1, Cita di Castello, 1911, t. 2, p. 312 and sq.

175. *Die Romfahrt Kaiser Heinrichs VII. im Bildercyclus des Codex Balduini Trevirensis*, ed. G. Irmer, Berlin, 1881, p. 103.

176. Jean d'Outremeuse, t. 6, p. 13 and sq., then 153–156, and Jacques d'Esch, pp. 16–17, then 55 and sq.

177. *Chronique du Religieux de Saint-Denis*, t. 1, pp. 490–492. See the general context in M. Lamy, Les Dominicains dans la tourmente: les suites de l'affaire Jean de Monzon, *Religion et société urbaine au Moyen Âge*, Mélanges Biget, Paris, Publ. de la Sorbonne, 2000, pp. 177–200.

178. *Chronique du Religieux de Saint-Denis*, t. 1, p. 682: *Quod tamen pro comperto non habui*.

179. In the first half of the fourteenth century, the predominant idea of a collusion between the pope and the OFP could not adapt to the existence of a sanction that the papacy would have imposed on this group.

180. Jacques d'Esch, pp. 16–17.

181. *Ordinarium juxta ritum sacri ofp*, ed. F. Guerrini, Rome, 1921; see the *missale conventuale* in the section *De officio ministrorum altaris et de sacra communione*, pp. 242–243, 247.

182. Herman Korner, *Chronica novella*, ed. J. Schwalm, Göttingen, 1895, p. 223.

183. On monopolizing the functions of the royal confessors, see X. de La Selle, *Le service des âmes à la cour. Confesseurs et aumôniers des rois de France du xiii*^e^ *au xv*^e^ *siècle*, Paris, 1995.

184. See l'*Histoire du christianisme*, VI: *Un temps d'épreuves (1274–1449)*, dir. M. Mollat, A. Vauchez, Paris, 1990, p. 332 and sq. then pp. 688–689. On the Germanic hostility toward the papacy, consult *Kaiser, Volk und Avignon. Ausgewählte Quellen zur antikurialen Bewegung in Deutschland in der ersten Hälfte des 14. Jhts.*, ed. O. Berthold, Berlin, 1960. We did not have access to this work.

185. See our work entitled *Jacobitus secundus Judas* listed in the bibliography.

186. On the ins and outs of the affair, see F. Autrand, *Charles V*, pp. 812–816.

187. Christine de Pizan, *Livre des faits*, pp. 137–139. Christine herself, concerned about writing for the Dauphin a mirror that exalted the monarchial harmony, avoids speaking of Charles the Bad (*le Mauvais*), confining herself exclusively to those who committed the crime; *Chronique des règnes...*, t. 2, p. 284: the confession of a du Tertre is only summarized. The work, due to the *chancelier* Pierre d'Orgemont, was integrated into the *Grandes Chroniques de France*.

188. Secousse, p. 373: *rex velit patefieri omnibus christicolis de bono jure ipsius et de injusticia et iniquitate dicti regis Navarre.*

189. *Chronique du Religieux de Saint-Denis*, t. 1, pp. 355–357 and p. 467.

190. Grégoire XI, *Lettres secrètes relatives à la France*, ed. L. Mirot and H. Jassemin, Paris, 1935, n°3439. See P. Jugie, *Le cardinal Gui de Boulogne (1316-1373), Biographie et étude d'une famille cardinalice*, thèse des Chartes, Paris, 1986, p. 308 and sq. (communicated by the author to whom we are very grateful).

191. C. Gauvard, La *Fama*, a founding word, p. 9.

192. *Chronique du Religieux de Saint-Denis*, t. 2, p. 88; Froissart, t. 3, p. 279 of Buchon's edition: "for they said that she wanted to poison the king and his children. And she had already completely bewitched the king because in his illnesses, he no longer could see the queen nor recognize any woman in the world except for this duchess" (*car on disoit qu'elle vouloit empoisonner le roi et ses enfans. Et jà l'avoit-elle bien ensorcelé car le roi en ses maladies ne vouloit point voir la roine ni reconnoitre ni nulle femme du monde fors celle duchesse*).

193. Id.

194. Honorat Bovet, *L'apparicion* . . . , p. 11, concerning these spreaders of lies who led the people astray: "And when they cannot succeed in curing the sick, / in order to cause peace and love to disappear / Among neighbors and dear relatives, / They find horrible and difficult cases / To trouble the hearts of the humble" (*Et quant ne puent à ce* [guérir les malades] *venir, / Pour paix et amour departir / Entre prouchains et parens chiers, / Treuvent cas orribles et fiers / Pour troubler les cuers des menus*).

195. *Chronique du Religieux de Saint-Denis*, t. 2, p. 545.

196. L'*Apparition* dates from 1398. It exists in a version dedicated to the Duc de Bourgogne, which lessens his involvement with the Orléans family.

197. Coville, p. 134 and sq. In November 1414, Jean the Fearless (*sans Peur*) addressed a copy to the Comte and the text was copied again in 1438.

198. Fauquembergue, *Journal*, t. 1, p. 17.

199. Id., p. 32.

200. Y. Grandeau, Le dauphin Jean de Touraine, p. 720.

201. Monstrelet, t. 3, p. 168: "the said Dauphin had been poisoned by some of those who then controlled the king because he was strongly allied with the Duc de Bourgogne as had been his brother" (*ledit dauphin avoit esté empoisonné par aucuns de ceux qui adonc gouvernoient le roy pour tant que icellui estoit fort alyé au duc de Bourgogne comme son frere precedent*). Jean de Touraine was the nephew of the Duc de Bourgogne; Grandeau, p. 721: "They poisoned the above named plunderers for the same reason that they poisoned our seigneur who was greatly feared by his brother" (*l'ont empoisonné les dessus dits rapineurs pour la mesme raison qu'ils empoisonnerent notre seigneur tres redouté son frere*). On the propaganda in letters under Charles VI, see B. Guenée, Les campagnes de lettres qui ont suivi le meurtre de Jean sans Peur, duc de Bourgogne (septembre 1419–février 1420), *ABSHF*, 1993, pp. 45–65.

202. R. Famiglietti, *Royal Intrigue, Crisis at the Court of Charles VI, 1392–1420*, New York, 1986, p. 180.

203. Fauquembergue, t. 1, p. 32, reproduces the arrest document of the royal prosecutor of the lampoons.

204. The article of the *DLF*, however, challenges this text, preserved in only one manuscript, which is a work of propaganda.

205. Adrien de But, p. 435.

206. Id., p. 446, addition to the original text, probably in light of the public wellbeing.

207. Basin, p. 35 and III, 5: *talium facinorum machinandi et patrandi assuefactio.*

208. *Recueil de pièces pour servir à l'histoire de Louis XI*, ed. Duclos, Paris, 1746, p. 360 and sq. See *Briefwechsel Karls des Kühnen (1433–1477), Inventar*, ed. W. Paravicini, Francfort, 2 vol., 1995, t. 1, p. 495, the list of the addressees of the letters.

209. Id., p. 496, excerpt from the Chronicle of Oudenbosch.

210. *Recueil de pièces*, p. 366.

211. Commynes, III, 9, p. 257 of Blanchard's edition. He does not speak explicitly of poison.

212. *Preuves des mémoires de Philippe de Comines*, ed. N. Lenglet du Fresnoy, Paris, 1747, pp. 199–200.

213. Stein, p. 464. The author describes the text as a call to arms.

214. Basin, t. 2, p. 134.

215. Jean de Roye, t. 2, p. 285.

216. See the documents assembled under n°CCIX in the *Preuves des mémoires de Philippe de Comines*, pp. 279–291, with the date of November 22, 1473. The king insists that the copies and *vidimus* were made by the Archbishop of Bordeaux and by the president of the Parlement of this town "to give value to and serve in time and place against the false and disloyal condemnation that the Duc de Bourgogne made by his false and disloyal lies" (*pour valoir et servir en temps et lieu contre la fausse et desloyale condamnation que le duc de Bourgogne a voulu faire par fausses et desloyales menteries*).

217. Jean de Roye, t. 1, pp. 303–309.

218. *Lettres de Louis XI*, n°1164 and PJ VI, t. 7, p. 317.

219. *Chronographia regum Francorum*, t. 3, p. 144 and Adam Usk, p. 60; it is necessary to observe that the death by poison of the Duke of Gloucester, imprisoned in Calais after an attempt against the king, his nephew, is reported by one French source, not by a pro-Lancaster English source, and that the *Chronique de la traïson et mort de Richard deux* does not speak of poison; all the narrative and judicial documents published in the *Chronicle of the Revolution, 1397–1400*, by Ch. Given Wilson, Manchester, 1993, refer to a murder by smothering under a featherbed; the second affair, reported only by Adam Usk, concerns the son of the son of the Duke of Gloucester also poisoned in his prison by a servant of Richard II (1399).

220. *Select cases; Richard II, etc.*, p. 113. See the very enlightening study of P. Strohm, *England's empty throne. Usurpation and the language of legitimation, 1399–1422*, New Haven and Londres, 1997, p. 65 and sq.

221. Henri de Mondeville, *Chirurgie*, p. 693.

222. Pietro d'Abano, *De venenis*, p. 33.

223. Brocardus, *Directorium ad passagium faciendum*, p. 431 then 439.

224. Eustache Deschamps, *Contre les empoisonneurs*, v. 25: "Watch out for their tricks... You in the West" (*Gardez vous de leurs agais... Vous, d'Occident*).

225. *Histoire des étrangers et de l'immigration en France*, s.d. Y. Lequin, Paris, Larousse, 1992, p. 178.

226. *Annales de Melk*, p. 511.

227. M. Aurell, *Les noces du comte...*, p. 112.

228. Rigault, p. 94. J. Favier, *Philippe le Bel*, pp. 410–411 then 456–461, shows the similarity of the ideological issues in the diverse affairs led by Guillaume de Nogaret.

229. P. Stafford, *Queen Emma and Queen Edith. Queenship and Women's Power in Eleventh Century England*, Oxford, 1997, p. 87 then 270, on the numerous political murders in Saxon England.

230. See D. C. Douglas, *William the Conqueror*, p. 415, n. 3. An idea that must be tempered by the fact that one of the accusers was a staunch Norman and that the other was Anglo-Breton; their movement failed because of two prelates who were of English origin (Id., p. 233).

231. J. C. Russell, *Twelfth Century Studies*, p. 85.

232. Jean de Salisbury, *Policraticus*, VIII, 19, t. 2, p. 372 in Webb's edition: *Siquidem Britannia venena semper exhorruit et in principes non novit.*

233. Matthieu Paris, t. 4, p. 61, suggests that the monks from Durham who were poisoned in Rome where they had gone to demand the confirmation of the election of an abbot who displeased the king died through the action of that king (1240).

234. See D. A. Carpenter, What happened in 1258? *War and Government in the Middle Adges, Essays in honour of J. O. Prestwich*, ed. J. Gillingham and J. Hold, Woodbridge, 1984, pp. 106–119. The Count of Gloucester was one of the barons who swore to defend English liberties; H. Ridgeway, King Henry III and the Aliens, 1236–1272, *Thirteenth Century England*, 1987, n 2, pp. 81–92.

235. Matthieu Paris, t. 5, p. 702 then 705.

236. Id., p. 708. However, it is necessary to point out that certain authors do not attribute the crime to the Poitevins and that the barons in their letter to the pope to whom they denounce the bad government of the kingdom do not accuse the Continentals of being poisoners (*Annales de Burton*, ed. R. Luard, *Annales monastici*, t. 1, Londres, 1864, p. 459).

237. Cited by K. J. Kesselfing, A draft of the 1531 "Acte for Poysoning," p. 899.

238. Pierre Gringore, *Jeu du Prince des sots, Œuvres complètes*, t. 2, p. 247.

239. De Gaulle, pp. 98–100.

240. Guillaume and Martin du Bellay, *Mémoires*, ed. V. Bourrilly and F. Vindry, Paris, 4 vol., 1912, t. 3, pp. 215, 218, 219.

241. See J.-F. Dubost, *La France italienne, xvi*[e]*–xvii*[e] *siècle*, Paris, Aubier, 1997, p. 320.

242. "True speech about what occurred in the town of Bruges in the year 1582 because King Philippe of Spain had once again committed new betrayals and murders in order to kill the Duc de Brabant, Anjou, Nassau . . . together with the Prince d'Orange with poison or another means" (*Discours véritable de ce qui est advenu en la ville de Bruges l'an 1582 parce que le roy Philippe d'Espagne a derechef praticqué nouveaux traistres et meurtriers pour oster la vie au duc de Brabant, Anjou, Nassau . . . ensemble au prince d'Orange par poison ou quelque autre sorte de meurtre*), Bruges, 1582.

243. P. Pluchon, *Vandou, sorciers empoisonneurs*, pp. 238–244.

244. J. de Maleyssie, Histoire du poison, chap. X. The author observes, p. 328, that the use of chemical weapons remains taboo: military parades exhibit nuclear missiles, not toxic weapons, which cannot be confessed, especially after the dreadful use of gas in the Great War. Poison remains in the domain of the occult.

Conclusion

In a short appendix on the poisonings attributed to William the Conqueror, D.C. Douglas says that "[t]he subject of medieval poisoning is inexhaustible," before he confesses that it is also a fascinating subject.[1] The reason why the subject is fascinating is precisely because it is multifaceted. And, since it is multifaceted, it always gives the impression of being partially concealed from the historian. The huge amount of inaccessible material includes not only facts and documents. It is also conceptual, for *veneficium* concerns numerous fields that extend widely beyond the field of the history of criminality. Even Christ was by some said to have been *veneficus*, because he dyed his clothes with his redeeming blood![2]

By adopting a panoramic approach that is inherently risky, we have sought to present varied points of view on a kind of homicide that is particular in its form, its methods, and its perception. This approach has produced several conclusions that the discovery of other cases and other texts could render questionable. That is why we decided to present this research as an essay, a genre that offers interpretations based on partial investigations and that permits extensions and revisions that are inevitable considering the scope of the subject. Furthermore, the word "essay" relates this work to the universe of poisoning because we can consider it as some kind of *proba*, an intellectual trial of a furtive historical subject that is difficult to keep up to date.

To keep up to date is indeed the appropriate expression for a matter that is in so many respects connected to opaqueness and secretness. The crime of poisoning is by nature a concealed crime. Such an acknowledgment, which is justified in the first place by the historiographical obscurity in which *toxicatio* remained for a long time, does not only state a legal formula used to define the crime of poisoning. It applies to many different aspects of the problem.

In the eyes of the people of the Middle Ages, *veneficium* was not solely a criminal *modus operandi*.[3] It became integrated with a cultural and historical behavior, beliefs, and representations, and it gives a rich point of view on medieval society, as does Louis d'Orléans' murder at the gate called Barbette on November, 23, 1407.[4]

Before we introduce the results of this essay, we need to present some of the questions that remain. The first one is quite banal. The very fact of looking at a topic leads to making it look more important in order to legitimize it. Yet, the frequency of poisoning cases in all kinds of sources is relatively low. The chronicles contain numerous references to deaths that were not linked to poison even when the circumstances of the death were mysterious. Judicial archives give very little space to *toxicatio* that juridical texts neglect, very different from cases of heresy or witchcraft. Indeed, it would be absurd to avoid an historical investigation of a topic because men of that time did not pay a lot of attention to it. But, the risk is always great when one decides to construct a theory about a problem that was more created than discovered. It can lead to one of these historiographic mirages that collapse because they have no ground to support them. Quite to the contrary, that is not the case with *veneficium*.

To paraphrase B. Guenée paraphrasing Chaucer,[5] one wonders if the field that has to be ploughed is not too vast, the plough too heavy, and the blade too light to dig furrows deep enough in an unstable soil. The *excusatio propter infirmitatem* expresses the feeling that if the crime *stricto sensu* and not its context had been the focus of attention in this work, whether the research would not have taken another direction. The same supposition could be made if the time selected had been the end of the Middle Ages instead of the entire period and also if the place researched had been only France instead of the West. Nevertheless, we are convinced that the breadth of this study that includes themes, chronology, and geography serves the topic better than would a narrower focus that would necessarily be more precise.

In addition, the historian's bias toward a cultural approach tempts him to lose sight of the factual dimension that cannot completely be put aside, at the risk of his becoming a novelist or a philosopher. Yet, it was the only way to avoid the positivist temptation, which is as vain as it is sterile. All the same, the preceding pages are riddled with indirect turns of phrase and expressions such as "taken for," "supposed to be," "reputed to have been," that may have been used too often. These expressions have not only been detrimental to the style, but they have also blurred the confused limits between the facts and the way they were perceived.

Another question comes from the fact that this approach had to intellectually link together elements that texts of the time do not always clearly connect. Indeed, the duty of the historian of ancient times consists as much in constructing interpretations as in recalling explicit conceptions of people who lived in the distant past. But, as Jacques Le Goff would say, in this game the risk is always to "over interpret" the facts and to use them artificially in demonstrations that ignore the contradictions in sources and to fill their silence with attractive conjectures. The guesses, the reconstitutions, and the hypotheses hold a place that hopefully no one will find excessive.

For instance, let us look at the following: one of the main ideas of the essay is that the crime of poisoning distinguished itself by being a murder with no blood in societies in which homicide normally equated murder with bloodshed. But this definition by default was probably not as clear for medieval minds. For example, needing a play on words, the Religious of Saint-Denis presents the King of Navarre as being thirsty for his cousins' blood (*sanguinem consanguineorum*), while in fact, he spends his time saving it by the use of poison.[6] According to the interpolator of the *Scandalous Chronicle* (*Chronique scandaleuse*), Charles de Guyenne's poisoner pronounced the words *peccavi tradens sanguineum justum* while hanging himself.[7] Where is the blood in this case? The homicidal act is often described with established formulas that convey only the outcome of the crime and not its modalities. There is another notion lacking in *veneficium*: violence. Violence is not as absent in the use of poison as is assumed when the cause of death is given. Mahaut d'Artois distinguishes "natural death" and "violent death," which he divides into death given by violence and death given by poison.[8] Chastellain writes that Henry VII "died violently" (*mourut violentement*).[9] Are blood, violence, and poison as different as we claimed for the needs of the demonstration? This last question concerns the dimension of "occult crime" that is important to us because of the many different meanings of the word "occult." However, it also presents the unresolved problem of the links that exist between medical knowledge, juridical science, and the perception of toxic criminal practice. Did the coherent image shaped by the pieces of the puzzle that we have put together ever exist in the minds of the contemporaries of Frederick II or Louis XI?

It was very tempting to construct some kind of continuum from one end of the Middle Ages to the other, and to assess in the same way facts from the sixth century and those from the fifteenth. The measurement of the continuum and the changes in a domain that deals with mental perceptions that evolve as time passes is never an easy task. But, *a contrario*, perception of evolution has always been the victim of the hypothetical documentary that sometimes makes us take revelations for revolutions. The paucity of crimes of poisoning during the Carolingian period is hard to explain. The increase in cases starting with the thirteenth century, and the emergence of an obsessive fear of this crime among the nobility who sought ways to protect themselves from it, is the result of multiple and complex phenomena that are difficult to rank: Can it be a consequence of contacts with the Orient? Is it the result of a cultural mutation that affects the question of the causes of death? Is it the result of the drama of a political hiatus that results from the abrupt disappearance of an authority figure? Is it due to the growth of the feeling that the Occident believed it was exposed to an underground threat of which heresy and witchcraft were other facets? The subtle blend of all these phenomena remains mysterious.

Notwithstanding these reservations and questions, several conclusions can be drawn. The first one, which is not surprising, is the difficulty in measuring this particular type of crime. The upsurge or the scarcity of *veneficium* is based on intuition, rather than on crime statistics, which, by the way, would reflect only crimes that were punished and not all crimes. One is led to suspect the relative absence of actual criminal poisoning. It contrasts with the perception of late Middle Ages when *toxicatio* was widely mentioned by the chroniclers and rumors, the exaggeration of reality.[10]

The second conclusion is that the medieval mind's perception of the crime by poison lacks clarity. *Venenatio* was clearly perceived as a special and distinct *modus necandi* noted by historical sources and sometimes mentioned by men of letters and preachers for narrative or edifying reasons. From time to time, it was also taken into account by jurists, and finally distinguished in legal texts but without being emphasized. The origin of this lack of visibility lies in the ambiguous vocabulary and the ambiguity of the law that places poisoning, from the Vulgate and the *Corpus juris civilis*, into the separate spheres of homicide and magic. The crime of poisoning is linked to homicide only when its ultimate consequences are considered. Consideration of the necessary preparations draws the crime close to the magical practices that surround the making of harmful substances. This heritage from early antiquity has deprived *veneficium* of a separate identity.

Another distortion between the facts and social representations is evident. The extant documents imply that poison is a weapon used in all social classes. The assumption that poisoning is confined to the elite classes has proved to be false. Besides the poisonings at court that play an important role in the chronicles and that Franc Gontier believes to be the sole venue for poisonings, there exist the poisonings in cottages or in the backs of shops revealed by judicial sources. The traditional sociology of *veneficium* overlaps the sociology of criminals created by the imagination of judges and the public in only one aspect: it spares no one, not even the most protected and cautious princes, and it kills *tam nobiles quam ignobiles*, as the narrator of the events of 1321 said. Furthermore, and the medieval situation is in no way remarkable, *toxicatio* occurred primarily in situations where strong bonds of intimacy and service could contribute to the carrying out of the crime. But the social representations of poisoners present a paradoxical image. Homicide by poisoning is an inside crime based on proximity to the victim; yet, it characterizes itself in the imaginary (of men since they are almost the only ones to discuss it), by exteriority, in so far as it is attributed to those who are different whether it be by sex, religion, customs, or country of origin. This attribution of *veneficium* implies a rejection that can be called one of identity. It enables the Occident to distinguish itself from neighboring civilizations that are stigmatized by their use of poison that they produce or make available.

Based on chivalric novels, the sword, the club, or the dagger are nothing more than tools to kill. Poison is very different. It is a weapon often obtained by stealth, in conditions where secret knowledge and magical rites play a part. It is made of substances that are not fully known and whose effects are unpredictable and ambiguous as well as often misunderstood. *Venenum* forces nature and distorts it at the same time. It is suspected more often at the end of the Middle Ages when people began to think more about the causes of death that had previously been comfortably attributed to divine will. Far from being a mark of credulity that positivist historiography denounced, the allegation of poisoning illustrates a greater desire to know and to understand in the society of the fourteenth and fifteenth centuries, which was better educated and more informed about medical matters.

The imaginary of poison, which is slightly dulled by the popularization of some substances sold by apothecaries and which is not completely dispelled by toxicological literature, reflects the horror that *veneficium* inspired. Indeed, we find a community of words in the language of poison specialists as well as that of the jurists who tried their hand at characterizing *toxicatio*. It is the vocabulary of the occult that proves useful for toxic properties as well as for carrying out the crime. Poisoning was considered a crime of secrecy, dissimulation, and ambush whose weapon was used clandestinely and secretly. Its use implied preparation, organization, and criminal deliberation that make premeditation inherent in *venenatio*. The intimacy and proximity necessary for its use connected it to treason and perfidy, in a world dependent on *fides*. The goals of its practitioners were to destroy from the inside the social units on which Occidental society was based, from the married couple to Christianity. Used rarely for murder between social equals, poison diverted and turned upside down social roles: the doctor poisoned instead of treating, the spouse contaminated instead of feeding, the servant poisoned instead of serving, the warrior poisoned instead of fighting, the host gave death instead of hospitality: poison was a bad gift that subtracted instead of adding.[11] And this inversion ended up affecting all society.

"The poisoning of the world" in the words of a poet of the 1300s emerged as a threat during the last centuries of the Middle Ages. The avowed fear of poison among the powerful was similar to the extreme fear of witchcraft. J. Chiffoleau has demonstrated the logic that linked the hunt for heretics to the hunt for witches and the evolution from the struggle against words harmful to the soul to combat against ethereal practices that were harmful to bodies.[12] Did not the use of poison constitute the last section of the infernal triptych, linked metaphorically to heresy (poison for the mind) and etymologically and organically to witchcraft, with its diabolical power? We are far from thinking like René Girard that "in the course of this period [the first half of the fourteenth century], the belief in occult forces was weakening," hence explaining the substitution of accusations[13] of poisoning for accusations of witchcraft. On the contrary, we believe that the former and the latter were part of a common "mythology of the occult."

The fear that *venenatio* inspired in the fourteenth century, or even the thirteenth century, triggered precautionary and repressive measures. They fell within a vast cultural, psychological, and ideological movement of the general exposure of the enemies of Christianity, who were considered fiends or allies of the *venenator*, who was the Devil. The pursuit of poisoners obviously took place against a background of the development of a judicial structure and the evolution of judicial procedures. This pursuit did not distinguish itself by its methods or by the punishments inflicted, and it cannot be compared quantitatively to the contemporary hunt for witches. However, it was not unrelated to the hunt for witches.

After all, the judicial dimension of poisoning is less interesting than its cultural dimension, so much so that the two dimensions have to be separated.[14] Even more than in Roman society, *toxicatio* moved in direct opposition to the values inherent in Occidental medieval society. Poisoning was a "nasty criminal case," the direct opposite of the "noble act of homicide." Poison was a fatal instrument of corrosion because it was insidious. It wormed its way into the social body of Christianity, which could also secrete its own toxic humor. Being held in such contempt and so loathed, it covered with infamy everyone who used it. Poison constituted a political and ideological weapon that made possible the elimination of an adversary or his cause and also justified massacres and pogroms. Poison unbalanced the established order when it was used as the weapon in a crime. Poison used to accuse another may also have been a means of social regulation by turning toward the outside the fury of disoriented peoples or by contributing to the purification of political society, even as a way to unite a community against a more or less imaginary enemy. In that sense we can say that the crime of poisoning takes a particular shape against the tormented background of the autumn of the Middle Ages.

NOTES

1. D. C. Douglas, *William the Conqueror*, p. 415, n. 3.
2. Bernardin de Sienne, *Sermons de Carême*, sermon XV for the Lenten Season.
3. R. W. Ireland,Medicine, necromancy and the law..., p. 60: "Poisoning has been too long ignored for it has been assumed that, as now, it is merely one *modus operandi* of homicide."
4. B. Guenée, *Un meurtre, une société: l'assassinat du duc d'Orléans, 23 novembre 1407*, Paris, Gallimard, 1992.
5. *Id., L'opinion publique...*, p. 17.
6. *Chronique du Religieux de Saint-Denis*, t. 1, p. 355.
7. Jean de Roye, t. 2, p. 285. Words probably taken from Scripture.
8. Godefroy Ménilglaise, p. 208.
9. Chastellain, t. 1, p. 26.
10. Fortunate expression de P. Pluchon, *Vaudou, sorciers empoisonneurs*, p. 163.
11. The expression *dare venenum* can be found and the same word *gift* means "gift " in English and in German "poison."
12. J. Chiffoleau, Sur la pratique et la conjoncture..., p. 376.
13. R. Girard, *Le bouc émissaire*, p. 28.
14. M. Sbriccoli, *Crimen laesae maiestatis...*, p. 169.

Glossary

Note: The following terms are in bold in the text.

aconite: the herb wolfsbane, or monkshood applied to any plant of the genus Aconitum, all the species of which are poisonous.

Al-Andalous: Arabic name given to the parts of the Iberian peninsula that were governed by the Muslims from the eighth to the fifteenth century.

antimony: a toxic element. Clinically, antimony poisoning is very similar to arsenic poisoning. In small doses, antimony causes headache, dizziness, and depression. Larger doses cause violent and frequent vomiting and lead to death in a few days.

bailliage: a regional court (generally in the North) that heard appeals from local seigneurial courts and cases involving nobles, minors, and those living in the church. The financial claims involved in a criminal case being heard by this court could not exceed a given sum, thus restricting their influence on many matters. See also *sénéchaussée.*

bezoars: a stony substance that is formed in the gastrointestinal tract of certain animals including human beings and to which were attributed curative properties and magical qualities.

camerlingue: name given to the official who holds the office of finance minister and serves as the head of the government in the Vatican between the death of the pope and the meeting of the cardinals to elect a new one.

cantharidin: a substance found in an emerald-green beetle in the family Meloidae, also called the Spanish Fly. The beetle contains up to 5 percent cantharidin that irritates animal tissues. The crushed powder is of yellowish brown to brown-olive color with iridescent reflections, of disagreeable scent, and bitter flavor.

cassidoine: precious stone found in Chalcedon used by the ancients to make vases.

ceruse: a pigment composed of white lead.

Chambre des Comptes: the department of government charged with overseeing the financial affairs of the royal court.

curopalate: name often given to the author of a ceremonial Byzantine treatise dating from the fourteenth century.

decretal: important papal documents that offer legal advice to papal judges.

diatesseron: a substance composed of four substances believed to have medical purposes: gentian roots, birthworts (Latin *aristolochia*), laurel leaves, and myrrh.

electuary: a pharmaceutical preparation of soft consistency composed of powders mixed with syrup, honey and pulp made from plants.

hellebore: any poisonous plant of the genus Heleborus of the buttercup family, having basal leaves and clusters of flowers.

In the early days of medicine, two kinds of hellebore were recognized: black hellebore, which included various species of Helleborus, and white hellebore, now known as Veratrum album ("false hellebore"). Although the latter plant is highly toxic, containing veratrine and the teratogens cyclopamine and jervine, it is believed to be the "hellebore" used by Hippocrates as a purgative. Black hellebore was used to treat paralysis, gout and other diseases, and insanity. Black hellebore is also toxic causing tinnitus, vertigo, stupor, thirst, a feeling of suffocation, swelling of the tongue and throat, emesis and catharsis, bradycardia (slowing of the pulse), and finally collapse and death from cardiac arrest.

Several legends surround the hellebore; in witchcraft it is believed to have ties to summoning demons. Helleborus niger is commonly called the Christmas rose due to an old legend that it sprouted in the snow from the tears of a young girl who had no gift to give the Christ child in Bethlehem. In Greek mythology, Melampus of Pylos used hellebore to save the daughters of the king of Argos from a madness induced by Dionysus that caused them to run naked through the city, crying, weeping, and screaming. During the Siege of Kirrha in 585 B.C., hellebore was reportedly used by the Greek besiegers to poison the city's water supply. The defenders were subsequently so weakened by diarrhea that they were unable to defend the city from assault. Some historians believe that Alexander the Great died because of a hellebore overdose, when he took it as medication.

hematite: a mineral occurring in brilliant black crystals and in earthy masses, the principal ore of iron.

***juge-mage*:** the magistrate charged with making judicial decisions in a town.

***juge ordinaire*:** judge of the courts of first instance within the royal seneschalsies of Beaucaire, Carcassonne, Toulouse, Rovergne, and Quercy. By 1350, the larger subordinate courts were recognized as the seats of *judices ordinarii*.

***languier*:** a structure in precious metal from which are hung snake tongues.

***lettre de commission*:** a demand for an inquiry.

lettre de rémission**:** a letter from the Prince in response to a plea for mercy by an accused party.

litharge: lead oxide produced by the cupellation of silver.

logothete: title borrowed by the West from Byzantium used especially in Sicily for the position of chancellor.

magnet stone: iron oxide

mithridatisme: immunity to mineral or plant poisons that is acquired by taking the substance in small doses over a period of time.

orpiment (arsenic sulfide): a mineral that was an important item of trade in the Roman Empire and used as a medicine in China although it is highly toxic. It was also used as a fly poison and to poison arrows. Because of its striking color, it was also a favorite with alchemists searching for a way to make gold, both in China and the West.

Orpiment was ground, processed, and used for centuries as a pigment in painting, being one of the few clear, bright yellow pigments available to artists up until the nineteenth century. Orpiment presented problems, however, such as its extreme toxicity and its incompatibility with other common pigments like lead and copper-based substances such as verdigris and azurite. The use of orpiment as a pigment matter ended almost entirely with the advent of the cadmium yellows and the various dye-based colors of the nineteenth century.

penitentials: short manuals that classified sins according to seriousness and made recommendations to the priests about what penance should be imposed.

privilège de for**:** right of the Church to establish its jurisdiction to judge the misdeeds of clerics and members of religious orders.

realgar: an arsenic sulfide mineral. It is a soft, sectile mineral occurring in monoclinic crystals, or in granular, compact, or powdery form, often in association with the related mineral, orpiment. It is orange-red in color, melts at 320 °C, and burns with a bluish flame releasing fumes of arsenic and sulfur.

Realgar was, along with orpiment, a significant item of trade in the ancient Roman Empire and was used as a pigment and a medicine. It was also used as a medicine in China and "is made up into household ornaments, such as wine pots, wine cups, images, paperweights, and various other kinds of ornaments and charms, to be kept near at hand in use, or worn about the person, with a view of warding off disease."

Realgar is also used by firework manufacturers to create the color white in fireworks, manufacturing shot, printing and dyeing calico, and depilating and tanning hides.

Realgar, orpiment, and arsenopyrite provide nearly all the world's supply of arsenic as a byproduct of smelting concentrates derived from these ores.

sandaraque: ancient name for realgar

sénéchaussée**:** a regional court (generally in the South) that heard appeals from local seigneurial courts and cases involving nobles, minors, and livings in the church. The financial claims involved in a criminal case being heard by this court could not exceed a given sum, thus restricting their influence on many matters. See also *bailliage*.

sigillated soil: yellowish-red soil with a fine texture used by the Turks to imprint official seals.

Solanaceae: a family of flowering plants, many of which are edible, while others are poisonous (some have both edible and toxic parts). The family includes the Jimson weed, eggplant, mandrake, deadly nightshade or belladonna, paprika, chile pepper, potato, tobacco, tomato, and petunia.

sublimé (anhydride arsenieux): the crystals, deposit, or material obtained when a substance is sublimated (to volatilize from the solid state to a gas, and then condense again as a solid without passing through the liquid state.

thériaque: a preparation known since Antiquity that contains more that fifty ingredients belonging to three realms of nature (including a strong dose of opium) and having the reputation of being effective against poison and certain discomforts.

tormentille: herbaceous plant from the Rosaceous family, a variety of potentilla reputed to have curative properties.

treacle: an extremely sweet substance such as molasses that was used as an antidote for poison.

Vif-argent sublimé: mercury.

Major Sources

Bibliographie de base

Abréviations usuelles :

ABSHF
Annuaire-bulletin de la Société de l'Histoire de France

AESC
Annales Économie-Société-Civilisation

BEC
Bibliothèque de l'École des chartes

JS
Journal des savants

MA
Le Moyen Âge

MEFR
Mélanges de l'École française de Rome

REJ
Revue des études juives

RHDFE
Revue historique de droit français et étranger

SHMESP
Société des historiens médiévistes de l'enseignement supérieur public

Histoire, anthropologie, ethnologie, imaginaire du poison

Boujot C., *Le venin,* Paris, Stock, 2001.

Cabanès A., Nass L., *Poison et sortilèges,* Paris, 1903.

Collard F., Le banquet fatal: la table et le poison dans l'Occident médiéval, *La sociabilité à table. Commensalité et convivialité à travers les âges,* Actes du colloque de Rouen (novembre 1990), Textes réunis par M. Aurell, O. Dumoulin et F. Thélamon, Rouen, Presses Universitaires de Rouen, 1993, p. 335–342.

Collard F., *Horrendum scelus.* Recherches sur le statut juridique du crime de poison au Moyen Âge, *Revue historique,* 1998, n° 300, p. 737–764.

Collard F., Quand l'épidémie sert d'alibi au crime. Dysenterie et empoisonnement au Moyen Âge, *Air, miasmes, contagion,* Actes de la Table ronde de Reims (1997), Langres, Guéniot, 2001, p. 189–197.

Collard F., Une arme venue d'ailleurs. Portrait de l'étranger en empoisonneur, *L'étranger au Moyen Âge,* Actes du XXXe Congrès de la SHMESP (Göttingen, mai 1999), Paris, Publications de la Sorbonne, 2000, p. 95–106.

Collard F., Des victimes désignées? Profils des empoisonnés au Moyen Âge, *Les victimes, des oubliées de l'histoire,* Actes du colloque de Dijon (octobre 1999), s.d., B. Garnot, Rennes, Presses Universitaires de Rennes, 2001, p. 445–453.

Collard F., *Venenosa mulier coronata.* Variations sur le thème de la reine empoisonneuse dans l'Occident médiéval, *Reines et princesses au Moyen Âge,* Actes du Ve colloque du CRISIMA (Montpellier, novembre 1999), M. Faure (éd.), Montpellier, 2001, p. 304–322.

Collard F., L'empereur et le poison: de la rumeur au mythe. Les enjeux historiographiques, politiques et idéologiques du prétendu empoisonnement d'Henri VII en 1313, *Médiévales,* 2001, n° 41, p. 113–131.

Collard F., Ouvrir pour découvrir. Réflexions sur les expertises de cadavres empoisonnés à l'époque médiévale, *Le corps à l'épreuve,* études réunies par D. Quéruel, E. Samama et F. Collard, Guéniot, Langres, 2002, p. 177–190.

Collard F., *In claustro venenum.* Quelques réflexions sur l'usage du poison dans les communautés religieuses médiévales, *Revue d'Histoire de l'Église de France,* 2002, n° 88, p. 5–19.

Collard F., *Jacobita secundus Judas.* L'honneur perdu des Prêcheurs après la mort d'Henri VII, *Religion et mentalités au Moyen Âge,* Mélanges en l'honneur d'Hervé Martin, Rennes, Presses Universitaires de Rennes, 2003, p. 221–234.

Collard F., *Veneficiis vel maleficiis.* Réflexion sur les relations entre le crime de poison et la sorcellerie dans l'Occident médiéval, *MA,* 2003, n° 109-1, p. 9–57.

Ireland R. W., Chaucer's toxicology, *Chaucer Review,* 1994, n° 29-1, p. 74–92.

Ireland R. W., Medicine, necromancy and the law : Aspects of medieval poisoning, *Cambrian Law Review,* 1987, n° 18, p. 52–61.

Kaufman D. B., Poisons and Poisoning among the Romans, *Classical Philology,* 1932, n° 27, p. 156–167.

Leleux Ch., *Les poisons à travers les âges,* Paris, 1923.

Lentsch R., La *proba.* L'épreuve des poisons à la cour des papes d'Avignon, *Les prélats, l'Église et la société,* XIe-XVe *s.,* Mélanges B. Guillemain, Bordeaux, 1994, p. 155–162.

Lewin L., *Die Gifte in der Weltgeschichte,* Heidelberg, 1920.

Maleyssie J. de, *Histoire du poison,* Paris, 1991.

Minois G., *Le couteau et le poison. L'assassinat politique en Europe (1400–1800)*, Paris, Fayard, 1997.

Obringer F., *L'aconit et l'orpiment. Drogues et poisons en Chine ancienne et médiévale*, Paris, 1997.

Pluchon P., *Vaudou, sorciers empoisonneurs. De Saint-Domingue à Haïti*, Paris, 1987.

Pogatscher H., *Von Schlangenhörnern und Schlangenzungen*, Rome, 1898.

Russell J. C., Allegations of poisoning in the Norman World, *Twelfth Century Studies*, New York, 1973, p. 83–93.

Troianos S. N., Zauberei und Giftmischerei in mittelbyzantinischer Zeit, *Fest und Alltag in Byzanz*, ed. G. Prinzing et D. Simon, Munich, 1990, p. 37–51.

Villeneuve R., *Poisons et empoisonneurs célèbres*, Paris, 1960, rééd. 1968.

Études sur des affaires d'empoisonnement spéciales

Albe E., *Autour de Jean XXII : Hugues Géraud, évêque de Cahors, l'affaire des poisons et des envoûtements*, Cahors-Toulouse, 1904.

Barber M., Lepers, jexs, moslems. The plot to overthrow Christendom in 1321, *History*, 1981, n° 216, p. 1–17.

Bériac F., La persécution des lépreux dans la France méridionale en 1321, *MA*, 1987, n° 93, p. 203–221.

Carbonelli C. G., *Gli ultimi giorni del conte rosso e i processi per la sua morte*, Pinerolo, 1912.

Courtray A.-M., *Une affaire mystérieuse, Pierre Gerbais accusé d'avoir empoisonné Hugues, sire de Grammont et de Corbières*, Extrait du *Bulletin de la Société Gorini* (1920–1924), Annecy, 1925.

Coville A., *Jean Petit et la question du tyrannicide au commencement du* XVe *siècle*, Paris, 1932.

Duplès-Agier H., Une accusation d'empoisonnement contre les Jacobins sous Charles VI (1390), *Revue des questions historiques*, 1866, p. 603–609.

Franke M. E., *Kaiser Heinrich VII. im Spiegel der Historiographie*, Cologne-Vienne, 1992.

Friedlander A., *The Hammer of the Inquisitors. Brother Bernard Délicieux and the Struggle Against the Inquisition in Fourteenth Century France*, Leiden, 2000.

Godefroy Ménilglaise M. de, Mahaut, comtesse d'Artois, *Mémoire de la société des antiquaires de France*, 1864, n° 28, p. 181–230.

Graus F., *Pest-Geissler-Judenmorde, Das 14. Jahrhundert als Krisenzeit*, Göttingen, 1987.

Knowles D., The case of saint William of York, *Cambridge historical Journal*, 1936, n° 5, p. 162–177.

Labande L.-H., Un complot des chanoines d'Avignon contre leur évêque (1305), *Annales d'Avignon et du comtat Venaisssin*, 1913, p. 129–144.

Langlois Ch.-V., La fin d'Hugues Géraud, évêque de Cahors, *Revue de Paris*, 1906, p. 531–552.

Mollat M., *Les affaires de Jacques Cœur. Journal du procureur Dauvet*, Paris, 2 vol., 1952.

Monfrin J., Étudiants italiens à la fin du XIVe siècle, *MEFR*, 1951, n° 63, p. 195–281.

Nelson J., La mort de Charles le Chauve, *Médiévales*, automne 1996, n° 31, p. 53–66.

Pasolini P. D., *Catherina Sforza*, Rome, 3 vol., 1893.

Provost A., *L'imagination au pouvoir. Recherches sur le procès de Guichard, évêque de Troyes (1308–1314)*, thèse de l'Université de Paris IV, 2000.

Rigault A., *Le procès de Guichard de Troyes*, Paris, 1896.
Stein H., *Charles de France, frère de Louis XI*, Paris, 1919.
Théry J., Les Albigeois et la procédure inquisitoire : le procès pontifical contre Bernard de Castanet, évêque d'Albi et inquisiteur (1307–1308), *Heresis*, 2000, n° 33, p. 7–48.
Vidal J.-M., La poursuite des lépreux en 1321, *Mélanges de littérature et d'histoire religieuse publiés à l'occasion du jubilé épiscopal de Mgr de Cabrières, évêque de Montpellier (1874–1899)*, Paris, t. 1, 1900, p. 483–518.

Histoire des sciences, de la médecine, des maladies

Agrimi J., Crisciani C., Savoir médical et anthropologie religieuse. Les représentations de la *vetula* (XIIIe-XVe siècle), *AESC*, 1993, p. 1281–1309.
Dall'Osso E., *L'organizzatione medico-legale a Bologna e a Venezia nei secoli XII-XIV*, Cesena, 1956.
Jacquart D., *La médecine médiévale dans le cadre parisien (XIVe-XVe siècles)*, Paris, Fayard, 1998.
Paravicini Bagliani A., *Medicina e scienze della natura alla corte dei papi nel Duecento*, Spolète, 1991.
Paravicini Bagliani A., *Le corps du pape*, Paris, Le Seuil, 1997 (1re éd. italienne 1994).
The regulation of Evil. Social and cultural attitudes to epidemics in the late Middle Ages, éd. A. Paravicini-Bagliani et F. Santi, Florence, 1998 *(Micrologus Library II)*.
Shatzmiller J., *Médecine et justice en Provence méridionale*, Aix-en-Provence, 1989.
Thorndike L., *An History of Magic and Experimental Science*, Londres, 8 vol., 1923–1958.
Thorndike L., *Science and Thought in the XVth Century*, New York, 1929.
McVaugh M., *Medicine before the Plague : Practitioners and their Patients in the Crown of Aragon (1285–1345)*, Cambridge, 1993.
Weill-Parot N., *Les "images astrologiques" au Moyen Âge et à la Renaissance. Spéculations intellectuelles et pratiques magiques (XIIe-XVe siècle)*, Paris, Champion, 2002.

Histoire de la criminalité, de la justice et du droit pénal

Bourin M., Chevalier B., Le comportement criminel dans les pays de la Loire moyenne d'après les lettres de rémission (vers 1380–vers 1450), *Annales de Bretagne*, 1981, n° 88, p. 245–263.
Carbasse J.-M., *Introduction historique au droit pénal*, Paris, 1990.
Carbasse J.-M., La peine en droit français des origines au XVIIe siècle, *Recueil de la Société Jean Bodin*, t. LVI : *La peine*, 2e partie, Bruxelles, 1991, p. 157–172.
Chiffoleau J., *Les justices du pape. Délinquance et criminalité dans la région d'Avignon*, Paris, 1984.
Chiffoleau J., Dire l'indicible. Remarques sur la catégorie du *Nefandum* du XIIe au XVe siècle, *AESC*, 1990, n° 45-2, p. 289–324.
Chiffoleau J., Sur la pratique et la conjoncture de l'aveu judiciaire en France du XIIIe au XVe siècle, *L'Aveu, Antiquité et Moyen Âge*, Actes de la Table ronde organisée par l'École française de Rome (mars 1984), Rome, 1986 (Coll. de l'École française de Rome, n° 88), p. 341–380.
Crime, Society and the Law in Renaissance Italy, ed. T. Dean et K. J. P. Lowe (ed.), Cambridge, 1994.

Esmein A., *Histoire de la procédure criminelle en France, et singulièrement de la procédure inquisitoriale depuis le* XIIIe *siècle jusqu'à nos jours*, Paris, 1882, réimpr. Francfort, 1969.
Gauvard C., *"De grace especial". Crime, État et société en France à la fin du Moyen Âge*, Paris, 2 vol., Publications de la Sorbonne, 1991.
Gauvard C., De la difficulté d'appliquer les principes du droit pénal en France à la fin du Moyen Âge, *Die Entstehung des öffentlichen Strafrechts*, s.d. D. Willoweit, Cologne-Weimar-Vienne, 1999, p. 91–120.
Gauvard C., La *Fama*, une parole fondatrice, *La renommée*, numéro spécial de *Médiévales*, 1993, n° 24, p. 5–13.
Gauvard C., Les sources judiciaires de la fin du Moyen Âge peuvent-elles permettre une approche statistique du crime?, *Commerce, finances et société* (XIe–XVIe *siècle)*, Mélanges Dubois, Paris, 1993, p. 469–488.
Gonthier N., *Le châtiment du crime au Moyen Âge*, Rennes, 1997.
Gundersheimer W. L., Crime and Punishment in Ferrara, 1450-1500, *Violence and Civil Disorder in Italian Cities, 1200–1500*, ed. L. Martines, Londres, 1972, p. 104–128.
Gyger P. J., *L'épée et la corde. Criminalité et justice à Fribourg (1475–1505)*, Lausanne, *Cahiers lausannois d'études médiévales*, 1999, n° 22.
Laingui A., Lebigre A., *Histoire du droit pénal*, Paris, 2 vol., s.d.
Lévy J.-Ph., *La hiérarchie des preuves dans le droit savant du Moyen Âge*, Paris, 1939.
Migliorino F., *Fama e infamia. Problemi della societa medievale nel pensiero giuridico nei secoli XII-XIII*, Catane, 1985.
Porteau-Bitker A., Criminalité et délinquance féminine dans le droit pénal des XIIIe et XIVe siècles, *RHDFE*, 1980, n° 58, p. 13–56.
Porteau-Bitker A. et Talazac-Laurent A., La renommée dans le droit pénal laïque du XIIIe au XVe siècle, *La renommée*, numéro spécial de *Médiévales*, 1993, n° 24, p. 67–80.
Sbriccoli M., *Crimen laesae maiestatis. Il problema del reato politico alle soglie della scienza penalistica moderna*, Milan, 1974.
Zorzi A., Giustizia criminale e criminalita nell'Italia del tardo medioevo : studi e prospettive di ricerca, *Societa e storia*, 1989, n° 46, p. 923–965.

Histoire sociale femmes, marginaux, juifs

Bériac F., *Histoire des lépreux au Moyen Âge*, Paris, Imago, 1988.
Blumenkranz B., *Juifs et chrétiens dans le monde occidental, 430–1096*, Paris, 1960.
Cutler A. et H., *The Jew as Ally of the Muslim. Medieval Roots of Anti-Semitism*, Notre-Dame, 1986.
Duby G., *Dames du* XIIe *siècle*. III : *Ève et les prêtres*, Paris, Gallimard, 1996.
Histoire des femmes, s.d., G. Duby, M. Perrot, t. 2, *Le Moyen Âge*, Paris, 1991.
Jordan W. C., *The French Monarchy and the Jews : from Philip Augustus to the Lest Capetians*, Philadelphie, 1989.
Kohn R., *Les juifs de la France du nord dans la seconde moitié du* XIVe *siècle*, Paris-Louvain, 1981.
Moore R. I., *La persécution. Sa formation en Europe*, Paris, Les Belles Lettres, 1991.
Nirenberg D., *Communities of violence. Persecution of minorities in the Middle Ages*, Princeton, 1996, tr. fr., Paris, PUF, 2001.

Pancer N., *Sans peur et sans vergogne. De l'honneur des femmes aux premiers temps mérovingiens,* Paris, Albin Michel, 2001.

Stafford P., *Queens, Concubines and Dowagers. The King's Wife in the Early Middle Ages,* Londres, 1983.

Trachtenberg J., *The Devil and the Jews,* New Haven, 1944.

Histoire des comportements et des déviances: magie, sorcellerie, hérésie

Blauert A., *Frühe Hexenverfolgungen, Ketzer, Zauberei-und Hexenproxesse des 15. Jahrhunderts,* Hambourg, 1989.

Boudet J.-P., La genèse médiévale de la chasse aux sorcières : jalons en vue d'une relecture, *Le Mal et le Diable. Leurs figures à la fin du Moyen Âge,* éd. N. Nabert, Paris, 1996, p. 35–52.

Cohn N., *Démonolâtrie et sorcellerie au Moyen Âge, fantasmes et réalités,* Paris, 1982.

Delumeau J., *La peur en Occident* (XIVe-XVIIIe *siècle),* Paris, 1978.

Glinzburg C., *Le sabbat des sorcières,* tr. fr., Paris, 1992 (éd. it. 1989).

Girard R., *Le bouc-émissaire,* Paris, 1982.

Kieckhefer R., *European Witch Trials : Their Foundations in Popular and Learned Culture, 1300–1500,* Londres, 1976.

Mercier F., *L'enfer du décor. La Vauderie d'Arras (1459–1491) ou l'émergence d'une nouvelle souveraineté autour des ducs Valois de Bourgogne,* thèse de l'Université de Lyon II, 2001.

Michelet J., *La sorcière,* Paris, Julliard, 1964.

Paravy P., À propos de la genèse médiévale de la chasse au sorcière : le traité de Claude Tholosan, juge dauphinois (1436), *MEFR,* 1979, n° 91, p. 333–379.

Peters E., *The Magician, the Witch and the Law,* Philadelphie, 1978.

Russel J. B., *Witchcraft in the Middle Adges,* New York, 1972.

Selected Bibliography

Quelques sources particulièrement sollicitées

Le crime de poison au Moyen Âge

Abréviations usuelles :

BEC
Bibliothèque de l'École des chartes

MEFRM
Mélanges de l'École française de Rome, Moyen Âge

MGH
Monumenta Germaniae historica

PL
Patrologie latine

RIS
Rerum italicarum scriptores

RHC
Recueil des historiens des croisades

RHGF
Recueil des historiens des Gaules et de la France

Traités des poisons

Ambroise Paré, *Discours a scavoir de la momie, du venin, de la licorne,* et *Traité des venins et morsures de chiens enragés et autres morsures et piqueures de bestes veneneuses,* in *Œuvres complètes,* t. 3, Paris, 1841.

Antonio Guaineri, *Opus praeclarum,* éd. de Lyon, 1525.
Arnaud de Villeneuve, *Tractatus de arte cognoscendi venena,* éd. de Milan, 1475 (avec le traité *De venenis* de Pietro d'Abano) et de Gênes, 1498.
Christoforus de Honestis, *Liber de venenis,* BNF, ms. lat. 6910, f. 87–113.
Frranciscus de Sienne, *Liber de venenis,* BNF, ms. lat. 6979.
Guido da Vigevano, *Texaurus regis Francie acquisitionis Terre Sancte de ultra mare necnon sanitatis corporis ejus et vite ipsius prolongacionis ac etiam cum custodia propter venenum,* BNF, ms. lat. 11015.
Jean Martin de Ferrare, *De venenis evitandis et eorum remediis libellus,* BNF, ms. lat. 6980.
Juan Gilles de Zamora, *Contra venena et animalia venenosa,* éd. M. Castro, *Archivo ibero-americano,* 1976, n° 36, p. 23–117.
Konrad Von Megenberg, *De mortalitate in Alammania,* éd. S. Krüger, *Festschrift H. Heimpel,* Göttingen, 1972, t. 2, p. 839–883.
Maïmonide, *Traité des poisons,* éd. I. M. Rabbinowicz, Paris, 1865.
Pestschriften aus den ersten 150 Jahren nach der Epidemie des schwarzen Todes, éd. K. Sudhoff, *Archiv für Geschichte der Medizin,* 1909 à 1925, nos 2 à 17.
Nicolas Falcucci de Florence, *De dispositionibus venenorum,* BNF, ms. lat. 6985.
Pietro d'Abano, *Tractatus de venenis,* éd. de Marburg, 1537; éd. partielle et commentaire par A. Benedicenti, Florence, 1949; tr. par Ogier, BNF, ms. fr. 14820.
Petrus Cararius, *Questio de venenis ad terminum,* éd. de Venise, 1566.
Sante Ardoini de Pesaro, *Opus de venenis,* éd. de Venise, 1492.

Sources narratives

Alain Bouchart, *Les grandes chroniques de Bretaigne,* éd. M.-L. Auger et G. Jeanneau, Paris, 3 vol., 1986–1998.
Benno ou Benzo, *De vita et gestis Hildebrandi,* éd. de Francfort, 1581.
Chronique des quatre premiers Valois, éd. S. Luce, Paris, 1862.
Chronique des règnes de Jean II et de Charles V, éd. R. Delachenal, Paris, 4 vol., 1917–1920.
Chronique du Religieux de Saint-Denis, éd. L.-F. Bellaguet, Paris, 6 vol., 1839–1852, réimpr. 1995.
Cornelius Zantfliet, *Chronique,* éd. Martène et Durand, *Veterum scriptorum... amplissima collectio,* t. 5, Paris, 1729.
Cronica de gestis principum a tempore Rudolfi regis usque ad tempora Ludowici imperatoris, éd. G. Leidinger, in *Bayerische Chroniken des XIV. Jahrhunderts, MGH, ss rr g in us. sch.,* 19, Hanovre-Leipzig, 1918.
Edmond de Dynter, *Chronica ducum Lotharingiae et Brabantiae,* éd. P. F. X. de Ram, Bruxelles, 4 vol., 1854–1857.
Enguerrand de Monstrelet, *Chronique,* éd. Douet d'Arcq, Paris, 6 vol., 1857–1862, réimpr. New York, 1966.
Georges Chastellain, *Chronique,* éd. Kervyn de Lettenhove avec les œuvres complètes, Bruxelles, 1863–1864.
Gesta Normannorum ducum, de Guillaume de Jumièges, Orderic Vital et Robert de Thorigny, éd. tr. E. van Houts, Oxford, 2 vol., 1992–1995.
Giovanni Villani, *Historie universali de suoi tempi,* éd. de Venise, 1559, éd. plus récente F. G. Dragomanni, 4 vol., Florence, 1844–1845 et G. Porta, Parme, 1991.

Grandes Chroniques de France, éd. J. Viard, Paris, 10 vol., 1920–1953 et éd. *RHGF* (1226–1328), XX et XXI, Paris, 1840–1855.
Grégoire de Tours, *Historia Francorum,* éd. B. Krusch et W. Levison, *MGH, Ss rr. mer.*, I, Hanovre, 1951, éd. R. Büchner, Darmstad, 1970, éd. R. Poupardin, Paris, 1913 et tr. R. Latouche, Paris, 2 vol, 1963–1965.
Guillaume de Malmesbury, *De gestis regum Anglorum,* éd. W. Stubb, Londres, 1887–1889 (Roll series, 90).
Guillaume de Nangis, *Chronique latine de 1113 à 1300,* et continuations jusqu'en 1368, éd. H. Géraud, Paris, 2 vol., 1843.
Guillaume de Tyr, *Historia rerum in partibus transmarinis gestarum,* éd. R. Huygens, Turnhout, 2 vol., 1986; éd. tr. dans le *RHC; Historiens occidentaux,* I et II, éd. non précisé, Paris, 1844; continuation française sous le titre *L'Estoire de Eraclés empereur,* dans le *RHC; Historiens occidentaux,* III, Paris, 1859.
Jacques du Clercq, *Mémoires,* éd. Michaud et Poujoulat, Paris, 1837, et éd. Buchon, 1826–1827.
Jean Froissart, *Chroniques,* éd. S. Luce, G. Raynaud et L. Mirot, Paris, 15 vol., 1869–1975 (Société de l'Histoire de France), et éd. Buchon, Paris, 1837.
Jean Juvénal des Ursins, *Histoire de Charles VI,* éd. J. A. Buchon, Paris, 1843, et éd. de 1614 et 1653, Paris.
Jean de Roye, *Chronique scandaleuse,* éd. Michaud-Poujoulat, Paris, 1837, et éd. B. de Mandrot, Paris, 2 vol., 1894–1896.
Jean de Saint-Victor, *Memoriale historiarum,* éd. partielle *RHGF,* XXI, Paris, 1855.
Matthieu Paris, *Chronica majora,* éd. H. R. Luard, Londres, 7 vol., 1872–1883, tr. A. Huillard-Bréholles, Paris, 9 vol., 1841.
Nicole Gilles, *Cronicques et annales de France,* éd. de Paris, 1566.
Orderic Vital, *Historia ecclesiastica,* éd. A. Le Prévost et L. Delisle, Paris, 5 vol., 1838–1855, et éd. M. Chibnall, Oxford, 6 vol., 1969–1980.
Philippe de Commynes, *Mémoires,* éd. J. Blanchard, Paris, 2001.
Philippe de Vigneulles, *Chronique,* éd. Ch. Bruneau, 4 vol., Besançon-Metz, 1927–1933.
Pierre le Baud, *Cronicques et ystoires des Bretons,* éd. Ch. de La Lande de Calan, Rennes, 1907–1922.
Ranulf Higden, *Polychronicon,* éd. C. Babington et J. R. Lumby, Londres, 9 vol., 1865–1886.
Robert Gaguin, *Historia Francorum,* éd. de Paris, 1500, et éd. de Francfort, 1577.
Thomas Basin, *Historia Ludovici undecimi,* éd. Ch. Samaran, Paris, 3 vol., 1963–1972.

Sources juridiques et judiciaires

Actes du Parlement de Paris (1254–1328), éd. E. Boutaric, 2 vol., Paris, 1863–1867, réimpr. 1975.
Actes du Parlement de Paris (1328–1350), éd. H. Furgeot, 3 vol., Paris, 1920–1975.
Archives nationales, *Parlement criminel,* registres X2a 1 à X2a 18, des origines à 1423, et *Trésor des Chartes,* registres JJ 68 à JJ 234 (1348–1501).
Andrea Barbazza, *Consilia,* éd. de Trente, 1517.
Azon, *Lectura sive commentarius in codicem justinianeum,* éd. de Paris, 1611.
Boniface VIII en procès. Articles d'accusation et dépositions des témoins, 1303–1311, éd. J. Coste, Rome, 1995.
Balde, *Commentarian libris codicis,* éd. de Venise, 8 vol., 1589.

Balde, *Consilia,* éd. de Francfort, 1589.
Bartole, *Commentaria in Digesti partes,* éd. de Turin, 1574.
Bartole, *Commentaria in Codicis partes,* éd. de Turin, 1574.
Burchard de Worms, *Corrector sive medicus,* livre XIX du *Décret,* éd. F. W. H. Wasserschleben, *Die Bussordnungen der abendländischen Kirche,* Halle, 1851, réimpr. Graz, 1958 p. 624–682, et éd. Migne avec l'ensemble du *Décret, PL* 140, Paris, 1853.
Die Bussordnungen der abendländischen Kirche, éd. F. W. H. Wasserschleben, Halle, 1851, réimpr. Graz, 1958.
Claude Tholosan, *Ut magorum et maleficiorum errores,* éd. P. Paravy, *MEFRM,* 1979, n° 91, p. 354–379.
Code théodosien, éd. J. Gothfried, Leipzig, 6 vol., 1743.
Confessions et jugements de criminels au parlement de Paris (1319–1350), transcrits par Étienne de Giens, greffier, éd. M. Langlois, Y. Lanhers, Paris, 1971.
Constitutiones regni Siciliae, éd. F. Huillard-Bréholles, in *Historia diplomatica Frederici secundi,* Paris, 5 vol., t. 4-1, 1854 et t. 6-2, 1861.
Contemporary narrative of the Proceedings against Dame Alice Kyteler for sorcery, éd. T. Wright, Londres, 1843.
Corpus juris canonici, éd. Friedberg, Graz, 1955.
Corpus juris civilis, éd. Krüger-Mommsen, Berlin, 3 vol., 1877–1895.
Digeste, éd. Mommsen-Krüger, Berlin, 2 vol., 1870.
Felino Sandeo, *Commentaria super toto quinto decretalium,* Turin, 1521.
Geoffroy de Salagny, *Commentaire sur l'Infortiat,* éd. de Lyon, 1552.
Hippolite de Marsiliis, *Commentaria super titulis ad legem Corneliam de sicariis et ad legem Pompeiam de pariciidiis et ad legem Corneliam de falsis,* Lyon, 1542.
Jean Bodin, *Fléaux des démons et sorciers,* Paris, 1579.
L'imaginaire du sabbat, édition critique des textes les plus anciens (1430–1440) réunis par M. Ostorero, A. Paravicini Bagliani, K. Utz Tremp, Lausanne, *Cahiers lausannois d'histoire médiévale,* 1999, n° 26.
Jacoppo Butrigario, *Lectura super prima parte Codicis,* éd. de Paris, 1516.
Jacques Fournier, *Registre d'inquisition,* éd. J. Duvernoy, Toulouse, 3 vol., 1975 (latin), Paris - La Haye, 1978 (français).
Pietro d'Ancharano, *Commentaria in Decretalium libris,* Bologne, 1581.
Procédures politiques du règne de Louis XII, éd. R. de Maulde, Paris, 1885.
Processus Bernardi Delitiosi, éd. A. Friedlander, Philadelphie, 1996.
Registre criminel du Châtelet, éd. H. Duplès-Agier, Paris, 2 vol., 1861–1864.
Quellen und Untersuchungen zur Geschichte des Hexenwahns und der Hexenverfolgung im Mittelalter, éd. J. Hansen, Bonn, 1901.
Siete partidas del rey Alfonso el sabio, éd. G. Lopez, Madrid, 5 vol., 1861.
Yves de Chartres, *Décret* et *Panormia,* Paris, 1647, et éd. Migne, *PL* 161, Paris, 1855.

Littérature politique

Brocardus, *Directorium ad passagium faciendum,* tr. sous le titre de *L'advis directif pour faire le passage d'oultremer,* éd. Ch. Kohler (fr. et lat.), in *RHC; Documents arméniens,* II, Paris, 1906, p. 367–517.
Christine de Pizan, *Le livre de la Cité des dames,* tr. E. Hicks et T. Moreau, Paris, Stock, 1986.
Christine de Pizan, *Livre des fais et bonnes mœurs du sage roy Charles V,* éd. S. Solente, Paris, 2 vol., 1940, et tr. E. Hicks et T. Moreau, Paris, Stock, 1997.

Gilles de Rome, *De regimine principum,* tr. fr. d'Henri de Gauchy, *Li livres du gouvernement des rois,* éd. S. P. Molenaer, New York, 1899.
Jean Gerson, *Œuvres complètes,* éd. Glorieux, Paris-Tournai, 10 vol., 1960–1973.
Jean Petit, *Apologie du tyrannicide,* éd. *in* Enguerrand de Monstrelet, *Chronique,* t. 1.
Jean de Salisbury, *Policraticus,* C. Webb, Oxford, 1909; tr. D. Foulechat, éd. Ch. Brucker, livres I-III, Genève, 1994 et IV-VIII, *Le moyen Français,* 1987, n° 21.
Poggio Bracciolini, *De infelicitate principum,* éd. D. Canfora, Rome, 1998.
Politische Propaganda Kaiser Friedrichs II. und seiner Gegner, éd. H. M. Schaller, Munich, 1965.

Quelques œuvres littéraires

Boccace, *Decameron,* éd. E. Pognon, Fribourg-Genève, 1978, et tr. s.d. C. Beck, Paris, 1994.
Le Chevalier au cygne et Godefroid de Bouillon, éd. Reiffenberg, Bruxelles, 4 vol., 1846–1854.
Ciperis de Vignevaux, éd. W. S. Woods, Chapel Hill, 1949.
Eustache Deschamps, *Œuvres complètes,* éd. Queux-Raynaud, Paris, 11 vol., 1878–1904 et éd. partielle par H. Millet, J.-P. Boudet *et al., Eustache Deschamps en son temps,* Paris, Publ. de la Sorbonne, 1997.
Geoffrey Chaucer, *Canterbury Tales,* éd. W. W. Skeat, in *Œuvres complètes,* Londres, 1912 et éd. modernisée D. Wright, 1964.
Gaydon, éd. Guessard et Luce, Paris, 1862.
Le jeu et la complainte de Pierre de la Brosse, éd. A. Jubinal, Paris, 1835.
Li bastard de Bouillon, éd. A. Scheler, Bruxelles, 1877.
Martin le Franc, *Le champion des dames,* éd. R. Deschaux, Paris, Champion, 5 vol., 1999.
La mort le roi Artu, éd. J. Frappier, Genève-Paris, 1964 (3e éd.).
Parise la Duchesse, éd. Guessard et Larchey, Paris, 1860 et éd. M. Plouzeau, Aix-en-Provence, 1986, 2 vol. (*Senefiance,* 17–18).
Roman d'Alexandre, tr. L. Harf-Lancner avec le texte édité par E. C. Armstrong *et al.,* Paris, 1994.
Ser Giovanni Fiorentino, *Il pecorone,* Turin, 1853.
Simon de Marville, *Vœux de l'épervier,* éd. G. Wolfram, F. Bonnardot, Metz, 1895.

Littérature d'édification, théologie

Ci nous dit, Recueil d'exemples moraux, éd. G. Blangez, Paris, 2 vol., 1978–1986.
Étienne de Bourbon, *Tractatus de diversis materiis praedicabilibus,* éd. J. Berlioz et J.-L. Eichenlaub, Turnhout, Brépols, 1998, et éd. partielle A. Lecoy de La Marche, Paris, 1877.
Grégoire le Grand, *Dialogues,* éd. A. de Voguë, tr. P. Antin, Paris, 1978–1980.
Jacques de Voragine, *Legenda aurea,* éd. Th. Graesse, Dresde, 1846, tr. J.-B. Rose, 2 vol., Paris, Flammarion, 1967.
Miracles de Notre-Dame de Rocamadour au XIIe *siècle,* éd.-trad. E. Albe, Paris, 1907.
Thomas d'Aquin, *Summa totius theologiae,* Rome, 4 vol., 1896.
La vie ancienne de saint Samson de Dol, éd. tr. P. Flobert, Paris, 1997.

Sources administratives, inventaires

Choix de pièces inédites relatives au règne de Charles VI, éd. L. Douët d'Arcq, Paris, 2 vol., 1863–1864.

Inventaire du trésor du Saint-Siège sous Boniface VIII (1295), éd. E. Molinier, *BEC*, 1882, n° 43, p. 19-310 et 626–646; 1884, n° 45, p. 31–57; 1885, n° 46, p. 16–44; 1886, n° 47, p. 646–667; 1888, n° 49, p. 226–237.

Die Inventare des päpstlichen Schatzes in Avignon, éd. Hoberg, Rome, 1944.

Leges palatinae regis Jacobi Majoricarum, éd. in *Acta Sanctorum,* Junii, III, Anvers, 1701.

Lettres de Louis XI, éd. J. Vaesen et E. Charavay, Paris, 11 vol., t. 7, 1478–1479, 1900.

Recueil de pièces servant de preuves aux mémoires sur les troubles excités en France par Charles II, éd. D. F. Secousse, Paris, 1755.

Statuta capitulorum generalium ordinis cisterciensis, éd. J. Canivez, Louvain, 8 vol., 1933–1941.

Index of Major Historical Figures

Abélard, 52, 77, 97, 111, 116–17, 136, 140, 144, 161, 163–64, 222, 252
Adaiulf, 181
Adèle de Pouille, 103, 108
Agnès Sorel, 4, 232
Albert, Duke of Austria, 69, 107
Alexander le Grand, 130, 224–26
Alexander V, 97, 230
Alexander VI, xvi, 3, 20, 51, 59, 97, 130, 230, 242
Alexis Comnène, 112, 164
Alphonse, comte de Saint-Gilles, 102, 161
Amédée VI, 103, 150
Amédée VII de Savoie, 20, 44, 59, 67, 70, 95, 129–30, 173, 182, 187, 229
Amédée VIII de Savoie, 41, 50, 229–30
Armagnacs, 221, 244–45
Arnaud de Villeneuve, 26, 52, 74
Assassins, 12, 14, 46, 108, 133, 138, 140, 241
Austria, Duchess of. 100
Ava de Ribagorça, Couness of Castille, 112, 145, 151, 199, 249

Bajazet, 57
Bar, Duchesse de, 4, 109
Barnabo Visconti, 3
Bartolomeo de Varignana, 193
Baudouin, Bastard of Bourgogne, 245
Benedict XI, 62, 74, 90, 99, 154, 169, 191, 196
Benedict XIII, 63–64, 83
Bernard de Castanet, 145, 191, 196, 207, 235, 280
Bernard de la Roche, 94, 103, 173, 192, 193, 229
Bernard Délicieux, 74, 154, 176, 191, 196, 242
Bernardin de Montepulciano, 137, 149
Bertrade de Montfort, 2, 67, 108, 141, 147
Bertrand Aimini, Bishop of Avignon, 128, 130, 196
Bianca Maria Visconti, 109
Black Prince (Prince Noir), 56
Blanche de Castille, 228
Blanche de Navarre, 44
Bohémond, 59, 102, 108
Boniface VIII, 26, 63–64
Bonne de Berry, 229
Bonne de Bourbon, 229
Boson, marquis de Provence, 107, 143
Brunehaut, 5, 100, 140

Cardinal de Boulogne, 261
Cardinal de Laon, 4, 197
Catherine Sforza, 43, 51, 57, 230
César Borgia, 230
Charles d'Anjou, 46, 138, 241
Charles de Guyenne, 29, 90, 129, 143–44, 246, 267
Charles de Tarente, 149
Charles de Valois, 100, 187, 189, 232
Charles d'Orléans, 26, 189
Charles the Foolhardy (le Téméraire), 175, 257, 245–47
Charles II the Bald (le Chauve), 2, 6, 8, 110, 137, 145, 172
Charles II de Navarre (Charles the Bad (le Mauvais), 41, 44, 47, 50–51, 60, 62, 94–95, 129, 135–36, 138, 145, 154, 243–44
Charles IV de Luxembourg, emperor, 103, 134, 189, 193
Charles V, 56, 63, 68–69, 95, 128, 131, 135–36, 147, 149, 175, 224, 244
Charles VI, 28, 51, 59, 82–83, 86, 89, 99, 111, 114, 122, 141, 145, 147, 175, 212, 214, 219, 221, 243–44, 261
Charles VII, 27, 36, 91, 140, 232
Charles VIII, 26, 70, 89, 147, 162, 186
Charlot, son of Robert de Béthune, 108, 148
Charoald, 184, 227
Childebert, 140
Claude Tholosan, 17, 19, 73, 178
Clement V, 26, 176, 179, 196, 230, 241
Clement VI, 63, 85
Clement VII, 65
Conan, comte de Bretagne, 149, 239
Conrad IV, 89, 240–41
Conradin, 89
Cunégonde, Queen of Bohemia, 100, 137

Dante, 231, 233, 253, 256
Déroud d'Amiens, 68–69
Djem, 57

Eadburh, 100, 145, 147, 250
Edmond de Kent, 228
Edward I, 70
Edward III, 228
Edward IV, 61
Emma, Lothaire's wife, 27, 100, 142, 263
Étienne, Patriarch of Jérusalem, 92
Eudes, King of the Francs, 125, 238

François Sforza, Duke of Milan, 51, 91, 138
Fredegonda, 140
Frédéric, son of Henri VII, 240
Frederick of Austria, 58, 61, 111
Frederick I Barbarossa, 47, 58, 222
Frederick II, 5, 13, 53, 65, 69, 99, 144, 156–57, 188, 196, 204, 233, 239–41, 267

Galéas Visconti, 249
Gaston Phoebus, 78, 94, 157
Gaston, son of Gaston III de Foix, 78, 94, 157
Gautier, comte du Mans, 88, 113, 136
Gilles de Bretagne, 41, 54, 133, 140, 154, 233
Godefroy de Bouillon, 112, 151, 185, 225
Gregory VII (Hildebrand), 92, 239, 242
Guichard de Troyes, 19, 44, 46, 48–49, 97, 141, 146, 148, 155, 159, 179, 182–83, 187–88, 190–91, 194, 196, 249
Guillaume, Bishop of Valence, 92, 154, 186
Guillaume de Tyr, 2, 27, 92, 95, 116, 120, 124–25, 285
Guinevere, 7–8, 56, 100, 185, 216, 226
Gundeberga, 181, 227

Helmigis, 53
Henri, Conrad's young brother, 240–41
Henri I of France, 173
Henry III of England, 110, 250–51
Henry IV, emperor, 49, 74, 175, 239, 248
Henry IV of England, 56
Henry V of England, 175
Henry VI, emperor, 103
Henry VI of England, 49

Henry VII, emperor, 52–53, 58–59, 66–67, 69, 90, 103, 110, 128, 136–37, 162, 225, 240–41, 249, 267
Henri VIII of England, 11, 203, 223, 250
Herbert de Vermandois, 3
Hercule, 26, 224, 226
Hugues d'Amboise, 56
Hugues de Grammont, 59, 181, 233
Hugues Géraud, 18, 44, 48, 82, 89, 97, 127, 129, 131, 136, 141, 160, 187–88, 194–95, 219, 230

Innocent IV, 240
Isabel of England, Frederick II's wife, 240

Jacqueline de Brabant, 100, 137
Jacques Coeur, 36, 232
Jacques Fournier, 20, 24, 45, 47, 74–75, 77, 84, 123, 153, 162, 168, 177, 217
Jean de Bavière, former Bishop of Liège, 3, 51
Jean de Berry, 162, 229
Jean de Chalon (Prince d'Orange), 45, 53, 247
Jean de Grandville, 20, 44, 95, 102, 117, 130–31, 136–37, 164, 189, 191–94, 229
Jean de Lusignan, 147
Jean de Marigny, 53
Jean de Touraine, 4, 58, 221, 245
Jean de Vliet, 203
Jean the Fearless (sans Peur), 78, 144, 221, 245
Jean VI1I, 93, 140
Jeanne de Bourgogne, Philippe VI's wife, 40, 53, 100, 147
Jeanne de Mortagne, 232
Jeanne de Navarre, 185, 187, 191
Jehan Bon, 202
Jehan Coustain, 41, 67, 94, 135–36, 148, 158, 176, 182, 195, 203, 233–34, 245
Jehan Hardy, 128, 203, 247
Jehan Lyon of Ghent, 4
John Lackland (sans Terre), xviii, 131
John XXII (Jacques Duèze), 26, 89, 93, 124, 127, 128–29, 160–61, 168–69, 176, 230, 260
John XXIII (Balthasar Cossa), 97, 230

Ladislas (ou Lancelot) of Hungary, 60
Lancelot of Naples, 51
Liutprand, Lombard king, 65, 120
Lothaire, King of the Francs, 100, 125, 142, 227, 238
Louis of Bavaria, emperor, 100, 242
Louis de Bourbon, 2, 229
Louis de France, Philippe III's son, 89, 100, 148, 231
Louis de Guyenne, 245
Louis de Nevers, 228–29
Louis d'Orléans, 113, 132, 136, 141, 143, 144–45, 154, 167, 244–45, 266
Louis V, 2, 89, 238
Louis VI, 27, 147, 224
Louis VII, 125, 227
Louis VIII, 3, 7, 131, 169
Louis IX (Saint Louis), 133, 151, 185, 223, 228, 231
Louis X, 66, 77, 147, 159, 175, 181, 186, 228, 232
Louis XI, xviii, 45, 62, 73, 78, 90, 94, 107, 113, 129, 143, 145, 149, 175–76, 179, 182, 202–03, 245–47, 267
Louis XII (Louis II d'Orléans), 147, 150
Louis XIV, xvi

Mahaut d'Artois, 63, 75, 77, 147, 159, 175, 181, 190, 196, 228–29, 267
Manfred, 89, 138, 241
Marachaire, 77, 156, 199
Marcatrude, 28, 108, 147, 198
Marche, Comtesse de la, 2, 27, 62, 66, 84, 120, 161, 149, 204, 223
Marie de Brabant, Philippe III's wife, 148, 199, 231, 251
Mélisende, Queen of Jérusalem, 101
Michelle de France, 90, 104, 176, 191
Mohammed, 223

Othe de Grandson, 185, 229
Otton III, 51

Philippe d'Alençon, Cardinal of Auch, 25
Philippe, duc de Brabant, 90, 111, 193
Philippe I, 5, 148
Philippe II Auguste, 58, 91, 112, 130, 133, 138, 224, 227
Philippe III, 94, 100, 108, 148, 231
Philippe IV, 155, 187
Philippe V, 66, 82, 158, 177, 192, 205–06, 228, 236
Philippe VI, 47, 71, 110, 115, 118, 121, 133
Philippe Hurepel, 228
Philippe le Bon, 4, 23, 94, 135, 148, 182, 198, 214, 234
Philippe le Hardi, duc de Bourgogne, 62, 150, 221, 244
Pierre de la Broce, 94, 131, 148, 169, 217, 231–33, 251
Pierre de Latilly, 97, 141, 232
Pierre de Rohan, marshal de Gié, 232
Pierre Gerbais, 94, 174, 176, 181, 187, 202, 233

Richard of Cornwall, 112, 151
Richard I of England, 91, 113, 133, 249
Richard II, 75, 79, 206, 248
Richard III of Normandie, 4, 99, 154, 252
Robert de Béthune, 63, 108, 148, 199, 228
Robert, duc de Normandie, 107, 199
Robert Guiscard, 63, 100, 103, 107, 112, 118, 145, 225–26
Robert Wourdreton, 41, 50–51, 59, 95, 113, 192
Romacharde de Coutances, 53, 56
Romilde, 199
Rosamund, 100, 107, 118, 199

Sabin, Bishop of Canossa, 10, 65, 116, 145, 199
Saint Benedict, 9, 15, 30, 59, 65, 86, 92, 136–37, 144, 154, 199, 222
Saint Georges, 30, 65, 75, 222
Saint John, 30, 65, 70, 86, 153, 222
Saint Marcel, 9, 70
Saint Mathias, 30, 80, 222
Saint Maurice, 70
Saint Patrick, 41
Saint Samson, 9, 65, 92, 116, 119, 124, 153, 222
Saint Thomas Becket, 30, 117
Saint William of York, 165, 209, 211, 279
Sédêchias, 137, 168
Séulfe, Archbishop of Reims, 3
Sichelgaïte, 98, 100, 108, 199
Sigebert, 140
Sigismond, emperor, 69, 103, 145
Sultan of Babylon, 151
Sultan of Constantinople, 53

Thibaud, duc de Lorraine, 65, 99
Thibaud IV, Count of Champagne, 131, 204, 228
Thierry (ou Théodoric) of Austrasie, 5, 134

Uther, King of Bretagne, 149

Valentine Visconti, 60, 83, 100, 103, 147, 150, 199, 244
Visconti (family), 54, 62, 65, 103, 107, 137, 150, 249

Wenceslas II, King of Bohemia, 69, 100
Wenceslas, King of the Romans, 59
William the Conqueror (Guillaume le Conquérant), 32, 94, 113, 205, 218, 238, 250, 265
William of Tyr, 110, 112
William of York, 52, 165, 181, 253

Yolande de Nevers, 108, 110, 148

About the Author and Translator

FRANCK COLLARD is Professor of Medieval History at the Universite de Paris X Nanterre. Apart from numerous published articles, he has also written *Pouvoirs et culture politique dans la France medievale, Ve-XVe siecle* (1999) and *Pouvoir et Poison. Histoire d'un crime politique de l'Antiquite a nos jours,* ed. Du Seuil, Paris (2007).

DEBORAH NELSON-CAMPBELL is Professor of French Studies and Director of the Center for the Study of Languages at Rice University. A scholar of medieval French and Occitan language and literature, she has published four books and numerous articles and book reviews mostly on French medieval topics, especially courtly narrative lyric poetry. She has taught at Rice University since 1971.

www.ingramcontent.com/pod-product-compliance
Ingram Content Group UK Ltd.
Pitfield, Milton Keynes, MK11 3LW, UK
UKHW020243290926
15470UKWH00002B/701

9 780313 346996